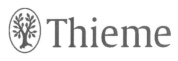

SPECT and SPECT/CT

A Clinical Guide

Chun K. Kim, MD
Clinical Director, Division of Nuclear Medicine and Molecular Imaging
Department of Radiology
Brigham and Women's Hospital
Associate Professor of Radiology
Harvard Medical School
Boston, Massachusetts

Katherine A. Zukotynski, MD
Associate Professor
Departments of Radiology and Medicine
McMaster University
Hamilton, Ontario, Canada

250 illustrations

Thieme
New York • Stuttgart • Delhi • Rio de Janeiro

Executive Editor: William Lamsback
Managing Editor: J. Owen Zurhellen IV
Editorial Assistant: Mary B. Wilson
Director, Editorial Services: Mary Jo Casey
Production Editor: Torsten Scheihagen
International Production Director: Andreas Schabert
International Marketing Director: Fiona Henderson
International Sales Director: Louisa Turrell
Director of Sales, North America: Mike Roseman
Senior Vice President and Chief Operating Officer:
 Sarah Vanderbilt
President: Brian D. Scanlan
Printer: Everbest Printing Co.

Library of Congress Cataloging-in-Publication Data

Names: Kim, Chun K., editor. | Zukotynski, Katherine A., editor.
Title: SPECT and SPECT/CT : a clinical guide / [edited by]
 Chun K. Kim, Katherine A. Zukotynski.
Description: First edition. | New York, NY : Thieme, [2017] |
 Includes bibliographical references and index.
Identifiers: LCCN 2016018886 (print) | LCCN 2016019458
 (ebook) | ISBN 9781626231511 (pbk.) |
 ISBN 9781626233393 (eISBN) | ISBN 9781626233393
Subjects: | MESH: Tomography, Emission-Computed,
 Single-Photon
Classification: LCC RC78.7.R4 (print) | LCC RC78.7.R4 (ebook) |
 NLM WN 206 | DDC 616.07/575–dc23
LC record available at https://lccn.loc.gov/2016018886

Copyright © 2017 by Thieme Medical Publishers, Inc.

Thieme Publishers New York
333 Seventh Avenue, New York, NY 10001 USA
+1 800 782 3488, customerservice@thieme.com

Thieme Publishers Stuttgart
Rüdigerstrasse 14, 70469 Stuttgart, Germany
+49 [0]711 8931 421, customerservice@thieme.de

Thieme Publishers Delhi
A-12, Second Floor, Sector-2, Noida-201301
Uttar Pradesh, India
+91 120 45 566 00, customerservice@thieme.in

Thieme Publishers Rio de Janeiro, Thieme Publicações Ltda.
Edifício Rodolpho de Paoli, 25º andar
Av. Nilo Peçanha, 50 – Sala 2508
Rio de Janeiro 20020-906 Brasil
+55 21 3172-2297 / +55 21 3172-1896

Cover design: Thieme Publishing Group
Typesetting by DiTech Process Solutions

Printed in China by Everbest Printing Co.   5 4 3 2 1

ISBN 978-1-62623-151-1

Also available as an e-book:
eISBN 978-1-62623-339-3

Important note: Medicine is an ever-changing science undergoing continual development. Research and clinical experience are continually expanding our knowledge, in particular our knowledge of proper treatment and drug therapy. Insofar as this book mentions any dosage or application, readers may rest assured that the authors, editors, and publishers have made every effort to ensure that such references are in accordance with **the state of knowledge at the time of production of the book.**

Nevertheless, this does not involve, imply, or express any guarantee or responsibility on the part of the publishers in respect to any dosage instructions and forms of applications stated in the book. **Every user is requested to examine carefully** the manufacturers' leaflets accompanying each drug and to check, if necessary in consultation with a physician or specialist, whether the dosage schedules mentioned therein or the contraindications stated by the manufacturers differ from the statements made in the present book. Such examination is particularly important with drugs that are either rarely used or have been newly released on the market. Every dosage schedule or every form of application used is entirely at the user's own risk and responsibility. The authors and publishers request every user to report to the publishers any discrepancies or inaccuracies noticed. If errors in this work are found after publication, errata will be posted at www.thieme.com on the product description page.

Some of the product names, patents, and registered designs referred to in this book are in fact registered trademarks or proprietary names even though specific reference to this fact is not always made in the text. Therefore, the appearance of a name without designation as proprietary is not to be construed as a representation by the publisher that it is in the public domain.

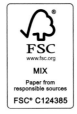

We dedicate this book to our respective families, who are our inspiration and the foundation of our being, as well as to our friends, who have been wonderful company along the road of life.

Contents

Preface

With the advent of hybrid imaging, the field of nuclear medicine has evolved significantly in recent years. In particular, single-photon emission computed tomography (SPECT) and SPECT/CT have come into their own as important diagnostic tools in routine clinical practice. Indeed, SPECT and SPECT/CT are often touted as game changers in the way clinical nuclear medicine is performed today. When we initially considered writing this book, we realized there were several books available covering the general topics of nuclear medicine and PET. However, we felt there was a lack of a concise book discussing the utility of SPECT and SPECT/CT in the imaging field and that this could be helpful primarily to residents, technologists and practicing physicians.

The goal of this book is to address a timely clinical need by providing a basic yet broad understanding of and practical approach to SPECT and SPECT/CT that will be useful to a spectrum of clinicians and technologists. The book begins with two chapters focusing on the technological foundation of SPECT and SPECT/CT as well as the radiochemistry used in association with these imaging techniques. This is followed by nine chapters, each of which details the utility of SPECT and SPECT/CT for imaging in a specific clinical context, including neuroscience, the thyroid and parathyroid glands, the cardiovascular system, the respiratory system, neoplastic disease, the skeletal system, infection/ inflammation, and pediatrics. Illustrative case examples focusing on each clinical area are included throughout the chapters. The final chapter of this book presents a compilation of interesting cases targeting topics not otherwise reviewed in the preceding chapters.

We have tried to write a book that is a concise, easy-to-read review of SPECT and SPECT/CT as it is currently used in the clinic. Information is presented in an accessible format with concise bullet points highlighting key imaging findings and teaching pearls throughout. We do not intend for this book to be a comprehensive reference on the topic; rather, we hope it will provide a strong foundation, improved understanding of these techniques, and focused high-yield material for successful clinical practice in the world of today.

Leading experts in the field of hybrid imaging have contributed to this book, and it is a pleasure to feature their work. We hope that you will enjoy reading our book and that you will find it to be a valuable addition to your library as well as a tool that will further your success!

Acknowledgments

We thank the leading experts in the field of hybrid imaging who made contributions; it was a genuine pleasure to review their work. We would like to give special thanks to the nuclear medicine teams at Harvard Medical School and McMaster University, without whom this book would not have been possible. We also thank the staff at Thieme Publishers for their support and for making the dream of our book a reality.

Contributors

Samuel E. Almodóvar, MD
Chief of Clinical PET
Assistant Professor of Radiology
Division of Molecular Imaging and Therapeutics
University of Alabama
Birmingham, Alabama

Kevin J. Donohoe, MD
Attending Physician
Division of Nuclear Medicine
Department of Radiology
Beth Israel Deaconess Medical Center
Assistant Professor of Radiology
Harvard Medical School
Boston, Massachusetts

Sharmila Dorbala, MD, MPH, FACC
Director, Nuclear Cardiology
Division of Nuclear Medicine and Molecular Imaging
Department of Radiology
Division of Cardiovascular Medicine
Brigham and Women's Hospital
Associate Professor of Radiology
Harvard Medical School
Boston, Massachusetts

Frederic H. Fahey, DSc, FSNMMI, FACR, FAAPM
Director of Nuclear Medicine
PET Physic
Boston Children's Hospital
Professor of Radiology
Harvard Medical School
Boston, Massachusetts

Elisa Franquet-Elía, MD
Research Fellow in Nuclear Medicine
Department of Radiology
Beth Israel Deaconess Medical Center
Boston, Massachusetts

Victor H. Gerbaudo, PhD, MSHCA
Senior Director, Nuclear Medicine, Molecular Imaging
  and Noninvasive Cardiovascular Imaging
  Administration
Associate Scientific Director, Advanced
  Multimodality Image Guided Operating Suite
Department of Radiology
Brigham and Women's Hospital

Assistant Professor of Radiology
Harvard Medical School
Boston, Massachusetts

Frederick D. Grant, MD
Division of Nuclear Medicine and Molecular Imaging
Department of Radiology
Boston Children's Hospital
Assistant Professor in Radiology
Harvard Medical School
Boston, Massachusetts

Stephen J. Horgan, MB, PhD
Cardiology Fellow
Department of Cardiovascular Medicine
Gagnon Cardiovascular Institute
Morristown Medical Center
Morristown, New Jersey

Hyewon Hyun, MD
Assistant Professor of Radiology
Harvard Medical School
Division of Nuclear Medicine and Molecular Imaging
Department of Radiology
Brigham and Women's Hospital
Boston, Massachusetts

Chun K. Kim, MD
Clinical Director, Division of Nuclear Medicine and
  Molecular Imaging
Department of Radiology
Brigham and Women's Hospital
Associate Professor of Radiology
Harvard Medical School
Boston, Massachusetts

Padma Manapragada, MD
Chief Resident
Division of Molecular Imaging and Therapeutics
Department of Radiology
University of Alabama
Birmingham, Alabama

Christopher J. Palestro, MD
Professor of Radiology
Hofstra North Shore–LIJ School of Medicine
Hempstead, New York

Paul J. Roach, FRACP, FAANMS
Head, Department of Nuclear Medicine
Royal North Shore Hospital–Sydney
Clinical Associate Professor of Medicine
Sydney Medical School
University of Sydney
Sydney, Australia

Geoffrey P. Schembri, MBBS, FRACP, FAANMS
Senior Staff Specialist
Department of Nuclear Medicine
Royal North Shore Hospital–Sydney
Sydney Medical School
University of Sydney
Sydney, Australia

Tarun Singhal, MD
Associate Neurologist
Department of Neurology
Brigham and Women's Hospital
Instructor in Neurology
Harvard Medical School
Boston, Massachusetts

Shankar Vallabhajoshula, PhD
Professor of Radiochemistry and Radiopharmacy
Weill Cornell Medical College of Cornell University
New York Presbyterian Hospital
New York, New York

Katherine A. Zukotynski, MD
Associate Professor
Departments of Radiology and Medicine
McMaster University
Hamilton, Ontario, Canada

Part I

The Fundamentals

1 Basic Principles of SPECT and SPECT/CT and Quality Control

Frederic H. Fahey

1.1 Introduction

Single-photon emission computed tomography (SPECT) can provide a tomographic representation of the in vivo distribution of gamma-emitting radiopharmaceuticals, irrespective of whether they are positron emitters or not. Early SPECT devices imaged a limited region of the body with high efficiency. However, by the mid-1980s, the rotating gamma camera had become the clinical SPECT device of choice with myocardial perfusion SPECT becoming the most commonly performed nuclear medicine procedure. In the past decade, there has been a renewed interest in dedicated, high-sensitivity SPECT systems with a smaller footprint for myocardial perfusion imaging. The higher sensitivity provided by these devices can yield similar clinical results to the rotating gamma camera in a shorter time, with less administered activity or a combination of the two. In addition, SPECT has recently been combined with computed tomography (CT), leading to hybrid SPECT/CT scanners that yield the anatomical imaging of CT with the functional capability of SPECT. This chapter majorly discusses the rotating gamma camera, as it is by far the most common SPECT device in the clinic, with a brief description of dedicated systems. This chapter also discusses hybrid SPECT/CT scanners.

1.2 Basic Principles

1.2.1 Tomography

Consider a simple, cylindrical object that is being imaged. The tomographic system (e.g., a SPECT or CT system) acquires "projection" data about the object (▶ Fig. 1.1). To first order, the data acquired at each location along the projection can be assumed to have originated along a ray intersecting at right angles to the detection device and extending back through the object. A complete set of projection data is acquired at evenly spaced angular intervals about the object. Depending on the particular tomographic imaging modality, a complete set may be considered a rotation over 180 or 360 degrees, as discussed in this chapter. The tomographic data set for a volume will consist

of projection data acquired for a series of parallel transverse planes or slices through the object. Although the acquisition of parallel rays within a projection may be reasonable for some applications and certainly provides a simple conceptual model, in many cases, it may be more efficient to acquire the data in either a fan-beam or cone-beam geometry. A complete set of projections acquired in fan-beam geometry can be reformatted into one consisting of parallel beams and thus can be considered to be equivalent. However, cone-beam geometries can provide some technical challenges, as discussed in this chapter.

Each one-dimensional (1D) projection can be stacked to form a two-dimensional (2D) image, where displacement across the projection is on the x-axis and the angle of orientation of that particular projection is on the y-axis (▶ Fig. 1.2). This representation of a complete set of projection data associated with a single slice through the object is known as the "sinogram" since such a representation of a point source results in a sine wave rotated 90 degrees. For a volume of data, each transverse slice would be represented by its own sinogram. The contour of a sinogram should normally be

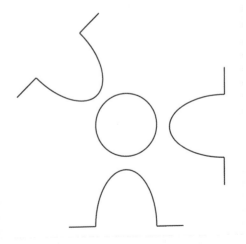

Fig. 1.1 Tomographic reconstruction generates an estimate of the underlying object from a series of projections acquired about the object. This figure shows three projections about a simple cylindrical object.

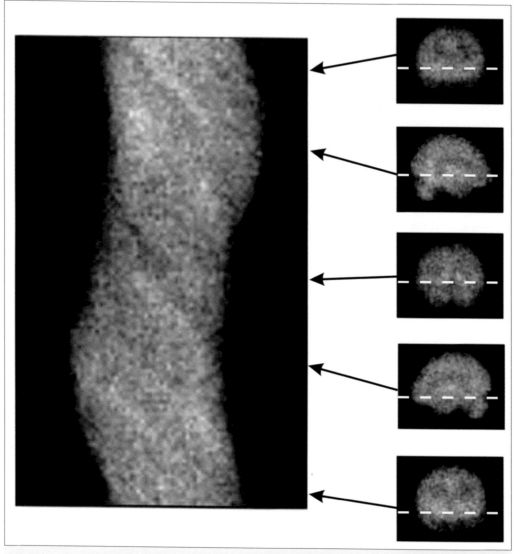

Fig. 1.2 The "sinogram" consists of a stack of the projections from a single transverse slice through the object where displacement across the projection and the angle of the projection are plotted horizontally and vertically, respectively. Five projections from a brain SPECT are shown on the right. The resultant sinogram from the slice indicated in the projections by the white dashed line is shown on the left. The arrows indicate where within the sinogram the projections at these five particular angles are located.

smooth and continuous. A break in the contour indicates patient motion (see ▶ Fig. 5.8 in Chapter 5).

The fundamental challenge of tomographic reconstruction is to estimate the internal structures of the object, given the set of projection data acquired about the object. With parallel-ray projection data, the events detected at a certain locus along the projection can be back projected across the object, assuming that the events must have originated along that ray (▶ Fig. 1.2). If this "simple back projection" is applied to all locations for all projections, the resultant reconstruction will provide a crude reconstruction of the data that is blurred considerably by streak artifacts. This is caused by the uneven sampling of frequency data, where high frequencies are sampled less often than low frequencies. Applying a "ramp filter," that is, one that weights the frequency components in a linear fashion, compensates for these streak artifacts but also leads to amplification of high-frequency noise in the reconstructed image. Therefore, a windowing filter (e.g., Butterworth, Hanning, Hamming, Shepp–Logan) is typically applied. A cutoff frequency is defined for the windowing function depending on the imaging task that effectively smooths the high-frequency noise while maintaining image quality with acceptable spatial resolution. This approach, referred to as filtered back projection, is relatively simple, fast, and robust and continues to be the standard reconstruction method for CT.

An alternative to filtered back projection is iterative reconstruction. In this approach, an initial guess of the object is assumed (e.g., that the object is uniform). From this initial guess, a set of projection data is generated using an a priori model of the imaging modality (▶ Fig. 1.3). This set of generated projections is compared to the set of acquired (real) projections. The differences between the

generated and real projections are back projected and added to the original guess, providing an update. This series of steps is repeated or "iterated" until an acceptable solution is reached. In determining the difference between the two sets of projections, a specific statistical criterion is applied. One commonly used criterion for iterative reconstruction is maximum likelihood. As a result, the reconstructed image is that which is most likely, in a statistical sense, to have led to the given set of projections. In addition, an optimization algorithm, such as expectation maximization, is utilized. As a result, the maximum likelihood expectation maximization (MLEM) algorithm is commonly used for the iterative reconstruction of medical image data.

Iterative reconstructions can lead to improvements in image quality relative to filtered back projection. In the first place, as the method does not directly rely on back projection, the streak

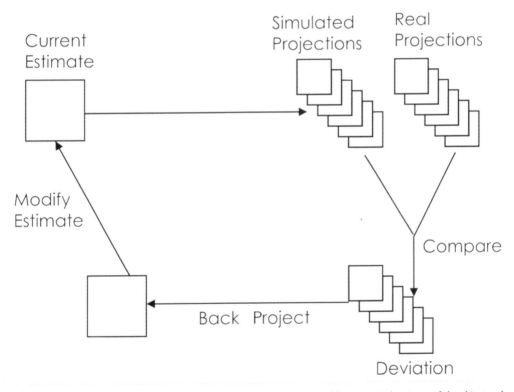

Fig. 1.3 In iterative reconstruction, a set of simulated projections is generated from an initial estimate of the object and a model of the imaging system. These simulated projections are compared to the set of real, acquired projections, and the deviation is back projected and added to update the estimate. This process is "iterated" until an acceptable reconstruction is reached based upon some convergence criteria. Current algorithms may take tens of iterations to converge on an acceptable result. However, methods such as the use of ordered subsets have been developed to provide a good result more quickly.

artifacts that can be encountered in filtered back projection are minimized considerably. Also, the Poisson statistical nature of the acquired projection data is specifically modeled into the MLEM algorithm. In addition, the iterative approach allows the incorporation of knowledge of the imaging process into the reconstruction process. These considerations can be incorporated directly into the model that is used for first generating the estimated projections from the current guess of the object being imaged and then reprojecting the difference between the two projection sets. This can include knowledge of photon attenuation, scattering within the patient, or the variation of spatial resolution across the field of view. This is in contrast to filtered back projection with its rather naive assumption that the data can be uniformly spread across the entire breadth of the patient. As a result, iterative reconstruction typically provides images that appear less noisy with fewer streak artifacts with the potential for higher spatial resolution. An example of streak artifact is shown in ▶ Fig. 8.4 in Chapter 8.

The MLEM can take tens of iterations, perhaps as many as 50 or 100, before obtaining an acceptable image. In general, the image will become sharper with more iterations but also noisier. In addition, acquiring many iterations can be time consuming, particularly for large data sets. Several approaches can be used to improve the image quality when more iterations are used or to reach an acceptable image with fewer iterations. A simple approach to reducing the image noise is to apply a postreconstruction regularization filter. The amount of smoothing applied can be varied depending on the acquisition modality and imaging task at hand.

In the traditional MLEM algorithm, the entire set of projections must be processed prior to generating an updated guess of the object. One way of obtaining an acceptable image with fewer iterations is to divide the set of projections into subsets of projections that are uniformly distributed about the patient. For example, assume that 100 projections (numbered 1 through 100) have been acquired about the patient and we want to divide this into 10 subsets. The first subset might contain projections 1, 11, 21, 31, ..., 81, 91. After applying the iterative algorithm to these 10 projections, the initial guess is updated. The next subset may contain projections 2, 12, 32, ..., 82, 92, and again updating the guess. After processing the full set of projections with 10 subsets, the initial guess has already been updated 10 times. As a result, fewer iterations are typically needed. The most commonly used algorithm for this approach is referred to as ordered subset expectation maximization (OSEM).

A rule of thumb indicates that OSEM yields similar image quality as MLEM when the product of the number of subsets and the number of iterations with OSEM equals the total number of iterations in MLEM. For example, OSEM reconstruction with 16 subsets and 3 iterations yields a similar image quality to MLEM with 48 iterations. It should be noted that processing more subsets does not take additional time. It only changes the order with which the data are processed. As a result, the ability to significantly reduce the number of iterations, in turn, leads to a substantial reduction in processing time. If OSEM with 16 subsets and 3 iterations provides an acceptable alternative to MLEM with 48 iterations, the data are reconstructed about 16 times faster. The ability to provide reconstructed data in a timely fashion may be the determining factor in it being applied routinely in the clinic.

1.2.2 Single-Photon Emission Computed Tomography

The rotating gamma camera—the SPECT device most commonly used in the clinic—consists of one or often two standard Anger gamma camera detectors mounted onto a gantry that allows the cameras to rotate around the patient (▶ Fig. 1.4). Much of the following discussion assumes the use of parallel-hole collimation as this is most commonly used clinically. Focused collimation is also discussed briefly. The patient is administered a radiopharmaceutical. After an appropriate uptake period, the patient is placed on the imaging table and the SPECT acquisition begins. A static gamma camera image is acquired at a particular angle. The camera then rotates to the next position and a second projection image is acquired. This process continues until a full set of projections is acquired about the patient. For brain and whole-body SPECT, the set of projections is traditionally acquired over 360 degrees, whereas 180-degree rotation is more common for myocardial perfusion SPECT.

With *parallel-hole collimation*, one can assume, to first order, that the gamma ray resulting from a particular emission event along the "line of origin" intersects the camera crystal at the point of detection and extends back through the patient. Therefore, the acquired image can be considered a 2D

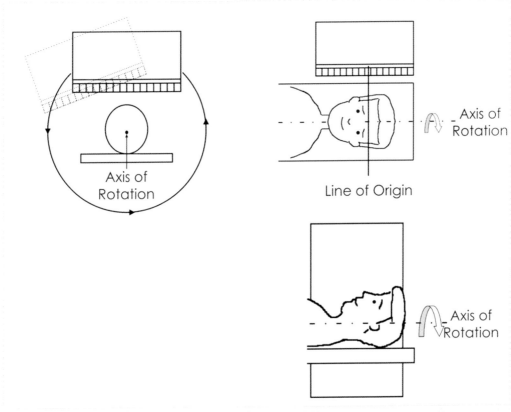

Fig. 1.4 The rotating gamma camera rotates about an axis of rotation that typically aligns with the long axis of the patient's body. With the use of parallel-hole collimation, a detected event is generally assumed to have been emitted along the "line of origin" shown in the upper right. The counts acquired at this location in the detector are thus back projected along this line.

projection image of the volume being imaged. Each horizontal row across the image represents the projection for that particular slice. Thus a single projection image represents a series of projections across all slices within the volume at a particular angle.

Although parallel-hole collimation is most commonly used in conjunction with the rotating gamma camera, *focused collimation* is sometimes used in special applications. *Fan-beam* or *cone-beam collimation* can provide enhanced sensitivity without sacrificing spatial resolution. This can be particularly useful when imaging a smaller region with a large field-of-view camera (▶ Fig. 1.5). For example, focused collimation has been applied to myocardial perfusion imaging, leading to three to four times the sensitivity with similar spatial resolution. The acquired projection data are subsequently reconstructed using either a fan-beam or a cone-beam algorithm. In modern cameras, the use

of sophisticated robotics can assure that the region of interest is maintained in the center of the reconstructed field of view.

Pinhole collimation has also been applied successfully in SPECT of small objects. In this case, the detected event is assumed to have been emitted from the ray that intersects the crystal at the point of detection and passes through the pinhole back through the object. The use of very small pinhole apertures and significant image magnification can lead to outstanding spatial resolution. For example, in preclinical SPECT of small animals, apertures less than 1 mm have been used, leading to reconstructed spatial resolution of less than 1 mm. In this instance, the limited sensitivity of using such a small pinhole aperture is overcome by using multiple pinholes and maintaining a very short object-to-aperture distance. Since the sensitivity of a pinhole collimator varies as the inverse square of this distance, reasonable levels of sensitivity can

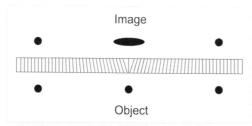

Fig. 1.5 Focused collimators can provide higher sensitivity without the usual loss of spatial resolution. The collimator shown in this figure is focused on the central portion with a parallel configuration on the periphery to minimize truncation of the object during reconstruction. In the focused, central portion of the collimator, the object is magnified and the gain in sensitivity is determined by this amount of magnification. In this simple 1D example, the gain in sensitivity would be about a factor of 3, but when expanded to 2D, it could be a factor of 5 or more.

be achieved with very short distances possible in small animal imaging. Although short object-to-aperture distances are not typically possible in clinical imaging, the use of multiple detectors with pinhole collimation has been applied to myocardial imaging, as discussed in this chapter.

1.2.3 Computed Tomography

CT, developed in the 1970s by Sir Godfrey Hounsfield, provides the ability to generate a cross-sectional representation of an object from a series of X-ray projections acquired about the object. This 3D representation greatly enhanced the image contrast by minimizing the ambiguity typically encountered in radiographs from over- and underlying tissues. The initial "first-generation" CT scanners required several minutes to acquire and reconstruct the data from a single slice. However, the technology developed quickly, and within just a few years, third-generation scanners could acquire data from a single slice on the order of a second. The introduction of helical and later multidetector CT allowed for the acquisition of an entire volume of the patient in less than a minute, thus making the modality truly 3D. CT could now provide high-resolution, high-quality anatomical representations of the patient in a matter of minutes. As a result, the clinical use of CT grew considerably from a few million CT procedures in the United States in 1985 to more than 80 million procedures by 2006.[1]

CT is a radiographic technique and thereby relies on the production of X-rays. As a result, the major components of the device are the X-ray tube and the detector matrix. Both of these are incorporated into a continuously rotating gantry that allows for the helical acquisition. The CT X-ray tube is essentially similar to a radiographic tube. Electrons are liberated from a heated cathode via thermionic emission and accelerated toward the tungsten anode. Upon striking the anode, a fraction of the electronic energy is converted into bremsstrahlung X-rays for imaging the patient. The number of electrons traversing the tube per second is characterized by the tube current, typically reported in milliamperes (mA). The number of X-rays produced is directly proportional to the number of electrons traversing the tube and striking the anode. As a result, the X-ray exposure and the radiation dose to the patient are directly proportional to the mA. For instance, doubling the mA will double the radiation dose. As the number of X-rays produced and radiation dose are also proportional to the duration of exposure, the product of this duration in seconds and the tube current is often represented in units of milliampere-seconds (mAs).

The tube voltage (in peak kilovoltage [kVp]) determines the energy of the electrons impinging on the anode and thereby affects the energy of the resultant X-rays. The bremsstrahlung X-rays are produced with a continuous energy spectrum, with the maximum energy depending upon the energy of the electrons and thus on the kVp. Characteristic X-rays of discrete energies below the electron energy can also be produced by X-ray fluorescence of the target material. Thus average or effective X-ray energy of the spectrum depends on kVp. As a result, the proper kVp is often selected such that it optimizes the image contrast for the task at hand. In addition, higher-energy electrons are more efficient at producing X-rays, and thereby the number of X-rays also increases with kVp. In fact, the number of X-rays produced and the radiation dose to the patient typically vary as the square of kVp.

As is traditional in radiography, a filter (typically copper or aluminum) is placed between the X-ray beam and the patient to absorb low-energy X-rays that have little potential of traversing beyond the first few centimeters within the patient and therefore would only contribute to the patient's surface dose without contributing to the generation of the image. In CT, a "bowtie" filter is also used to minimize the exposure on the periphery of the projection while maintaining adequate exposure at the center. Both of these types of filters can affect the energy spectrum of the X-rays impinging upon the patient.

The original commercial CT scanners could only image a single slice at a time. The patient was then indexed and a subsequent slice was acquired. Although the time necessary to acquire a single slice was quite short, perhaps less than 1 second, each slice was imaged independently, and thus it may take a reasonable amount of time to image a specified volume of the patient. Two advancements in the 1980s led to a more efficient imaging of a volume of the patient. In the original scanners, the gantry would complete a single rotation during the acquisition of a single slice. The gantry would then need to reset in order to acquire the next slice. To address this limitation, the helical approach to CT scanning was developed, whereby a gantry was developed using slip-ring technology that could rotate continuously during the acquisition. In addition, the bed moved during the acquisition and thus the path of the X-ray tube formed a helix around the patient. In this manner, an entire volume of the patient could be scanned in a single acquisition without having to reset the gantry along the way. In addition, multiple CT slices could be acquired simultaneously by providing several rings of detectors in the axial or z-direction. In the past, the third-generation CT detector assembly comprised a 1D array of small radiation detectors. In the multidetector design, the array now comprised a 2D matrix, both in the azimuthal direction about the ring and also in the z-direction into the ring. The number of available rings in a multidetector CT design soon went from 4 slices to 16, 32, or 64 slices or even more. These advancements allowed for a volume of the patient to be imaged more efficiently and faster and thereby led to a subsequent increase in the clinical utilization of CT. More recently, the incorporation of a second X-ray source into the gantry design has led to even faster acquisition of the CT data.

For helical CT, the "pitch" describes the speed of the imaging table, defined by the length that the table traverses in a single rotation of the CT gantry relative to the nominal beam width. As a result, if the distance the table traversed during a gantry rotation matches the beam width, this is characterized as a pitch of 1.0 to 1 (1.0:1). If the table travels 50% faster, the pitch would be 1.5:1, indicating stretching of the helix and slight undersampling within the acquisition.

As with all medical imaging, the evaluation of image quality depends on the clinical task at hand. In some instances, spatial resolution, that is, the ability to discern small lesions or represent fine detail, is of clinical importance, whereas, in other cases, outstanding contrast resolution is essential. As a result, the three parameters of image quality of importance are *spatial resolution*, *image contrast*, and *noise*.

The *spatial resolution* is typically defined by the X-ray focal spot size and the detector dimensions in both the transverse and axial or z-direction. The smaller the detector and focal spot size, the higher the spatial resolution. In addition, a thinner slice thickness would reduce the partial volume effect in the axial or z-direction.

As discussed previously, the choice of kVp can affect *image contrast*; thus the kVp should be determined based on the clinical task.

Quantum noise within the CT image depends on the number of detected X-ray quanta incorporated into a CT transverse image. As described previously, the number of X-rays produced depends on both kVp and mAs. The fraction of those detected further depends on the size of the patient, the slice width, the pitch, and smoothing during image reconstruction. In other words, practically all aspects of the CT acquisition affect quantum noise in the CT image. The magnitude of the quantum noise is often parameterized by the "noise index," which is defined by the standard deviation of the pixel values within a standard uniform CT phantom.

1.3 Instrumentation

1.3.1 Single-Photon Emission Computed Tomography

The large majority of current SPECT devices are dual-detector rotating gamma cameras with very large field-of-view ($30 \times 50\,cm$) camera heads. The two detectors provide twice the sensitivity and also allow for simultaneous acquisition of anterior/posterior whole-body imaging. The SPECT gantry provides not only rotation about the patient but also radial motion of the detector heads. As is the case in planar imaging, keeping the detectors as close to the patient as possible improves the spatial resolution of the projection data and ultimately the reconstructed data. Current SPECT systems have sensors that can detect the body surface and thus provide noncircular orbits (NCOs) of the detectors, maintaining the distance from the collimator face and the patient to within a few centimeters.

In brain and whole-body SPECT, acquiring projections over 360 degrees is preferred. Due to photon attenuation, conjugate projections are not equivalent. For example, it is clear that the anterior view of a bone scan is different from the posterior view. Therefore, the inclusion of the opposite views provides additional information to reconstruct the process. As a result, a dual-detector SPECT system is commonly used to acquire the conjugate views, simultaneously increasing the overall sensitivity of the acquisition by a factor of 2. Conversely, since the heart is located in the left anterior thorax, there is limited value in the data added from the right posterior projections. Thus the cardiac SPECT data are traditionally acquired only over 180 degrees. In this case, a dual-detector system with opposed detectors is of limited value. So dual-detector systems can typically be configured with the detectors at 90 degrees to each other as an option, allowing projection data across 180 degrees with a 90-degree rotation, which still allows for twice the efficiency.

Since the dual-detector gamma camera system can be used for a variety of applications, including both planar imaging and SPECT, multiple parallel-hole collimator sets are typically available, including several low-energy sets (e.g., ultra-high resolution, high resolution, general purpose, or high sensitivity) as well as medium- and high-energy sets. In some instances, focused collimators may be available for myocardial imaging (▶ Fig. 1.5). In the example shown in ▶ Fig. 1.5, the collimator is focused on the central field of view for improved sensitivity but has parallel holes on the field-of-view periphery to minimize the truncation artifact that can arise from focused SPECT. The use of focused collimators for high sensitivity still allows the camera to be utilized for other planar and SPECT applications as well as myocardial imaging.

Over the past decade, several SPECT devices specifically designed for myocardial imaging have been developed. In general, these devices provide high-sensitivity imaging with a small footprint that makes them attractive for busy, outpatient cardiac imaging centers. Several such devices are shown in ▶ Fig. 1.6. In some cases, the device is simply a multidetector gamma camera system with smaller detectors and a fixed 90-degree geometry. For the most part, these operate exactly like the conventional rotating gamma camera systems.

Alternatively, the system shown in ▶ Fig. 1.6a has three compact camera heads and keeps the patient erect, which allows for a small footprint and targeted imaging of the myocardium. Other systems may use a larger number of smaller detectors that specifically scan the patient over the region of the heart. Owing to the small size of each detector, semiconductor

radiation detectors may be used rather than the conventional sodium iodide scintillating crystal. For example, the device shown in ▶ Fig. 1.6 c has 10 cadmium zinc telluride (CZT) semiconductor detectors, each scanning a fan beam independently over the myocardium. The device shown in ▶ Fig. 1.6b consists of 19 stationary detectors, each utilizing a parallel-hole collimator. In this case, neither the cameras nor the collimators move. Instead, 19 projections are simultaneously acquired and later reconstructed. All of these dedicated SPECT devices have considerably higher sensitivity with comparable or better spatial resolution than a dual-detector SPECT system. Therefore, the study can be acquired in either a shorter time to improve workflow, with less administered activity to reduce patient radiation dose, or a combination of the two.

1.3.2 Hybrid Single-Photon Emission Computed Tomography/Computed Tomography

The initial motivation for a hybrid SPECT/CT scanner was to provide a rapid and accurate method of attenuation compensation, particularly for thoracic SPECT. In the early 1990s, Hasegawa et al developed a SPECT/CT prototype that utilized a single high-purity germanium semiconductor detector for both the SPECT and CT components of the scanner.[2] In the late 1990s, a commercial SPECT/CT scanner was developed that utilized a low-power X-ray tube that acquired SPECT and CT data simultaneously. Although the CT image quality was quite limited and certainly not adequate for diagnostic CT, it was clearly sufficient for attenuation compensation and provided anatomical correlation for the SPECT findings, which was found to be of considerable clinical value.

Hybrid positron emission tomography PET/CT was introduced around the turn of the 21st century and its clinical acceptance was overwhelming. In fact, within 5 years, only hybrid PET/CT scanners were commercially available and PET-only scanners could no longer be purchased. One notable difference between PET/CT scanners and early SPECT/CT scanners was the incorporation of high-quality, state-of-the-art CT. The phenomenal success of PET/CT led to the further advancement of hybrid SPECT/CT scanners. Both conventional dual-detector rotating gamma cameras and dedicated cardiac SPECT devices have been incorporated into hybrid SPECT/CT devices. Although the use of SPECT/CT has not been as

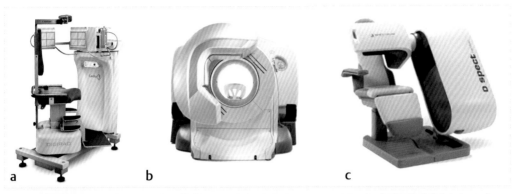

Fig. 1.6 Three SPECT systems dedicated to cardiac imaging. Each provides high-sensitivity imaging of the myocardium as well as a small footprint, thus making it suitable for placement in either a hospital or outpatient clinic. (**a**) This device consists of three compact gamma cameras. The patient sits upright and is rotated in front of the three cameras. (**b**) This device consists of 19 stationary cadmium zinc telluride (CZT) detectors, each associated with a pinhole collimator providing 19 simultaneous projections of the myocardium. (**c**) This device has 10 individual collimated CZT detectors, each scanning the myocardium in a fan beam.

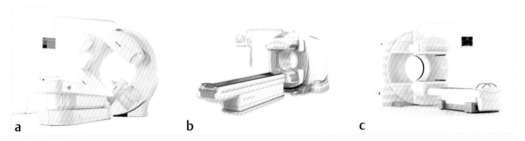

Fig. 1.7 Three current, commercially available SPECT/CT systems. In all three cases, the CT is combined with a dual-detector rotating gamma camera SPECT system. (**a**) This system uses a cone-beam, flat-panel approach to the CT acquisition. (**b, c**) These systems utilize standard third-generation CT systems behind the SPECT component of the instrument.

universally applied as PET/CT, it is considered very useful for a number of clinical applications.

Two approaches have been used in commercial SPECT/CT scanners. In many instances, the CT component is a state-of-the-art multidetector, helical CT gantry, although it may have a smaller number of CT slices available. For example, although a 2-, 8-, or 16-slice CT scanner may be available for SPECT/CT, 32 slices or more are common with PET/CT. However, even with the limited number of slice capability, this may still be considered a diagnostic CT scanner. Alternatively, lower-level cone-beam CT capability using flat-panel detectors may be provided, which may be considered quite adequate for attenuation correction and anatomical localization but may not be considered a fully diagnostic CT scanner. In general, the SPECT component is in the front part of the device and the CT is in the back (▶ Fig. 1.7).

1.4 Quality Control

As medical imaging equipment becomes more sophisticated, the necessity for a comprehensive and consistent quality control (QC) program becomes essential. In general, this includes routine calibration and periodic testing of the equipment. Without such a program, there is considerable potential for a significant loss of performance or quantitative accuracy, as well as the possibility of artifacts that can either obscure or mimic pertinent pathology. Notable artifacts may also result from departures from proper image acquisition and processing, or variants within the patient. In the context of hybrid imaging, artifacts can result from improper alignment between the two modalities. This section reviews routine calibrations and testing procedures for SPECT, CT, and hybrid SPECT/CT scanners. Model QC programs are provided. Examples of artifacts that may result in the clinical application of SPECT and SPECT/CT are also discussed.

1.4.1 Single-Photon Emission Computed Tomography

It has been clear since the earliest days of SPECT that the technology was not very forgiving regarding small variations in performance. For example, slight spatial nonuniformities in camera sensitivity on the order of just a few percent that would perhaps be barely visible on a planar image could render a SPECT study uninterpretable or lead to artifacts that could mimic pathology. As a result, it is well accepted that attention to detail is essential in QC, data acquisition, and reconstruction in order to provide SPECT images of appropriate quality for clinical use. SPECT QC has two components: calibration and testing. The SPECT camera must undergo routine calibration in order to compensate for certain variations in the data acquisition and reconstruction processes. Subsequently, the system should be tested, initially upon acceptance of new instrumentation and later on a routine basis, to assure proper operation of the system. Finally, the resulting clinical images must be reviewed with a skeptical eye always on the lookout for artifacts or other anomalies that may adversely affect the clinical interpretation of the images.

SPECT calibration entails the characterization of the spatial uniformity of the camera sensitivity, the alignment of the center of rotation (COR) with that of the reconstruction matrix, and the proper registration of detector heads for multidetector systems. These calibrations must be performed routinely to assure proper SPECT performance.

However, the frequency with which these calibrations should be performed depends on the stability of the specific system in that the basic assumption is that the performance of the camera on the day of the clinical study is essentially the same as it was on the day the calibration was performed. In most cases, these calibrations can be performed on a monthly or perhaps a quarterly basis, although there may be instances where semiannual calibration is acceptable for some calibrations, whereas others may need to be performed biweekly. Routine proper testing of the SPECT system after calibration can assist the user in determining the stability of that system and thereby establishing the proper frequency for calibration.

The rotating gamma camera SPECT system is particularly susceptible to artifacts from inadequate calibration for spatial variation in camera performance. For example, if there is a uniformity variation in camera sensitivity that leads to a small region of lower counts, then that region will have lower counts in that location in all projections as the camera rotates about the object. When these data are reconstructed, this nonuniformity will lead to a ring of lower counts (i.e., a "cold" ring) with the radius of the ring equal to the distance the nonuniformity is from the center of the reconstruction matrix. If the nonuniformity is caused by a region of higher sensitivity, then the ring will be "hot," that is, a ring of higher counts. It is possible to have several such nonuniformities within the camera's field of view, leading to a number of rings forming a "bull's-eye" artifact with the center of the bull's-eye being the center of the reconstruction matrix. Images with ring and bull's-eye artifacts are shown in ▶ Fig. 1.8.

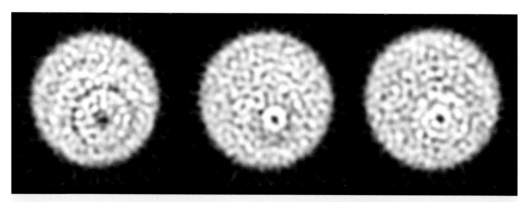

Fig. 1.8 Transverse images from a cylindrical phantom filled with a uniform concentration of radioactivity. The "ring" artifacts seen in these images are caused by inadequate uniformity calibration of the system.

It is practically impossible to design a gamma camera that does not have some level of nonuniformity that could potentially yield SPECT artifacts. Therefore, it is necessary to accurately characterize these nonuniformities in order to compensate for them during data acquisition. This characterization is accomplished by acquiring very high count uniformity (or "flood") images. The number of counts necessary for these calibrations must be high enough so that the quantum noise in the calibration data does not lead to artifacts in their own right. It has been determined that these floods must have between 100,000 and 200,000 to meet this criterion for the 128 × 128 acquisition matrix that is typically used in SPECT. These high-count calibration floods are not to be confused with the 10- to 20-million count uniformity "floods" images acquired as part of daily testing of the gamma camera. This calibration generates regional corrections of uniformity variations that are applied on the fly while the gamma camera images are being acquired. If properly applied with a well-performing gamma camera system, this calibration should eliminate the potential for SPECT-ring or bull's-eye artifacts.

Uniformity calibration can also be applied using flood images acquired extrinsically, that is, with the collimator in place. Some manufacturers utilize a combination of intrinsic and extrinsic floods because intrinsic uniformity is more likely to change quickly (possibly on the order of weeks and months), whereas collimator uniformity tends to be more stable. In addition, extrinsic uniformity calibration would need to be acquired for every collimator set used for SPECT. Some users may use three or four collimator sets for SPECT. Using the combination approach, the intrinsic calibration flood may be acquired more frequently, for example, on a monthly basis, and the extrinsic floods may only need to be acquired quarterly or semiannually.

In SPECT reconstruction, the projection data are oriented to the center of the gantry referred to as the "center of rotation." The COR defines where the axis about which the device rotates is referenced in the reconstruction matrix. In general, the reconstruction algorithm assumes that the COR also aligns with the center of the computer matrix. For example, if the data are being reconstructed into a 128 × 128 matrix with x and y locations defined from 0 to 127, then the COR is assumed to align with location (63.5, 63.5), that is, the center of the matrix. If this alignment is slightly off, then the back-projected data will be askew, leading to a blurring in the reconstructed data. In fact, inadequate COR calibration is the most common cause of loss of SPECT spatial resolution. Therefore, the COR needs to be routinely specified through calibration. ▶ Fig. 1.9 shows a transverse slice of a brain SPECT study. The image on the left is reconstructed correctly, but in the middle and right images, the COR has been miscalibrated by 3 and 6 mm, respectively.

For multidetector SPECT, the assumption is that the projection image acquired with one detector at a particular angular position is identical in scale,

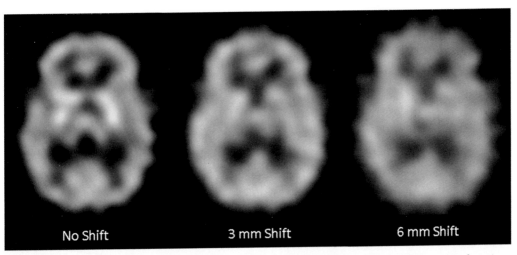

No Shift   3 mm Shift   6 mm Shift

Fig. 1.9 Three reconstructions of a brain SPECT scan. In the image on the left (labeled "No Shift"), the center of rotation (COR) has been properly specified. In the middle and right images, the COR has been misspecified by 3 and 6 mm, respectively. The blurring of the data by poor COR calibration is clearly demonstrated.

location, and orientation to the image acquired with another detector in the same position. In this way, the data from the multiple detectors can be combined without having to correct the projection data prior to reconstruction. For both COR and multidetector calibration, a known object is imaged by both detectors at multiple projection angles. The object for calibration may, for example, be a set of point sources in a known configuration. Because the calibration algorithm knows how the sources are configured, it can shift the projections to assure that the COR aligns with the center of the computer matrix and adjust the image size, location, and orientation for each detection such that they properly align at all projection angles. This calibration should be performed routinely. Although the frequency may depend on the stability of the specific SPECT system, it is typical that this calibration is performed monthly or quarterly. One further calibration may be necessary to assure proper alignment when the

SPECT data are acquired with noncircular orbits. This calibration maintains proper COR and multidetector calibration even when the detectors are at varying distances from the axis of rotation.

It is prudent to routinely test the SPECT image quality by imaging a standard phantom that tests for spatial resolution, contrast, and uniformity artifacts. Such a phantom typically consists of a fillable structure with features of known size and configuration, such as Plexiglas rods and spheres of different diameters and spacing. The phantom should also have a considerable-sized region of uniform activity in order to evaluate the presence of ring artifacts that can result from inadequate uniformity calibration. The SPECT QC phantom should be imaged at least quarterly using the same imaging setup (e.g., same collimator and radius of rotation), acquisition parameters (e.g., total counts per projection), and reconstruction method so that the current results can be compared to those acquired previously. ▶ Fig. 1.10

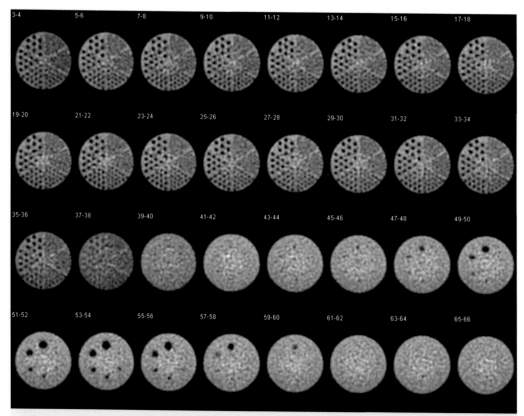

Fig. 1.10 The transverse slices from a SPECT acquisition of a standard phantom used for tomographic quality control. The phantom consists of a Plexiglas cylinder filled with liquid of a uniform radioactivity concentration. This phantom also has a section of Plexiglas rods of varying sizes and spacing, as well as six Plexiglas spheres of varying diameter that can be used to assess spatial resolution and contrast, respectively. The uniform portions of the phantom can also be used to evaluate the presence of ring artifacts. The images shown indicate that this SPECT system is in good working order.

shows images from a QC phantom when the scanner is performing appropriately.

1.4.2 Hybrid Single-Photon Emission Computed Tomography/Computed Tomography

A QC program considered proper for a clinical CT scanner should also be implemented for the CT component of a hybrid SPECT/CT system.[3] This is of particular importance if the CT images acquired with the device are to be used for diagnostic purposes. On a daily basis, the water phantom should be acquired, and the mean and standard deviation of CT numbers for water should be evaluated. In addition, the water phantom should be evaluated for artifacts. The video monitor used for diagnosis should be evaluated at least monthly. On an annual basis, other factors, such as the alignment light accuracy, image thickness, table travel accuracy, beam width, and low-contrast performance, should be evaluated. In addition, the alignment of the SPECT and CT scanners should be checked on a regular basis and corrected if necessary.

1.5 Radiation Dosimetry and Dose Optimization

The clinical benefits of SPECT and more recently SPECT/CT have been well established. In fact, chapters of this book clearly describe the application of SPECT and SPECT/CT in a wide variety of clinical applications. On the other hand, the application of SPECT and SPECT/CT involves the use of radiopharmaceuticals and X-rays, and thereby the patient is exposed to ionizing radiation. Such exposure may carry with it some small risk of adverse health effects. In 2006, the U.S. National Academy of Sciences released its report entitled *Health Risks from Exposure to Low Levels of Ionizing Radiation,* also referred to as the BEIR (Biological Effects of Ionizing Radiation) VII Phase 2 Report.[4] In this report, it was stated that induction of solid tumors was consistent with the "linear no-threshold" model of radiocarcinogenesis, whereas the induction of leukemia was more consistent with a linear-quadratic model. In either case, the report indicated that any exposure to ionizing radiation could carry some risk, although, for small exposures, this risk could be quite small. In addition, the risk of each exposure was independent and not affected by previous exposures to radiation. BEIR VII also indicated that the risk from adverse effects could be higher in children than in adults by a factor of 2 or 3. Also, young girls may be at a 30 to 40% higher risk than young boys, mostly due to the potential induction of breast cancer. Although the induction of cancer at higher radiations doses is well established, there is considerable uncertainty in the estimates for whole-body doses less than 200 mGy. The magnitude of the risk at these low doses could be a bit higher or a bit lower than that estimated by BEIR VII, or perhaps there is no risk at all. However, many would consider it prudent from a radiation safety point of view to consider the recommendations of BEIR VII, particularly in children.

The radiation dose to the patient resulting from the administration of a radiopharmaceutical can be estimated using the formalism described in MIRD Report 21.[5] The basic MIRD equation is given by

$$D(r_T) = \sum_S \tilde{A}(r_S)S(r_T \leftarrow r_S),$$

where $D(r_T)$ is the radiation dose to a particular target organ from a series of specified source organs. The time-integrated activity, $\tilde{A}(r_S)$ in units of becquerel-second (Bq-s), is determined by the amount of the administered activity that went to a certain source organ and how long it stayed there. Thus $\tilde{A}(r_S)$ depends directly on the amount of administered activity but is modified by the fraction that is distributed in the source organ and its effective mean-life within that source organ. The "S factor" (in mGy per Bq-s) defines the radiation dose to the target organ per unit time-integrated activity in the source organ. More specifically, S is given by

$$S(r_T \leftarrow r_S) = \sum_i \Delta_i \phi_i / M_T,$$

where Δ_i is the mean energy of the ith radiation (e.g., gamma ray, X-ray, or beta particle) emitted by the radionuclide of interest (most radionuclides emit more than one radiation), the absorbed fraction ϕ_i defines the fraction of that energy emitted by the source organ that is absorbed by the target organ, and M_T is the mass of the target organ. The S factor equation is summed over all radiations emitted by the radionuclide of interest as indicated by $\sum_i$. The S factor thereby depends on the physical aspects of the radionuclide plus a size- and shape-dependent model of the patient that yields both the absorbed fraction and the organ masses. Finally, the symbol $\sum_S$ indicates that the entire equation is summed over all source organs to yield the total radiation dose to the target organ.

In CT, the patient is irradiated by an X-ray tube that rotates around the patient. A particular portion of the patient can receive dose from the primary X-ray beam if it is within the collimated field of view and from the scattered X-rays if it is not within the field of view. Thereby, portions of the patient being imaged will receive the highest radiation dose, and other regions will receive less dose, depending on how far removed they are from the field of view. The resulting radiation dose to the patient will depend on the energy of the X-rays, the intensity of the X-ray fluence, and the duration of the exposure, as well as the size of the patient and the composition of the tissue being irradiated. The number of X-rays irradiating the patient is determined by the tube current (mA), scan duration, and tube voltage (kVp). The radiation dose varies linearly with the current-duration product (mAs) and roughly as the square of the kVp. The radiation dose also varies indirectly with the pitch/table speed. In some instances, the quotient of the mAs and the pitch (i.e., mAs/pitch) is referred to as the effective mAs.

The parameter of dose most commonly used in CT, referred to as the CT dose index (CTDI), is based on estimates made with one of two standard phantoms, 16- or 32-cm Plexiglas cylinders. Typically, the 16-cm phantom is used for head or pediatric estimations and the 32-cm phantom is used for whole-body estimations. A 100-mm, pencil-shaped ionization chamber is often used for the measurements from a single-slice CT acquisition; thus this measurement is referred to as $CTDI_{100}$, which depends on all the factors previously discussed, including mAs, kVp, and collimation. Both CTDI phantoms have five holes in which to place the dosimeter: one in the center and four on the periphery. The weighted combination of these measurements is given by $CTDI_w$:

$$CTDI_W = \frac{2}{3}\,CTDI_{100}^{Surface} + \frac{1}{3}\,CTDI_{100}^{Center}$$

For the same CT acquisition parameters, $CTDI_w$ would be higher when using the 16-cm phantom than when using the 32-cm phantom due to less attenuation for the central measurement for the smaller phantom. This also demonstrates why the CT dose for younger patients, such as children, is generally higher than that for adults for the same acquisition parameters. For helical CT, the pitch is incorporated to yield $CTDI_{vol}$:

$$CTDI_{Vol}\,(in\ mGy) = CTDI_W / pitch.$$

As expected, $CTDI_{vol}$ is indirectly proportional to pitch.

It is noted that, by definition, the CTDI parameters, including $CTDI_{vol}$, do not vary as a function of the axial extent of the scan. On the other hand, the energy deposited within the patient is clearly affected by this extent and thereby, perhaps, the associated potential risk. For this reason, the dose length production (DLP) is defined by

$$DLP\ (in\ mGy\ cm) = CTDI_{vol} \times L,$$

where L is the axial length of the scan in centimeters. In general, both the $CTDI_{vol}$ and the DLP are reported for each CT data acquisition and are now routinely incorporated in the DICOM radiation dose structure report for each patient. However, it is important to remember that these parameters do not directly relate to the radiation dose received by a particular patient but by the standard CTDI phantom, given the CT acquisition parameters used for the scan.

There has been recent interest in the optimization of SPECT and SPECT/CT protocols allowing for the acquisition of high-quality diagnostic information that addresses the clinical question at hand while maintaining the radiation dose (and thereby the radiation risk) to the patient at the lowest level possible. The Alliance for Radiation Safety in Pediatric Imaging has worked with a number of professional organizations, such as the Society of Pediatric Radiology, the Society of Nuclear Medicine and Molecular Imaging, and the American College of Radiology, to promote the Image Gently campaign (www.imagegently.org). For nuclear medicine, this has led to the development of the North American Consensus Guidelines for Administered Activities in Children and Adolescents. Also, the European Association of Nuclear Medicine has developed its Pediatric Dosage Card to provide guidance for pediatric nuclear medicine. More recently, these two organizations have worked together to harmonize these two sets of guidelines. In addition, the Japanese Society of Nuclear Medicine has also published guidelines for pediatric nuclear medicine.[6] For adult nuclear medicine, the Image Wisely Campaign provides useful information for nuclear medicine practitioners, referring physicians, and patients (www.imagewisely.org).

1.6 Conclusion

Over the past 30 years, SPECT has developed into an essential medical imaging modality due to its ability to provide an accurate 3D representation of the in vivo radiopharmaceutical distribution within the patient. In fact, the most common radiopharmaceutical procedure in the United States is myocardial perfusion SPECT. More recently, SPECT has been combined with CT to combine the anatomical and physiological imaging capabilities of the two modalities. SPECT requires attention to detail in regard to QC, data acquisition, and reconstruction in order to provide images of high diagnostic quality. In addition, procedures should be optimized to provide such high-quality image information while keeping the radiation dose to the patient as low as possible. This chapter provides the basic information necessary for nuclear medicine practitioners to best understand these challenges in the context of their particular clinical practice.

References

[1] National Council on Radiation Protection and Measurements (NCRP). Ionizing radiation exposure of the population of the United States. NCRP Report No. 160. Bethesda, MD: NCRP;2006

[2] Hasegawa BH, Stebler B, Rutt BK, et al. A prototype high-purity germanium detector system with fast photon-counting circuitry for medical imaging. Med Phys. 1991; 18 (5):900–909

[3] American College of Radiology. Computed Tomography Quality Control Manual. Reston, VA: American College of Radiology; 2012

[4] Committee to Assess Health Risks from Exposure to Low Levels of Ionizing Radiation; Board on Radiation Effects Research; Division on Earth and Life Studies; National Research Council. Health Risks from Exposure to Low Levels of Ionizing Radiation: BEIR VII, Phase 2. Washington, DC: The National Academies Press; 2006

[5] Bolch WE, Eckerman KF, Sgouros G, Thomas SR. MIRD pamphlet no. 21: a generalized schema for radiopharmaceutical dosimetry—standardization of nomenclature. J Nucl Med. 2009:50(3):477–484

[6] Fahey FH, Bom HH, Chiti A, et al. Standardization of administered activities in pediatric nuclear medicine: a report of the first nuclear medicine global initiative project, part 1-statement of the issue and a review of available resources. J Nucl Med. 2015:56(4):646–651

2 Radiopharmaceuticals for Clinical SPECT Studies

Shankar Vallabhajoshula

2.1 Introduction

George de Hevesy in the 1920s coined the terms *radioindicator* and *radiotracer* and introduced the *tracer principle* into biomedical sciences. A radiotracer can be defined as a specific radiolabeled molecule (or probe) that resembles or traces the in vivo behavior of a natural molecule and can be used to provide information about a specific biological process. One of the most important characteristics of a true radiotracer, however, is the ability to study the components of a homeostatic system without disturbing their natural function. Occasionally, the term *radioligand* is also used in the context of imaging studies. A radioligand is defined as any radiolabeled molecule that binds with another molecule or substance (binder) in a predictable way under controlled conditions.

All radiolabeled compounds or substances used for the purpose of diagnosis or therapy, however, have been defined as *radioactive drugs* or *radiopharmaceuticals* by the U.S. Food and Drug Administration (FDA). A radiopharmaceutical is a natural or synthetic chemical compound containing a radionuclide or a radioisotope. While the chemical compound with structural or chemical properties determines the in vivo distribution and physiological behavior of the radiopharmaceutical, the radionuclide provides the desired radiation characteristics for imaging or therapy. From a regulatory point of view, a radiopharmaceutical must be sterile, pyrogen free, safe for human use, and efficacious for a specific indication. FDA-approved radiopharmaceuticals for routine clinical single-photon emission computed tomography (SPECT) studies are listed in ▶ Table 2.1. Radiopharmaceuticals usually have no pharmacological effects, as they are used in minute quantities. Thus there is no dose–response relationship in this case, which differs significantly from conventional drugs.

2.2 Radiopharmaceutical

2.2.1 Ideal Properties of Diagnostic Radiopharmaceuticals

- The radionuclide used to label the chemical compound should
  - preferably be a pure gamma (γ) emitter with energy in the range of 100 to 250 keV for optimum performance of a gamma camera.
  - have a physical half-life ($t_{1/2}$) suitable for diagnostic use.
  - result in low radiation dose to the patient and nuclear medicine personnel.

Table 2.1 FDA-approved radiopharmaceuticals

Radiopharmaceuticals/Kits	Manufacturer	Trade names
Molybdenum Mo-99 generator	Mallinckrodt (Covidien) Lantheus Medical Imaging	Ultra-TechneKow DTE TechneLite
Technetium-99 m macroaggregated albumin	DRAXIMAGE	
Technetium-99 m sulfur colloid	Pharmalucence	
Technetium-99 m pentetate, DTPA	DRAXIMAGE	
Technetium-99 m succimer, DMSA	GE Healthcare	
Technetium-99 m medronate	Bracco Diagnostics DRAXIMAGE GE Healthcare Pharmalucence	MDP-Bracco MDP-25 MDP Multidose
Technetium-99 m oxidronate	Mallinckrodt	Technescan HDP
Technetium-99 m exametazime	GE Healthcare	Ceretec
Technetium-99 m bicisate	Lantheus Medical Imaging	Neurolite
Technetium-99 m disofenin	Pharmalucence	Hepatolite

Table 2.1 (*continued*) FDA-approved radiopharmaceuticals

Radiopharmaceuticals/Kits	Manufacturer	Trade names
Technetium-99 m mebrofenin	Bracco Diagnostics Pharmalucence	Choletec
Technetium-99 m mertiatide	Mallinckrodt	Technescan MAG3
Technetium-99 m sestamibi	Lantheus Medical Imaging Cardinal Health Mallinckrodt DRAXIMAGE Lantheus Medical Imaging Pharmalucence	Cardiolite
Technetium-99 m tetrofosmin	GE Healthcare	Myoview
Kit for labeling technetium-99 m RBCs	Mallinckrodt	UltraTag
Technetium-99 m pyrophosphate	Mallinckrodt	
Technetium-99 m tilmanocept	Navidea Biopharmaceuticals	Lymphoseek
Thallium-201 chloride	Mallinckrodt GE Healthcare Lantheus Medical Imaging	
Gallium-67 citrate	Amersham GE Mallinckrodt Lantheus Medical Imaging	Neoscan
Indium-111 pentetate (DTPA)	GE Healthcare	
Indium-111 oxyquinoline (oxine)	GE Healthcare	
Indium-111 pentetreotide	Mallinckrodt	OctreoScan
Indium-111 capromab Pendetide	EUSA Pharma	ProstaScint
Iodine-123 sodium iodide capsules	Cardinal Health Mallinckrodt	
Iodine-123 iobenguane, MIBG	GE Healthcare	AdreView
Iodine-123 ioflupane	GE Healthcare	DaTscan
Iodine I-131 sodium iodide	Mallinckrodt DRAXIMAGE	HICON

- The radiopharmaceutical should
  - have an in vivo biodistribution providing high target/background ratio.
  - be easy to prepare with very high (> 90%) radiochemical purity (RCP).
  - be stable in vivo without metabolite formation or release of free radiochemical impurities.

2.2.2 Mechanisms of Radiopharmaceutical Localization

The uptake and retention of radiopharmaceuticals by different organs and tissues involve many different mechanisms, as summarized in ▶ Table 2.2. The mechanisms of radiopharmaceutical localization may be substrate nonspecific (not participating in any specific biochemical reaction) or substrate specific, depending on the chemistry of the radiopharmaceutical. As the radiopharmaceutical may undergo metabolism in vivo, the observed biodistribution (based on imaging) would include the distribution of the intact parent radiopharmaceutical and also of its radiolabeled metabolites. In addition, the patient's medication and several other factors may significantly alter the biodistribution of the radiopharmaceutical.

Table 2.2 Mechanisms of radiopharmaceutical localization

	Mechanism	Radiopharmaceutical
1	Isotope dilution	^{99m}Tc-Red blood cells (RBC)
2	Capillary blockade	^{99m}Tc-Macroaggregated albumin (MAA)
3	Phagocytosis	^{99m}Tc-Sulfur colloid (SC)
4	Cell migration	^{111}In-oxine-White blood cells (WBC), ^{99m}Tc-HMPAO-WBCs
5	Cell sequestration	^{99m}Tc-RBCs (heat damaged)
6	Simple diffusion	^{133}Xe gas, ^{99m}Tc-DTPA aerosol, and Technegas
	Diffusion and mitochondrial binding	^{99m}Tc-sestamibi (Cardiolite) and ^{99m}Tc-tetrofosmin (Myoview)
	Diffusion and intracellular binding	^{99m}Tc-Exametazine (HMPAO; Ceretec) ^{99m}Tc-Bicisate (ECD; Neurolite) ^{99m}Tc-DMSA
	Diffusion and increased capillary permeability	^{67}Ga-citrate
7	Active transport	
	Na$^+$/I$^-$ NIS	^{123}I and ^{131}I Sodium iodide (I$^-$)
	Na$^+$-K$^+$-ATPase pump	^{201}Tl-Thallous chloride (Tl+)
8	Ion exchange with Ca^{2+} in hydroxyapatite	^{99m}Tc-Medronate (MDP) ^{99m}Tc-Oxidronate (HDP)
9	Glomerular filtration	^{99m}Tc-Pentetate (DTPA)
10	Tubular secretion	^{99m}Tc-Merteatide (MAG3)
11	Tissue hypoxia and acidic pH	^{67}Ga-citrate
12	Specific receptor binding	
	Hepatocyte anionic receptor	^{99m}Tc-DISIDA or Disofenin (Hepatolite) ^{99m}Tc-Mebrofenin (Choletec)
	Somatostatin (SSTR2) receptor	^{111}In-Pentetreotide (Octreotide; OctreoScan)
	Dopamine transporter (DaT)	^{123}I-Ioflupane (DaTscan)
	Norepinephrine and serotonin transporters and energy-dependent type I amine uptake mechanism	^{123}I and ^{131}I-Metaiodobenzylguanidine (MIBG)

2.3 Radionuclides Used for SPECT Radiopharmaceuticals

The most common radionuclides used for diagnostic SPECT studies are summarized in ▶ Table 2.3. Technetium-99 m (^{99m}Tc) is the most ideal radionuclide for SPECT radiopharmaceuticals because it decays by isomeric transition (IT) to ^{99}Tc, with γ photons of 140 keV in high abundance (89%). Among the radionuclides that decay by electron capture (^{123}I, ^{67}Ga, ^{111}In, ^{201}Tl), ^{123}I has an ideal γ energy (159 keV) with a high photon abundance (83%). The three metallic nuclides (^{67}Ga, ^{111}In, and ^{201}Tl) have longer half-lives (~3 days) and deliver more radiation dose to the patient than ^{99m}Tc- or ^{123}I-labeled radiopharmaceuticals. It is important to remember that the γ photons from ^{201}Tl are in low abundance and not useful for imaging studies. However, ^{201}Tl decays to ^{201}Hg, and the low-energy characteristic X-rays (~80 KeV) emitted as a result of this process are useful for imaging.

Table 2.3 Radionuclides useful for SPECT imaging studies

Element	Z_1	Natural isotopes		Radioisotope	Decay	Half-life	γ-Emission	
		Isotope	Abundance (%)				Energy (KeV)	Abundance (%)
Technetium	43			^{99m}Tc	IT	6.0 h	141	89.0
Iodine	53	^{127}I	100	^{123}I	EC	13.1 h	159	83.0
				^{131}I	$β^-$, γ	8.0 d	528	1.40
							364	81.0
							637	7.0
Gallium	31	^{69}Ga	60.1	^{67}Ga	EC	3.26 d	93	36.0
		^{71}Ga	39.9				185	20.0
							300	16.0
							394	4.5.0
Indium	49	^{113}In	4.3	^{111}In	EC	2.83 d	173	91.0
		^{115}In	95.7				247	94.0
Thallium	81	^{203}Tl	29.524	^{201}Tl	EC	3.046 d	167	10.0
		^{205}Tl	70.476				69–80	100
							X-rays	

[1]Atomic Number (Z).

2.3.1 Production of Radionuclides

Radionuclides used for SPECT studies are produced in a nuclear reactor or a cyclotron. The nuclear reactions commonly used to produce radionuclides are shown in ▸ Table 2.4. In a nuclear reaction, when the atoms of a stable element (target) are bombarded by a subatomic particle (bombarding particle or projectile), the nucleus absorbs the subatomic particle and becomes unstable or excited (parent nucleus). Spontaneous decay results in the emission of radiation and/or particle(s) to form a product, which is usually a more stable nuclide. The equation for a nuclear reaction is written as follows:

$$T(P, R)Y,$$

where T represents the target nuclide; P is the projectile, the incident or bombarding particle; R represents the radiation (subatomic particle or γ photons) emitted by the compound nucleus; and, finally, Y represents the product unstable radionuclide. The P and R in parenthesis, written as (P, R), represent the nuclear reaction. A number of reactions, such as (p, n), $(p, α)$, (d, n), and $(n, γ)$, are some of the common nuclear reactions used to produce artificial radioisotopes.

2.3.2 Nuclear Reactor Produced Radionuclides

When a large fissile atomic nucleus, such as uranium-235 or plutonium-239, absorbs a thermal neutron (energy < 0.25 eV), it may undergo nuclear fission (f). The heavy nucleus splits into two or more lighter nuclei (the fission products), releasing kinetic energy, gamma radiation, and free neutrons. A portion of these neutrons may later be absorbed by other fissile atoms and trigger further fission events, which release more neutrons, and so on. This is known as a nuclear chain reaction. A nuclear reactor is a device used to initiate and control a sustained nuclear chain reaction. The fuel cells containing enriched ^{235}U (as ^{235}UF$_6$ or ^{235}UO$_2$) pellets are surrounded by a moderator (graphite or heavy water) to slow down the energetic fission neutrons. Control rods capable of absorbing neutrons but not undergoing a nuclear reaction (such as cadmium and boron) are used to sustain the chain reaction.

When the reactor is in operation, the nuclear reaction (n, f) produces a number of neutron-rich fission fragments $(Z = 28–65)$, which decay by $β^-$, or γ-emission. Radionuclides such as ^{99}Mo and ^{131}I accumulate in the fuel rods to enormous activities (thousands of gigabecquerels [GBq]). All the fission fragments can be separated chemically and

Table 2.4 Production of radionuclides useful for SPECT studies

Method	Radionuclide	Nuclear reaction	Specific activity (mCi/µmol)
Reactor-produced radionuclides	^{99}Mo	^{235}U (n, f) ^{99}Mo ^{99}Mo (n, γ) ^{99}Mo	1000
	^{131}I	^{235}U $(n, f)^{131}$I ^{130}Te (n, γ) ^{131}Te $(t_{1/2} = 25$ m$) \rightarrow ^{131}$I	>16,000
Cyclotron-produced radionuclides	^{67}Ga	^{68}Zn $(p, 2n)$ ^{67}Ga ^{66}Zn (d, n) ^{67}Ga.	>67
	^{111}In	^{111}Cd (p, n) ^{111}In ^{112}Cd $(p, 2n)$ ^{111}In	
	^{201}Tl	^{203}Tl $(p, 3n)$ ^{201}Pb $\rightarrow$ ^{201}Tl	>200
	^{123}I	^{127}I $(p, 5n)$ ^{123}Xe $\rightarrow$ ^{123}I ^{124}Xe $(p, 2n)$ ^{123}Cs $\rightarrow$ ^{123}Xe $\rightarrow$ ^{123}I ^{124}Xe (p, pn) ^{123}Xe $\rightarrow$ ^{123}I	>237,000

purified to yield no-carrier-added (NCA), high-specific-activity radionuclides.

A nuclear reaction in which a neutron is captured or absorbed by the nucleus of a stable atom leading to a nuclear transformation is called *neutron activation*. The most common nuclear reaction is (n, γ), in which the target nucleus with a mass number A captures a neutron to become an unstable excited radioisotope of target nucleus with a mass number A + 1. The excited nucleus emits a gamma photon, and the product radionuclide decays by β-emission to reach a ground state. As the product nuclide is an isotope of the target element, the product cannot be separated and purified to avoid the contamination of the carrier. As a result, radioisotopes produced using (n, γ) reaction are generally very low in specific activity.

It is possible to produce carrier-free, high-specific-activity nuclides in a reactor. Certain (n, γ) reactions produce a short-lived radioisotope of the target element, which decays by β-emission to another unstable radioactive nuclide with relatively longer half-life compared to that of the intermediate. ^{131}I can be produced by neutron activation of enriched ^{130}Te isotope.

2.3.3 Cyclotron-Produced Radionuclides

A cyclotron is a particle accelerator in which charged particles (protons, deuterons, and α particles) are accelerated using a high-frequency alternating potential difference between two hollow **D**-shaped sheet metal electrodes called "dees" placed inside a vacuum chamber in a magnetic field. The resulting high-energy charged particle beam is directed toward a target (atoms of a stable element), chosen in such a way that the desired radionuclide is produced. Most modern-day medical cyclotrons are called *negative-ion machines* because they generate positive particle beams with high energies (10–75 MeV) and currents (50–150 µA). When the target atoms are bombarded by a positive charge, the product is a proton-rich (neutron-deficient) radionuclide of a different element that decays by electron capture or positron emission. As a result, the radioisotopes produced in a cyclotron have high specific activity and are carrier free. Common radionuclides produced in a cyclotron are summarized in ▶ Table 2.3.

Specific Activity

Specific activity is defined as the amount of radioactivity per unit mass of an element, molecule, or compound, where the mass is the combined mass of the radioactive and the nonradioactive (stable or cold) species. Units of specific activity include mCi/mg, Ci/mmol, or GBq/µmol. Since 1 mol represents 6.02×10^{23} atoms or molecules (Avogadro's number), one µmol consists of 6.02×10^{17} atoms or molecules. The theoretical specific activities of several radionuclides are shown in ▶ Table 2.3.

Carrier Free

Carrier free means that the radioactive species is not contaminated with a nonradioactive counterpart, which is known as a carrier. When radionuclides are produced using a cyclotron, the target element is converted into a different element (with a higher atomic number). As a result, cyclotron-produced radionuclides are theoretically *carrier free*. In reality, it is very difficult to eliminate the contamination of natural carbon, fluorine, or other trace metals during the synthesis procedure. Thus a more appropriate concept is NCA, which means a stable, nonradioactive species is not intentionally added. In certain cases, carrier may be added intentionally during radioisotope production to facilitate chemical and biochemical reactions. Such preparations should specifically be reported as *carrier added*.

2.3.4 Radionuclide Generators

A radionuclide generator is a device used to produce a daughter radionuclide from a parent radionuclide via radioactive decay, and the daughter radionuclide is then separated from the parent radionuclide. In this serial radioactive decay process, the daughter is continuously produced by the decay of the parent while the daughter activity is also decaying. At equilibrium, the parent and daughter activities appear to decay with the same rate, even if the two radionuclides have different half-lives. Two different equilibrium conditions (transient or secular) may exist, depending on how short lived the daughter radionuclide is compared to the parent. If the parent is short lived compared to the daughter, then there is no equilibrium at all. If the parent and daughter radionuclides are different elements, they can be separated chemically, and the daughter radioactivity can be obtained in high specific activity. Such a parent–daughter (mother–daughter) radionuclide pair is ideal to build a generator system to produce daughter radionuclide.

^{99m}Tc Generator

^{99}Mo is one of the fission products of ^{235}U fission in a nuclear reactor. It is known as fission moly and is produced with a very high specific activity compared to ^{99}Mo produced by neutron activation. Most commercial generators are made with fission moly. The generator is based on a solid column method in which 5 to 10 g of preheated alumina (Al_2O_3) is loaded into a plastic or glass column. The ^{99}Mo activity (2–32 Ci) in the form of molybdate ion (MoO_4^{2-}) is adsorbed on the column. The column is thoroughly washed to remove undesirable contaminants. The amount of ^{99}Mo activity on the column, along with the date and time of calibration

(TOC), is provided for each generator. Commercial generators are sterilized and well shielded with lead or depleted uranium.

Once the generator is washed and calibrated, at time T_0, there is no ^{99m}Tc activity on the column. As ^{99}Mo ($t_{1/2} = 66$ hours) decays, ^{99m}Tc activity ($t_{1/2} = 6$ hours) is produced and builds up in the column as a function of time. Unlike molybdenum, technetium does not bind to alumina; it is immediately converted to ^{99m}Tc pertechnetate ion (^{99m}TcO4$^-$), which is the most stable chemical form of technetium, with an oxidation state of +7. Typically, > 75% of ^{99m}Tc activity can be eluted with 3 to 10 mL of physiological saline solution.

Small amounts of ^{99}Mo activity may occasionally *break through* (leakage or partial elution) from the column into the ^{99m}Tc pertechnetate solution. The maximum ^{99}Mo contamination allowed is 0.15 µCi/mCi or 0.15 kBq/MBq of ^{99m}Tc pertechnetate solution at the time of elution. Each ^{99m}Tc dose to a patient should not contain > 5 µCi of ^{99}Mo activity. As a chemical impurity, Al ion concentration should be < 10 to 20 µg/mL of eluent.

Both ^{99}Mo (13%) and ^{99m}Tc decay to long-lived ^{99}Tc, which, in turn, decays slowly by β-emission to stable ^{99}Ru. Since ^{99m}Tc and ^{99}Tc are isomers and chemically the same element, the presence of ^{99}Tc may act as a carrier in the preparation of ^{99m}Tc radiotracers. When the generator is eluted once a day (every 24 hours), the number of ^{99m}Tc atoms is 27% of total ^{99}Tc atoms. If the generator is eluted after 4 days, the number of ^{99m}Tc atoms is 5% of the total ^{99}Tc atoms.

2.4 Preparation of Radiopharmaceuticals

2.4.1 General Methods of Radiolabeling

Depending on the type of radioisotope chosen and the method used to prepare a radiopharmaceutical, two different methods are generally used, as summarized in the following:

1. *Isotope exchange*: A radiopharmaceutical can be prepared by direct exchange (isotopic substitution) of one or more stable atoms of an element in a molecule with one or more nuclides of a radioisotope of the same element. The radiolabeled molecule and the unlabeled molecule are chemically identical and behave in vivo in a similar manner. This method of radiolabeling is generally used to prepare radioiodinated

radiopharmaceuticals in which the stable ^{127}I atom is replaced by a ^{123}I or ^{131}I atom.

2. *Introduction of a foreign element, such as a radiometal*: A radiopharmaceutical can be prepared by the introduction of a foreign element or radionuclide in a chemical compound. Most of the radiopharmaceuticals are prepared based on this method. This method involves attaching a radionuclide, such as ^{99m}Tc and ^{111}In, to an organic molecule known as a chelating agent. One or more atoms (such as ^{16}O, ^{14}N, and ^{32}S) in the chelating agent donate a pair of electrons to the radiometal atom to form coordinate covalent bonds. As a result, the chemical and biological properties of the radiometal–chelate complex are different compared to the chelating agent. Certain peptides and macromolecules, such as monoclonal antibodies, can be labeled with radiometals based on the metal chelation method described previously. This technique, however, requires conjugation of a bifunctional chelate (BFC) to the peptide or protein first, and then subsequent chelation of the radiometal by the BFC molecule. The radiometal is not directly incorporated into the peptide or protein molecule.

2.4.2 ^{99m}Tc Radiopharmaceuticals

Chemistry of Tc-99m

^{99m}Tc is a second-row group VII transition metal and capable of multiple oxidation states (- 1 to + 7). In aqueous solution, the pertechnetate anion, ^{99m}TcO$_4^-$, is the most stable chemical species, with a + 7 oxidation state. Because its size and charge are similar to those of iodide (I$^-$), the in vivo distribution of pertechnetate is similar to that of the iodide ion. As pertechnetate is chemically stable and inert, it cannot bind directly to any organic molecule or chelate. Following reduction by appropriate reducing agents, ^{99m}Tc pertechnetate can be transformed into lower oxidation states that are chemically more reactive. Several reducing agents have been investigated, with stannous chloride (SnCl$_2$) being the most widely employed for preparing complexes of Tc(V) and Tc(I), while boron hydrides are used to prepare organometallic Tc(I) complexes. During reduction by the stannous ion (Sn^{2+}) in an appropriate buffer and pH, the presence of a ligand stabilizes Tc in its lower oxidation state. In a specific Tc complex, the oxidation state of Tc, however, depends on the chelate and pH. As a transition metal, Tc can adopt a large number of coordination geometries, depending on the donor atoms and the type of chelating agent. Several donor atoms, such as N, S, O, and P, geometrically arranged in a chelating molecule can form coordination complexes with technetium. A number of ligands (e.g., DTPA, MAG3, DMSA), iminodiacetic acid derivatives (e.g., diisopropylacetanilido iminodiacetic acid [DISIDA] and bromine-substituted acetanilido iminodiacetic acid [BrIDA]), and phosphates and phosphonates (e.g., PYP, MDP, and EHDP) have been labeled with ^{99m}Tc and routinely used for diagnostic imaging studies in nuclear medicine.

^{99m}Tc-labeled radiopharmaceuticals are generally prepared using cold lyophilized kits typically formulated with a coordinating ligand (or a chelating agent); a reducing agent (stannous chloride); and adjuvants, such as ancillary chelating agents, buffers, and antioxidants. The optimum formulation is determined for each specific type of cold kit.

^{99m}Tc pertechnetate eluted from a generator is used to prepare all other ^{99m}Tc-labeled radiopharmaceuticals. Preparation of certain ^{99m}Tc radiopharmaceuticals requires ^{99m}Tc pertechnetate containing minimal amounts of ^{99}Tc atoms. It is important to remember that ^{99m}Tc is never "carrier free." Eluting the generator twice, with the second elution made only a few hours after the first elution, will provide optimal labeling yields and a more favorable ratio of ^{99m}Tc to ^{99}Tc.

Sodium Pertechnetate Tc-99 m Injection

^{99m}Tc is a sterile solution of ^{99m}Tc (and ^{99}Tc) as sodium pertechnetate in 0.9% sodium chloride (normal saline) injection obtained by the elution of the ^{99}Mo → ^{99m}Tc generator. The pertechnetate ion distributes in the body similarly to the iodide ion but is not organified when trapped in the thyroid gland. Pertechnetate tends to accumulate in intracranial lesions with excessive neovascularity or an altered blood–brain barrier. It also concentrates in the thyroid gland, salivary glands, gastric mucosa, and choroid plexus. However, in contrast to the iodide ion, the pertechnetate ion is released unchanged from the thyroid gland.

Tc-99 m Albumin Aggregated Injection (^{99m}Tc-MAA)

^{99m}Tc-MAA is a sterile aqueous suspension of ^{99m}Tc labeled to macroaggregates of human albumin. Macroaggregated albumin (MAA) cold kits contain lyophilized material of MAA particles, stannous chloride, and human albumin sealed under nitrogen. Approximately 90% of particles are in the range of 10 to 90 μm, and none can exceed 150 μm. Because the kit is designed as a multidose vial and contains 4 to 6 million particles, the appropriate amount of ^{99m}Tc pertechnetate must be added to the vial in order to have a single 3.0 mCi dose of ^{99m}Tc-MAA contain 200,000 to 500,000 particles. It is important to remember that the number of particles per dose will increase with time. The number of particles may need to be decreased for pediatric subjects and for those patients who have right-to-left cardiac shunts.

Within 1 to 5 minutes of intravenous injection, > 90% of ^{99m}Tc-MAA particles are trapped in the arterioles and capillaries of the lung by a purely mechanical process, which is a function of regional pulmonary blood flow. Particles < 10 μm are taken up by the reticuloendothelial system. Elimination of the labeled particles from the lungs occurs with a biological half-life of approximately 6 hours.

Tc-99 m Sulfur Colloid Injection (^{99m}Tc-SC)

^{99m}Tc-SC is a sterile colloidal dispersion of sulfur particles labeled with ^{99m}Tc pertechnetate and a cold kit containing three components:

1. A reaction vial containing a lyophilized mixture of 2.0 mg of sodium thiosulfate, 2.3 mg of disodium edetate (Al3 + chelator), and 18.1 mg of gelatin (protective colloid).
2. A solution *A vial* with 1.8 mL of 0.148 M HCl.
3. A solution *B vial* with 1.8 mL of a buffer containing anhydrous sodium phosphate (44.28 mg) and sodium hydroxide (14.22 mg).

After mixing the contents of the vial with 1 to 3 mL of ^{99m}Tc pertechnetate (~ 200 mCi) and hydrochloric acid, the mixture is heated at 100°C for 5 minutes. The vial is cooled and the buffer is added to the vial. During the reaction, elemental sulfur atoms are released to form colloid particles (< 1.0 μm). Gelatin provides a protective coating of the particles and controls the size of particles. Also during the reaction, ^{99m}Tc (nonreduced form) interacts with sulfur atoms, forming ^{99m}Tc-heptasulfide (Tc$_2$S$_7$). ^{99m}Tc-SC filtered through a 0.1- or 0.22-μm membrane filter is used in lymphoscintigraphy to localize the sentinel node in breast cancer and melanoma.

Following intravenous administration, ^{99m}Tc-SC is rapidly cleared by the reticuloendothelial system from the blood with a nominal clearance half-life of approximately 2.5 minutes. Approximately 80 to 90% of the injected colloidal particles are phagocytized by the Kupffer cells of the liver, 5 to 10% by the spleen, and the rest by the bone marrow.

Tc-99 m Pentetate Injection (^{99m}Tc-DTPA)

^{99m}Tc-DTPA is a sterile aqueous solution prepared by adding 2 to 8 mL ^{99m}Tc pertechnetate (200–500 mCi) to a kit (vial) containing a lyophilized mixture of the pentetate (or DTPA), stannous chloride, and other chemicals, such as calcium chloride and para-aminobenzoic acid (PABA; a free radical scavenger).

Following intravenous administration, ^{99m}Tc-DTPA rapidly distributes itself throughout the extracellular fluid space, from which it is promptly cleared from the body by glomerular filtration. There should be little or no binding of the chelate by the renal parenchyma. Depending on the preparation, the plasma protein binding of ^{99m}Tc may be 3 to 10%. The images of the kidneys obtained in the first few minutes after administration of ^{99m}Tc-DTPA represent the vascular pool within the kidney. ^{99m}Tc-DTPA is also used for the preparation of ^{99m}Tc-DTPA aerosol for lung ventilation studies.

Tc-99 m Succimer Injection (^{99m}Tc-DMSA)

^{99m}Tc-DMSA is a sterile aqueous solution prepared by adding ^{99m}Tc pertechnetate (40 mCi in 1–6 mL) to a kit containing a lyophilized mixture of DMSA (1.0 mg), stannous chloride dihydrate (0.42 mg), ascorbic acid (0.7 mg), and inositol (50 mg) sealed under nitrogen. Following incubation at room temperature (RT) for 10 minutes, the resulting product with a pH of 2.0 to 3.0 is stable for 4 hours. Ascorbic acid helps the formation of ^{99m}Tc (III)-DMSA complex with optimal renal cortical uptake.

After intravenous administration, ^{99m}Tc-DMSA is distributed in the plasma, apparently bound to plasma proteins. There is negligible activity in the red blood cells. The activity is cleared from the plasma, with a half-time of approximately 60 minutes, and concentrates in the renal cortex. Approximately 16% of the activity is excreted in the urine within the first 2 hours. At 6 hours, approximately 20% of the dose is concentrated in each kidney. It is used as an aid in the scintigraphic evaluation of renal parenchymal disorders. A different preparation of ^{99m}Tc (V)-DMSA (not approved by FDA) localizes differently, with little kidney uptake, and is taken up by a variety of tumors.

Tc-99 m Medronate Injection (^{99m}Tc-MDP)

^{99m}Tc-MDP is a sterile aqueous solution prepared by the addition of ^{99m}Tc pertechnetate (< 500 mCi/ 2–8 mL) to a lyophilized kit containing medronic acid or methylene diphosphonate (10–20 mg) and stannous chloride (0.17–1.21 mg). To protect the relatively labile complex from degradation by oxygen and free radicals, kits may also contain ascorbic acid, PABA, or gentisic acid as stabilizers.

During the initial 24 hours following intravenous injection of ^{99m}Tc-MDP, approximately 50% is retained in the skeleton and approximately 50% is excreted into the bladder. In humans, blood levels fall to 4 to 10% of the injected dose by 2 hours and to 3 to 5% by 3 hours. It exhibits a specific affinity for areas of altered osteogenesis. Uptake of ^{99m}Tc-MDP in bone binds to hydroxyapatite and appears to be related to osteogenic activity and skeletal blood perfusion.

Tc-99 m Oxidronate Injection (^{99m}Tc-HDP)

^{99m}Tc-HDP is a sterile aqueous solution prepared by adding ^{99m}Tc pertechnetate (300 mCi/3–6 mL) to a kit containing a lyophilized mixture of oxidronate sodium (3.15 mg), stannous chloride dehydrate (0.297 mg), gentisic acid (0.84 mg), and sodium chloride (30 mg). The clinical pharmacology and mechanism of bone localization are similar to those of ^{99m}Tc-MDP.

Tc-99 m Exametazime Injection (^{99m}Tc-HMPAO)

^{99m}Tc-HMPAO is a sterile aqueous solution prepared by adding ^{99m}Tc pertechnetate (10–54 mCi/ 1–2 mL) to a kit vial containing a sterile lyophilized mixture of exametazime or hexamethylpropyleneamine oxime (HMPAO; 0.5 mg), stannous chloride dehydrate (7.6 µg), and sodium chloride (4.5 mg). This product a not very stable and must be injected within 0.5 hours. Because the kit contains very small amount of stannous chloride, ^{99m}Tc

pertechnetate with minimal ^{99}Tc contamination must be used. In order to prepare a stabilized product, the kit also contains two additional vials: one with methylene blue solution (1%) and the other with phosphate buffer. First, 0.5 mL of methylene blue is mixed with 4.5 mL of phosphate buffer. Within 2 minutes after the preparation of ^{99m}Tc-HMPAO, 2 mL of the methylene blue/phosphate buffer mixture is added. The product is stable for 4 hours. However, the patient dose needs to be injected through a 0.45-µm membrane filter to remove any particles. The European kits contain cobaltous chloride as the stabilizer.

Because ^{99m}Tc-HMPAO has two chiral carbon atoms, it can form up to four stereoisomers: two *meso* isomers (that are identical) and two *D,L* isomers (also known as enantiomers). The *meso* isomers have poor brain uptake. The commercial kit contains *D,L* racemate, and ^{99m}Tc-HMPAO is neutral and lipophilic. But it is unstable and is converted to a hydrophilic complex mediated by reducing agents.

Following intravenous administration, a maximum of 3.5 to 7.0% of administered activity localizes in the brain as a function of cerebral perfusion. Over the next 2 minutes, 15% of the activity is washed out, and the remaining activity is trapped in the neuronal cells. The brain retention is due to the intracellular conversion to a nondiffusible hydrophilic complex mediated by intracellular glutathione.

Tc-99 m Bicisate Injection (^{99m}Tc-ECD)

The kit for the preparation of ^{99m}Tc-ethyl cysteinate dimer (^{99m}Tc-ECD) contains two vials: vial A contains a lyophilized mixture of bicisate dihydrochloride, also known as ethyl cysteinate dimer (ECD; 0.9 mg), stannous chloride dihydrate (72 µg), disodium edetate dihydrate (0.36 mg), and mannitol (24 mg), adjusted to pH 2.7 and sealed under nitrogen, and vial B contains 1.0 mL of phosphate buffer at pH 7.6. In order to prepare ^{99m}Tc-ECD, ^{99m}Tc pertechnetate (100 mCi in 2.0 mL) is first added to the vial containing phosphate buffer. Then 3.0 mL saline is added to the ECD vial and, within 30 seconds, 1.0 mL is removed from the ECD vial and added to the vial containing ^{99m}Tc pertechnetate in buffer. The mixture is allowed to incubate for 30 minutes at room temperature.

^{99m}Tc-ECD is a sterile, stable, neutral, and lipophilic complex, which can cross the blood–brain barrier and intact cell membranes by passive diffusion. The ECD ligand exists as *L,L* and *D,D* isomers, but only the *L,L* isomer exhibits brain retention. The uptake in the brain is approximately 4.8 to 6.5% of the injected dose at 5 minutes after injection and is stable for approximately 6 hours. The activity in blood clears very rapidly, and 5% of the injected dose remains in circulation at 1 hour. It is excreted primarily through the kidneys. Within 2 hours, 50% of the injected dose is excreted, and by 24 hours 74% is found in the urine. Localization of the parent compound in the brain, in part, depends on both perfusion of the region and uptake of [99mTc]-ECD by the cell. Once in the brain cells, the parent compound is metabolized to polar, less diffusible compounds.

Tc-99 m Disofenin Injection ([99mTc]-DISIDA)

[99mTc]-DISIDA is a sterile aqueous solution prepared by adding [99mTc] pertechnetate (20–100 mCi in 4–5 mL) to a kit containing disofenin or DISIDA (20 mg) and stannous chloride dehydrate (0.6 mg) at pH 4 to 5, sealed under nitrogen. The mixture is allowed to incubate for 5 minutes at RT. [99mTc]-DISIDA is a hexacoordinate complex in which the Tc atom is complexed by two disofenin molecules resulting in a net negative charge (1–).

Following intravenous administration, [99mTc]-DISIDA is rapidly cleared from circulation. Approximately 8% of the injected dose remains in circulation at 30 minutes, and 9% is excreted in the urine over a period of 2 hours. The remainder of the activity is essentially quantitatively cleared through the hepatobiliary system. The uptake in the liver is by active transport at the anionic receptor site on the hepatocyte membrane, where it competes with bilirubin. As the serum bilirubin level increases, the blood clearance gets progressively delayed.

Tc-99 m Mebrofenin Injection ([99mTc]-BrIDA)

[99mTc]-BrIDA is a sterile aqueous solution prepared by adding [99mTc] pertechnetate (up to 100 mCi in 1–5 mL) to a kit containing mebrofenin or methyl- and bromine-substituted acetanilido iminodiacetic acid (45 mg), stannous fluoride dihydrate (1.03 mg), methylparaben (5.2 mg), and propylparaben (0.58 g), sealed under nitrogen. The mixture is allowed to incubate for 15 minutes at RT. [99mTc]-BrIDA is a hexacoordinate complex in which the [99mTc] atom is complexed by two mebrofenin molecules, resulting in a net negative charge (1–).

Following intravenous administration in normal subjects, [99mTc]-BrIDA is rapidly cleared from the circulation. The percent injected dose remaining in the blood at 10 minutes was 17%, and 1% was excreted in the urine during the first 3 hours. The mechanism of liver uptake is similar to that of [99mTc]-DISIDA.

Tc-99 m Mertiatide Injection ([99mTc]-MAG3)

[99mTc]-MAG3 is a sterile aqueous solution prepared by adding [99mTc] pertechnetate (20–100 mCi in 4–10 mL) to a kit containing a lyophilized mixture of betiatide or N-[N-[N-[(benzoylthio) acetyl] glycyl] glycyl] glycine (1.0 mg), stannous chloride dihydrate (0.2 mg), sodium tartrate dihydrate (40 mg), and lactose monohydrate (20 mg), sealed under argon. Following addition of [99mTc] pertechnetate, air (2.0 mL) is introduced into the vial to oxidize the excess stannous chloride. The vial is incubated for 10 minutes at 100°C (in boiling water). During the reaction, [99mTc] first binds to tartrate, and during the heating process, the betiatide molecule loses the protective benzoyl group, and [99mTc] is then transferred to the MAG3 molecule, resulting in a [99mTc]-MAG3 complex with a negative charge (1–). The vial is cooled for 10 minutes before use.

Following intravenous injection, [99mTc]-MAG3 binds to plasma proteins. However, the binding is reversible, and the tracer is rapidly excreted by the kidneys via active tubular secretion and glomerular filtration. In normal individuals, 89% of the tracer was plasma protein bound but was rapidly cleared from the blood. The percentage of injected dose excreted in the urine within the first 3 hours was nearly 90% of the dose.

Tc-99 m Sestamibi Injection ([99mTc]-Sestamibi)

[99mTc]-Sestamibi is a sterile aqueous solution prepared by adding [99mTc] pertechnetate (25–150 mCi in 1–3 mL) to a sterile kit containing a lyophilized mixture of tetrakis or 2-methoxy isobutyl isonitrile copper tetrafluoroborate (1.0 mg), stannous chloride dihydrate (25–75 µg), sodium citrate dihydrate (2.6 mg), L-cysteine hydrochloric acid monohydrate (1 mg), and mannitol (20 mg), sealed under nitrogen. The vial is incubated at 100°C for

10 minutes and then allowed to cool for 15 minutes. During the reaction process, the reduced ^{99m}Tc first forms ^{99m}Tc-citrate and ^{99m}Tc-cysteine complexes. During the heating process, the copper–MIBI complex is broken, and then the free MIBI ligands displace the citrate and cysteine from the ^{99m}Tc complexes to form ^{99m}Tc-sestamibi, in which ^{99m}Tc is coordinated with six MIBI ligands, with a net positive charge (1 +).

Following intravenous administration, ^{99m}Tc-sestamibi rapidly clears from circulation. At 5 minutes postinjection, approximately 8% of the injected dose remains in circulation. Myocardial uptake, which is coronary flow dependent, is 1.2% of the injected dose at rest and 1.5% of the injected dose at exercise. The myocardial biological half-life is approximately 6 hours after a rest or exercise injection. The biological half-life for the liver is approximately 30 minutes after a rest or exercise injection.

^{99m}Tc-Sestamibi is a cationic complex that has been found to accumulate in viable myocardial tissue in a manner analogous to that of thallous chloride ^{201}Tl. However, animal studies have shown that myocardial uptake is not blocked when the sodium/potassium pump mechanism is inhibited. Studies of subcellular fractionation and electron micrographic analysis of heart cell aggregates suggest that myocardial uptake is by passive diffusion, and cellular retention occurs specifically within the mitochondria as a result of electrostatic interactions.

Tc-99 m Tetrofosmin Injection (^{99m}Tc-Tetrofosmin)

^{99m}Tc-Tetrofosmin is a sterile aqueous solution prepared by adding ^{99m}Tc pertechnetate (up to 200 mCi in 4–8 mL) to a sterile kit (stored at 2–8°C) containing a lyophilized mixture of tetrofosmin or 1,2-bis[bis(2-ethoxyethyl)phosphine] ethane (0.23 mg), stannous chloride dihydrate (30 µg), disodium sulfosalicylate (0.32 mg), sodium D-gluconate (1.0 mg), and sodium bicarbonate (1.8 mg), sealed under nitrogen. Following addition of ^{99m}Tc pertechnetate, air (2.0 mL) is removed from the vial and incubated at RT for 15 minutes. During the reaction process, the reduced ^{99m}Tc first forms ^{99m}Tc-gluconate and is then transferred to tetrofosmin to form a lipophilic ^{99m}Tc-tetrofosmin complex with a net positive charge (1 +).

Following intravenous administration, ^{99m}Tc-tetrofosmin rapidly clears from the blood, liver, and lung. At 5 minutes postinjection, only 5% of the injected dose is in the blood and liver. The initial myocardial uptake is rapid and coronary flow dependent. The first-pass extraction fraction in the myocardium is 0.45, and there is minimal clearance at 3 hours, with a typical myocardial uptake of up to 1.2% of the injected dose.

^{99m}Tc-Tetrofosmin is a cationic complex that has been found to accumulate in viable myocardial tissue by passive diffusion, and cellular retention may occur within the cytoplasm or in mitochondria as a result of electrostatic interactions.

Technetium Tc-99 m Tilmanocept (Lymphoseek)

The kit for the preparation of Lymphoseek contains two vials: vial A contains tilmanocept powder (250 µg), stannous chloride dihydrate (0.075 mg), trehalose dihydrate (20 mg), glycine (0.5 mg), and sodium ascorbate (0.5 mg), and vial B contains 4.6 mL of sterile buffered saline (diluent for the Lymphoseek vial). Prior to the preparation of Lymphoseek, determine the planned injection technique and the number of injections that will be used for a given patient.

Lymphoseek is a sterile aqueous solution prepared by adding ^{99m}Tc pertechnetate (2.5 mCi in 0.35 or 0.7 mL) to *vial A* containing tilmanocept powder. Remove an equal volume of air and incubate at RT for 15 minutes. Reconstitute the Lymphoseek vial with the diluent (vial B) to a final volume of 0.5, 2.5, or 5.0 mL. Total injection volume (depending on the number of syringes) for a patient should be between 0.1 and 1.0 mL.

Lymphoseek accumulates in lymphatic tissue and selectively binds to mannose-binding receptors (CD206) located on the surface of macrophages and dendritic cells. ^{99m}Tc-Tilmanocept is a macromolecule consisting of multiple units of DTPA and mannose, each covalently attached to a 10-kDa dextran backbone. The mannose acts as a ligand for the receptor, and the DTPA serves as a chelating agent for labeling with Tc-99 m. Human studies have demonstrated that Lymphoseek has been detectable in lymph nodes within 10 minutes and for up to 30 hours after injection. The drug half-life at the injection site is 1.8 to 3.1 hours. The amount of the accumulated radioactive dose in the liver, kidney, and bladder reached a maximum 1 hour postadministration of Lymphoseek and was approximately 1 to 2% of the injected dose in each tissue.

Lymphoseek may pose a risk of hypersensitivity reactions due to its chemical similarity to dextran.

Tc-99m-Labeled Aerosols

An aerosol is a relatively time-stable two-phase system consisting of particles (liquid or solid) suspended in gas (air). The particles are deposited predominantly in the alveolar region by diffusion. The percentage of particles remaining in the lung after inhalation (called the deposition fraction) depends mainly on the particle size ($0.1–2.0\,\mu m$) and shape. The composite property of a particle is therefore expressed as its aerodynamic diameter. Smaller particles have a higher deposition fraction, while particles larger than $1\,\mu m$ are deposited in the lower respiratory tract, and particles larger than $5\,\mu m$ impact remain in the upper airways.

^{99m}Tc-DTPA is the most commonly used radiopharmaceutical for the preparation of liquid aerosols. Several nebulizers producing liquid aerosols are available on the market. ^{99m}Tc-DTPA is prepared according to the procedure described in the package insert. The activity of ^{99m}Tc-DTPA introduced into a nebulizer is 30 to 40 mCi, from which the patient receives approximately 0.5 to 1.0 mCi to the lungs. ^{99m}Tc-DTPA aerosol is hydrophilic and is cleared from the alveolar region by transepithelial diffusion. The biological half-life varies from 80 ± 20 minutes in healthy nonsmokers to 45 ± 8 minutes in healthy passive smokers and 24 ± 9 minutes in healthy smokers. Resorbed ^{99m}Tc-DTPA is excreted via glomerular filtration in the kidneys.

Technegas is an aerosol comprising extremely small ^{99m}Tc-labeled solid graphite (carbon) particles generated at high temperature. Technegas particles have a diameter of approximately 0.005 to 0.2 μm and are hydrophobic, but they tend to grow by aggregation and should therefore be used within 10 minutes of generation. The graphite particles are slowly cleared from the alveolar region by resorption, with a biological half-life of 135 hours. Using Technegas has minimized the problem of hotspots in patients with obstructive lung disease, and it is considered better than the best liquid aerosols.

2.4.3 Radioiodinated SPECT Agents

Iodine belongs to the family of group 7A elements, known as *halogens*. Among the radioisotopes of iodine, ^{123}I and ^{131}I have physical characteristics suitable for developing radiopharmaceuticals for SPECT. Radioactive isotopes of iodine are generally available as sodium radioiodide (NaI).

A number of radioiodinated radiopharmaceuticals have been prepared for clinical use. The free molecular iodine (I_2) has the structure of $I^+–I^-$ in aqueous solution. The hydrated iodonium ion, H_2OI^+, and the hypoiodous acid, HOI, are believed to be the highly reactive electrophilic species. In an iodination reaction, iodination occurs by (1) electrophilic substitution of a hydrogen ion by an iodonium ion in a molecule of interest or (2) nucleophilic substitution (isotope exchange) where a radioactive iodine atom is exchanged with a stable iodine atom that is already present in the molecule. The most widely used methods for preparing iodinated radiopharmaceuticals are (1) isotopic exchange (involves exchanging radioactive iodine atom with a stable iodine atom in the molecule) and (2) an electrophilic substitution involving substituting I^+ for hydrogen in an aromatic compound activated by an electron-donating group, such as hydroxyl (OH) or amine (NH_2) in the aromatic ring. Different reagents (e.g., chloramine-T, lactoperoxidase, and iodogen) have been used as oxidizing agents to facilitate radioiodination reactions. The two FDA-approved agents are $^{123/131}$I-labeled *meta*-iodobenzylguanidine (MIBG) and ^{123}I-FP-CIT (DaTscan).

Sodium Iodide I-123 and I-131 Capsules or Solution

^{123}I and ^{131}I radionuclides are available as radioiodide (NaI) in hard capsules and as a solution in various amounts of activity for diagnostic and therapeutic procedures involving the thyroid gland. For example, ^{123}I capsules are available in strengths of 3.7 and 7.4 MBq (100 and 200 μCi) I-123 at TOC. I-123 radioiodide preparations may have radionuclidic impurities, such as I-125 and Te-121. The radioiodide dosage forms have been formulated to stabilize radioiodine in a nonvolatile reduced state as iodide (I^-) using adjuvants such as sodium bisulfite, disodium phosphate, and disodium EDTA. It has been reported in the literature that radioactive iodine uptake tests may show falsely reduced uptake due to incomplete dissolution of iodide from the capsule following oral administration.

Radioiodide is readily absorbed from the upper gastrointestinal tract. Following absorption, the iodide is distributed primarily within the extracellular fluid of the body. It is trapped and organically bound by the thyroid and concentrated by the stomach, choroid plexus, and salivary glands. It is excreted by the kidneys. The extent of urinary excretion depends on thyroid function. The iodide uptake by the thyroid gland is a result of an active transport mechanism mediated by the sodium/iodide symporter (NIS), a transmembrane glycoprotein that transports two sodium cations (Na^+) for each iodide anion (I^-) into the cell. NIS-mediated uptake of iodide into follicular cells of the thyroid gland is the first step in the synthesis of thyroid hormone.

Iobenguane I-123 and I-131 Injection

Iobenguane I-123 injection (AdreView) is a sterile, pyrogen-free radiopharmaceutical for intravenous injection. Each milliliter contains 0.08 mg of iobenguane sulfate, 74 MBq (2 mCi) of I-123, 23 mg of sodium dihydrogen phosphate dihydrate, 2.8 mg of disodium hydrogen phosphate dihydrate, and 10.3 mg (1% v/v) of benzyl alcohol with a pH of 5.0 to 6.5.

Iobenguane sulfate I-131 injection is a sterile, pyrogen-free radiopharmaceutical for intravenous injection. Each milliliter contains 0.69 mg of iobenguane sulfate, 85.1 MBq (2.30 mCi) of I-131 (as iobenguane sulfate I-131 at calibration), 0.36 mg of sodium acetate, 0.27 mg of acetic acid, 4.2 mg of sodium chloride, 0.56 mg of methylparaben, 0.056 mg of propylparaben, and 0.01 mL of benzyl alcohol.

Iobenguane is rapidly cleared from the blood and accumulates in adrenergically innervated tissues. Retention is especially prolonged in highly adrenergically innervated tissues (e.g., the adrenal medulla, heart, and salivary glands). In normal individuals, the majority of the dose (70–90%) is excreted unaltered by the kidneys via glomerular filtration. Iobenguane is similar in structure to the antihypertensive drug guanethidine and to the neurotransmitter norepinephrine (NE). Iobenguane is, therefore, largely subject to the same uptake and accumulation pathways as NE. Iobenguane is taken up by the NE transporter in adrenergic nerve terminals by type I (active transport) mechanism and stored in the presynaptic storage vesicles. Iobenguane accumulates in adrenergically innervated tissues, such as the adrenal medulla, salivary glands, heart, liver, spleen, and lungs, as well as tumors derived from the neural crest. It is indicated for use in the detection of primary or metastatic pheochromocytoma or neuroblastoma as an adjunct to other diagnostic tests.

Ioflupane I-123 Injection (DaTscan)

DaTscan is a sterile, pyrogen-free sterile solution supplied in single-use vials in which each milliliter contains 0.07 to 0.13 µg of ioflupane, 74 MBq (2 mCi) of I-123 (as ioflupane I-123), 5.7 mg of acetic acid, 7.8 mg of sodium acetate, and 0.05 mL (5%) of ethanol. The pH of the solution is between 4.2 and 5.2. The active drug substance in DaTscan is ioflupane or N-ω-fluoropropyl-2 β-carbomethoxy-3 β-(4-[^{123}I]iodophenyl)nortropane.

Following intravenous administration, only 5% of the injected dose remained in whole blood at 5 minutes postinjection. Uptake in the brain reached approximately 7% of injected dose at 10 minutes postinjection and decreased to 3% after 5 hours. DaTscan is a radiopharmaceutical indicated for striatal dopamine transporter (DaT) visualization using SPECT brain imaging to assist in the evaluation of adult patients with suspected parkinsonian syndromes (PSs). In these patients, DaTscan may be used to help differentiate essential tremor from tremor due to PS (idiopathic Parkinson's disease, multiple system atrophy, and progressive supranuclear palsy). Since ioflupane binds to the dopamine transporter (DaT) in the brain, drugs that bind to the DaT with high affinity (e.g., amphetamine and cocaine) may interfere with the image quality.

2.4.4 Radiopharmaceuticals Based on Group IIIA Radiometals

Gallium (Ga), indium (In), and thallium (Tl) are members of group IIIA in the periodic table. Each of these metals can assume different oxidation states by losing one, two, or three valence electrons. In acidic aqueous solution (pH < 3.0), both gallium and indium exist in a soluble ionic form (3$^+$). As the pH is raised above 3.0, these two metals readily form hydroxides with very low solubility products. To prevent precipitation, these metals must be complexed with a suitable ligand such as citrate, acetate, or oxine (or hydroxyquinoline) to prevent precipitation. With chelating agents such as DTPA, these metals form highly stable complexes at neutral pH.

The most relevant oxidation state for Tl is 1$^+$, which typically forms thallous hydroxide (Tl(OH)$_2^+$). The principal chemical form used as a radiopharmaceutical is ^{201}Tl chloride, which exists as a monocation and hence acts as a potassium ion (K^+) analogue.

Ga-67 Citrate Injection (^{67}Ga-Citrate)

^{67}Ga-citrate is available as a sterile aqueous solution containing 3 to 12 mCi of ^{67}Ga in multidose vials. It is prepared by neutralizing acidic, NCA ^{67}Ga chloride with sodium hydroxide in the presence of sodium citrate (4%), producing a 1:1 complex. Each milliliter of the isotonic solution contains 2 mCi of ^{67}Ga (0.0083 µg), 1.9 mg of sodium citrate dihydrate, and 7.8 mg of sodium chloride. The final formulation has a pH of 5.5 to 8.0 and contains 0.9% benzyl alcohol as a preservative.

Following intravenous injection, NCA ^{67}Ga is bound to plasma protein transferrin, and ^{67}Ga-transferrin complex is transported to various organs, tissues, and tumor sites. The highest tissue concentration of ^{67}Ga other than tumors and sites of infection is the renal cortex. After the first day, the maximum concentration shifts to bone and lymph nodes and, after the first week, to liver and spleen. Ga-67 is excreted relatively slowly from the body. The average whole-body retention is 65% after 7 days, with 26% having been excreted in the urine and 9% in the stools. The mechanism of concentration of tumor uptake and localization at the site of infection is unknown, but investigational studies have shown that pH of the tumor tissue and transferrin receptors on tumor cells play a significant role. Intracellularly, ^{67}Ga accumulates in lysosomes and is bound to a soluble intracellular protein.

In-111 Pentetreotide Injection (OctreoScan)

OctreoScan is a kit for the preparation of ^{111}In-pentetreotide, a diagnostic radiopharmaceutical. The kit (stored at 2–8°C) consists of two components:

1. A lyophilized mixture containing 10 µg of pentetreotide (DTPA-conjugated octreotide), 4.9 mg of anhydrous sodium citrate, 0.37 mg of anhydrous citric acid, 2 mg of gentisic acid, and 10 mg of inositol.
2. A 10-mL vial of ^{111}In chloride sterile solution (1.1 mL) containing 3.3 mCi of ^{111}In chloride in 0.02 N HCl at TOC. The vial also contains ferric chloride (3.5 µg/mL), which may increase the labeling yield.

OctreoScan is prepared by adding ^{111}In chloride solution to the vial containing pentetreotide and incubating the mixture at RT for 30 minutes. The final product has a pH between 3.8 and 4.3 and is stored at or below 25°C. OctreoScan is indicated for localization of primary and metastatic neuroendocrine tumors (NETs) expressing somatostatin receptors (SSTRs).

Within an hour of injection, most of the dose of ^{111}In-pentetreotide distributes from plasma to extravascular body tissues and concentrates in tumors containing a high density of SSTRs. Radioactivity is cleared rapidly from the body, primarily by renal excretion. Only one-third of the injected dose remains in the blood pool at 10 minutes after administration, and by 20 hours, approximately 1% of the injected dose is in the blood pool. While five subtypes of receptors (SSTR1–SSTR5) have been identified on most of the NETs, small cell lung cancers, and medullary thyroid carcinoma, SSTR2 is the predominant one in NETs. So it is the presence as well as the density of SSTR2 that provides the molecular basis for a number of clinical applications of OctreoScan.

In-111 Oxyquinoline Solution (^{111}In-Oxine)

^{111}In-Oxine is supplied as a sterile, nonpyrogenic, isotonic aqueous solution with a pH range of 6.5 to 7.5. Each milliliter of the solution contains 1 mCi of ^{111}In (> 50 mCi/µg of ^{111}In, NCA at TOC), 50 mg of oxyquinoline, 100 mg of polysorbate 80, and 6 mg of HEPES (N-2-hydroxyethyl-piperazine-N'-2-ethane sulfonic acid) buffer in 0.75% sodium chloride solution. ^{111}In-Oxine is a diagnostic radiopharmaceutical intended for radiolabeling autologous leukocytes. During the labeling process, ^{111}In-oxine diffuses into the leukocytes and dissociates within the cell. While the free oxine diffuses out, the free intracellular ^{111}In binds to nuclear and cytoplasmic proteins.

In-111 Pentetate Injection (^{111}In-DTPA)

^{111}In-DTPA injection is a sterile aqueous solution of ^{111}In^{3+} complexed to disodium pentetate in a 1:1 molar ratio. ^{111}In forms an eight-coordinate complex with DTPA. It is supplied as a single-use vial with 1.5 mL of isotonic solution containing ^{111}In (1.0 mCi/mL at TOC), 20–50 µg of pentetic acid, and sodium bicarbonate.

^{111}In-DTPA is a diagnostic drug for intrathecal administration; some of the radiopharmaceutical is absorbed from the subarachnoid space, and the remainder flows superiorly to the basal cisterns within 2 to 4 hours and subsequently will be apparent in the sylvian cisterns and the interhemispheric cisterns and over the cerebral convexities. In normal individuals, the radiopharmaceutical will have ascended to the parasagittal region within 24 hours, with simultaneous partial or complete clearance of activity from the basal cisterns and sylvian regions. Approximately 65% of the administered dose is excreted by the kidneys within 24 hours and 85% in 72 hours.

Tl-201 Thallous Chloride Injection (^{201}Tl-Chloride)

^{201}Tl-chloride is a sterile aqueous solution that contains ^{201}Tl (1 mCi/mL at TOC) in 0.9% sodium chloride solution, pH adjusted to 4.5 to 7.0, and preserved with 0.9% benzyl alcohol. Multidose vials in 2, 4, 8, and 9 mCi sizes are available.

After intravenous administration, ^{201}Tl-chloride clears rapidly from the blood, with maximal concentration by normal myocardium occurring at approximately 10 minutes. Blood clearance of Tl-201 is primarily by the myocardium (3–6%), thyroid, liver, kidneys, and stomach, with the remainder distributing fairly uniformly throughout the body. Five minutes after intravenous administration, only 5 to 8% of injected activity remains in the blood. Approximately 4 to 8% of the injected dose is excreted in the urine in the first 24 hours. The whole-body disappearance half-time was 9.8 ± 2.5 days.

^{201}Tl as a monocation (Tl$^+$) is transported into the myocardial cells by active transport and accumulates in viable myocardium via Na$^+$/K$^+$-ATPase (or sodium pump) in a manner analogous to that of potassium ion (K$^+$), and the myocardial distribution of ^{201}Tl correlates well with regional perfusion.

2.5 Radiolabeled Cells

2.5.1 In-111-Labeled White Blood Cells (^{111}In-WBC)

The routine method of labeling WBCs (or leukocytes) first requires separation of leukocytes from the whole blood. Whole blood (43 mL) is mixed with ACD (citric acid, sodium citrate, and dextrose) solution (7 mL) and hetastarch (6%, 10 mL) in a 60-mL syringe. In order to get good labeling, the patient's blood must have at least 2 million granulocytes per milliliter. The

syringe is allowed to stand upright for 1 to 2 hours. The top leukocyte-rich plasma is then separated and centrifuged (at 450g for 10 minutes) to obtain a leukocyte pellet (LP). The leukocyte-poor plasma (LPP) is used subsequently to resuspend the labeled WBC preparation. The LP is resuspended in 2 mL of normal saline and incubated with ^{111}In-oxine (0.5–1.0 mCi in 1.0 mL) for 15 to 30 minutes at RT. Subsequently, 10 to 15 mL of LPP is added to the In-111-labeled cell mixture and centrifuged at 450g for 10 minutes. The ^{111}In-labeled LP is then resuspended in 5 to 10 mL of normal saline or LPP for reinjection into the patient. The usual adult dose is 0.3 to 0.5 mCi. The recommended maximum amount of time between drawing blood and reinjection of labeled cells must be less than 5 hours because of potential reduction in granulocyte chemotaxis during prolonged storage.

2.5.2 Tc-99m-Labeled White Blood Cells (^{99m}Tc-WBC)

The LP from the whole blood, prepared as described previously, is mixed with 20 to 30 mCi (in 5 mL) of freshly prepared ^{99m}Tc-HMPAO and incubated for 15 to 30 minutes at RT. Following centrifugation at 450g, the ^{99m}Tc-labeled LP is resuspended in LPP. The usual adult dose is 5 to 10 mCi. The plasma half-life of ^{99m}Tc-leukocytes is approximately 4 hours compared with 6 hours for ^{111}In-leukocytes.

2.5.3 Tc-99m-Labeled Red Blood Cells (^{99m}Tc-RBC)

RBCs can be labeled with Tc-99 m either in vivo or in vitro. Both methods are based on the principle of pretinning the RBCs first with either stannous pyrophosphate (Sn-PYP) or stannous citrate, followed by incubation with ^{99m}Tc pertechnetate. During the incubation period, ^{99m}Tc pertechnetate diffuses into the RBCs, gets reduced by Sn^{2+} ion, and gets bound to hemoglobin. The in vivo method requires first an intravenous administration of Sn-PYP (10–20 µg/kg/1–2 mL) 20 to 30 minutes prior to the intravenous administration of ^{99m}Tc pertechnetate (15–25 mCi). In the in vitro method, RBCs are labeled in whole blood (1–3 mL coagulated with ACD solution or heparin) using the UltraTag RBC kit (Covidien). For splenic sequestration studies, ^{99m}Tc-RBCs typically are damaged by heating for 20 minutes in a water bath at 49 to 50°C.

2.6 Quality Control of Radiopharmaceuticals

Quality control (QC) testing of radiopharmaceuticals is absolutely critical to ensure their safety and effectiveness. The package insert (approved by FDA) for each radiopharmaceutical would provide the necessary information regarding preparation of QC testing of the final drug product formulation. In addition, the U.S. Pharmacopeia is the official compendium for all FDA-approved radiopharmaceuticals. The most important QC parameters and testing procedures are summarized as follows:

- *Radionuclide identity:* The most common method to identify a radionuclide is by half-life or by the type and energy of radiations it emits. Radionuclide identity tests are not required for FDA-approved SPECT radiopharmaceuticals.
- *Radionuclidic purity:* This is defined as a ratio, which is expressed as a percentage of the radioactivity of the desired radionuclide in a radiopharmaceutical, to the total radioactivity in the final drug product. Since radionuclidic impurities in a radiopharmaceutical can contribute an unnecessary radiation dose to the patient, the levels of impurities must be as low as possible. Since the radionuclidic impurities may have longer half-lives, the percentage of impurities increases with time. The most common radionuclidic impurities present in SPECT radiopharmaceuticals are summarized in ▶ Table 2.5. For most of the radiopharmaceuticals, radionuclidic purity is tested by the manufacturer. The only radionuclide test performed in radiopharmacy is the ^{99}Mo breakthrough test on the ^{99m}Tc pertechnetate eluate from the generator.
- *Radiochemical purity (RCP):* The RCP value of a radiopharmaceutical is defined as the ratio, expressed as a percentage, of the radioactivity in the desired chemical form to the total radioactivity in the final formulation of the drug product. The acceptable RCP for several radiopharmaceuticals is shown in ▶ Table 2.6. With ^{99m}Tc-labeled radiopharmaceuticals, free ^{99m}Tc pertechnetate is the main radiochemical impurity. The other two impurities are ^{99m}Tc-reduced hydrolyzed (^{99m}Tc-RH) species and ^{99m}Tc-stannous colloids (^{99m}Tc-SnC). These impurities are undesirable since their biodistribution differs from that of the radiopharmaceutical of interest.

Paper chromatography and silica gel instant thin-layer chromatography (SG-ITLC) methods are commonly used in radiopharmacy to determine both the RCP and radiochemical impurities. A small sample (1–3 µL) of the radiopharmaceutical is spotted at the origin of a chromatographic stationary phase (paper or SG), which is then placed in a solvent (at the bottom of a chamber). Various radiochemical species either stay at the origin or migrate with the mobile phase, depending on the relative solubility of the chemical species in the solvent. The radioactivity distribution on the strip is then measured by cutting the strip and counting, or by using a radiochromatogram scanner. The relative front (R_f) of a radiochemical component is the distance the component travels from the origin relative to the solvent front (S_f). For example, with paper (Whatman 31ET) or SG-ITLC, and acetone as the solvent, ^{99m}Tc-DTPA stays at the origin ($R_f =$ 0.0), whereas ^{99m}TcO$_4^-$ migrates with the solvent S_f ($R_f = 1.0$). The chromatographic conditions and the expected R_f values for different radiochemical species for ^{99m}Tc radiopharmaceuticals are summarized in ▶ Table 2.6.

Table 2.5 Radionuclidic impurities in SPECT radiopharmaceuticals

Radiopharmaceutical	Radionuclidic impurity		
	Radionuclide	$t_{1/2}$ (d)	Limits at TOC
^{99m}Tc Pertechnetate	^{99}Mo	2.75	≤0.15 µCi ^{99}Mo/mCi of ^{99m}Tc
^{67}Ga-Citrate	^{66}Ga	0.395	0.02%
	^{65}Zn	244.0	0.20%
^{111}In-Oxine	^{114m}In	49.50	≤1.0 µCi of ^{114m}In per mCi ^{111}In
^{201}Tl-Chloride	^{200}Tl	1.087	≤1.0%
	^{202}Tl	12.23	≤1.0%
	^{203}Pb	2.161	≤0.25%

Table 2.6 Chromatographic methods for the determination of radiochemical species in ^{99m}Tc-labeled radiopharmaceuticals

Radiopharmaceutical	Stationary phase	Mobile phase	R_f values of ^{99m}Tc chemical species			Minimum RCP (%)
			^{99m}Tc-labeled complex of interest	^{99m}Tc-RH and ^{99m}Tc-SnC	Free ^{99m}TC	
^{99m}Tc Pertechnetate	SG	Acetone	N/A	N/A	1.0	95
^{99m}Tc Pertechnetate	SG	0.9% NaCl	N/A	N/A	1.0	95
^{99m}Tc-DTPA ^{99m}Tc-MDP ^{99m}Tc-HDP	Whatman 31ET or SG	Acetone	0.0	0.0	1.0	90
^{99m}Tc-DTPA ^{99m}Tc-MDP ^{99m}Tc-HDP	Whatman 31ET or SG	0.9% NaCl	0.9	0.0	1.0	90
^{99m}Tc-DISIDA ^{99m}Tc-BrIDA	ITLC-SA (salicycle acid)	20% NaCl	0.0	0.0	1.0	90
^{99m}Tc-DMSA	ITLC-SA	Acetone	0.0	0.0	1.0	85
^{99m}Tc-MAG3	Pall solvent saturation pads	Chloroform:acetone:Tetrahydrofuran (1:1:2)	0.0–0.5	0.0–0.5	0.5–1.0	90
^{99m}Tc-HMPAO	Pall solvent saturation pads	Ether	1.0	0.0	0.0	
^{99m}Tc-HMPAO	ITLC-SG	Methylethyl ketone	0.8–1.0	0.0	0.8–1.0	80
	ITLC-SG	0.9% NaCl	0.0	0.0	0.8–1.0	
	Whatman 31ET	50% Acetonitrile	0.8–1.0	0.8–1.0	0.8–1.0	
^{99m}Tc-Sestamibi	Baker flex aluminum oxide TLC plate	Ethanol	1.0	0.0	0.0	90

Abbreviations: ITLC, instant thin-layer chromatography; TLC, thin-layer chromatography; NaCl, sodium chloride; SG, silica gel.

2.7 Radiopharmaceuticals: Special Topics

2.7.1 Radiation Dosimetry

As early as 1971, the International Commission on Radiological Protection (ICRP) started work on doses to patients from radiopharmaceuticals (Publication 17, ICRP, 1971). Since then, a number of ICRP publications (Publication 53, ICRP, 1987; Publication 62, ICRP, 1991; Publication 80, ICRP 1998; and Publication 106, ICRP, 2008) have been updating the dosimetry estimates. As a result, the radiation dosimetry values reported in the package inserts may be different from the values published in Publication 106.

The absorbed dose to a target organ or tissue (T) from a radionuclide in a single source organ (S) is given by

$$D(T \leftarrow S) = \tilde{A}_S \times S(T \leftarrow S),$$

where $\tilde{A}_S$ is the time-integrated or cumulated activity, which is equal to the total number of nuclear transformations in S, and S (T ← S) is the absorbed dose in T per unit cumulated activity in S. The special unit for radiation dose to any tissue or organ is the gray (Gy) and generally expressed as mGy/MBq. Radiation exposure of the different organs and tissues in the body results in different probabilities of harm and different severities. To reflect the combined detriment from stochastic effects due to the equivalent doses in all the organs and tissues of the body, the equivalent dose in each organ and tissue is multiplied by a tissue weighting factor, and the results are summed over the whole body to give the effective dose (ED). The special unit for ED is the sievert (Sv), which replaced the old unit rem. The ED and the *critical organ* (the organ receiving the highest radiation absorbed dose) dose for several radiopharmaceuticals are summarized in ▶ Table 2.7.

2.7.2 Pediatric Dosing

Radiation absorbed doses for a given amount of radiopharmaceutical dose are higher in children (▶ Table 2.8) than in an adult because the radioactivity is concentrated in a smaller mass of the organs. The dose adjustments for pediatric subjects may be calculated based on several different factors, such as age (year), weight (kg), body

Table 2.7 Radiation dosimetry of SPECT radiopharmaceuticals

Radiopharmaceutical	Adult dose (mCi)	Effective dose		Critical organ radiation dose		
		mSv/MBq	mSv/mCi	Critical organ	mGy/MBq	cGy (rads)/mCi
[99m]Tc-pertechnetate	1.0–35.0	0.016	0.588	Stomach wall	0.0676	0.25
^{99m}Tc-MAA	3.0–4.0	0.010	0.377	lung	0.0594	0.24
^{99m}Tc-SC	1.0–8.0	0.009	0.30	Liver	0.091	0.338
^{99m}Tc-MDP	10.0–20.0	0.004	0.159	Urinary bladder wall	0.035	0.13
^{99m}Tc-HDP	10.0–20.0	0.004	0.159	Bone surface	0.087	0.322
^{99m}Tc-DTPA	3.0–20.0		0.159	Urinary bladder wall	0.033	0.115
^{99m}Tc-MAG3	5.0–10.0	0.005	0.172	Urinary bladder wall	0.138	0.51
^{99m}Tc-DMSA	1.0–5.0			Renal cortex	0.189	0.70
^{99m}Tc-HMPAO	7.0–25.0	0.010	0.3737	Gall bladder wall	0.051	0.19
^{99m}Tc-ECD	10.0–30.0	0.006	0.213	Urinary bladder wall	0.073	0.27
^{99m}Tc-DISIDA	1.0–8.0	0.009	0.319	Upper large intestinal wall	0.108	0.40
[99m]Tc-BrIDA	2.0–10.0	0.009	0.319	Upper large intestinal wall	0.068	0.25
[99m]Tc-Pertechnegas	1.0–2.0	0.0146	0.540	Urinary bladder wall	0.123	0.48
[99m]Tc-Sestamibi	10.0–30.0	0.007	0.260	Upper large intestinal wall	0.049	0.18
[99m]Tc-Tetrofosmin	5.0–24.0	0.006	0.233	Gall bladder wall	0.033	0.123
[67]Ga-Citrate	3.0–8.0	0.086	3.178	Bone surfaces	0.324	1.20
[111]In-Pentetreotide	6.0	0.069	2.54	Spleen	0.665	2.46
[201]Tl-Chloride	2.0–4.0	0.102	3.774	Testes	0.560	2.07
[123]I-NaI capsules (35% thyroid uptake)	0.2–0.4	0.233	8.621	Thyroid	3.514	13.0
[131]I-NaI solution (25% thyroid uptake)	0.005–2.0	2.22	82.14	Thyroid	340.0	1300
[123]I-Ioflupane	3.0–5.0	0.0213	0.819	Brain striata	0.23	0.86

▶

Table 2.7 (*continued*) Radiation dosimetry of SPECT radiopharmaceuticals

Radiopharmaceutical	Adult dose (mCi)	Effective dose		Critical organ radiation dose		
		mSv/MBq	mSv/mCi	Critical organ	mGy/MBq	cGy (rads)/mCi
^{123}I-MIBG	0.14 mCi/kg	0.0132	0.488	Urinary bladder wall	0.095	0.35
^{131}I-MIBG	0.5–1.0	0.19	7.00	Urinary bladder wall	0.757	2.8
^{111}In-WBCs	0.3–0.5	0.59	21.83	Spleen	5.946	22.0
^{99m}Tc-WBCs	5.0–10.0			Spleen	0.184	0.68
^{99m}Tc-RBCs		0.0085	0.315	Heart	0.023	0.085
^{99m}Tc-RBCs (heat damaged)		0.041	1.517	Spleen	0.56	2.10

Table 2.8 Effective dose to pediatric subjects from SPECT radiopharmaceuticals

Radiopharmaceutical	Effective dose (mSv/mCi)		
	Adult	10-y-old	1-y-old
^{99m}Tc-DTPA	0.18	0.30	0.60
^{99m}Tc-DMSA	0.33	0.56	1.37
^{99m}Tc-HMPAO	0.34	0.63	1.81
[99m]Tc Pertechnetate	0.48	0.96	2.92
^{99m}Tc-DISIDA	0.63	1.07	3.70
[111]In-Octreoscan	2.00	3.70	10.4
[67]Ga-Citrate	3.70	7.40	23.7
[123]I-Sodium iodide	5.60	13.0	51.8
^{111}In-WBCs	23.6	45.9	125.0

surface area (BSA in m^2), or even height (cm). The most common methods are based on adjustment using either body weight or BSA (estimated by height–weight monogram). Pediatric doses, however, should be based finally on the principle of giving minimum radioactivity that will result in a satisfactory imaging procedure regardless of a dose adjustment calculation.

Age-based dose adjustment:

$$\text{Pediatric dose} = \text{Adult dose} \times \left[\frac{\text{Child age (year)} 1}{\text{Child age(year)} + 7} \right]$$

BSA-based dose adjustment:

$$\text{Pediatric dose} = \text{Adult dose} \times \left[\frac{\text{Child BSA(m}^2)}{\text{std. adult BSA (1.73 m}^2)} \right]$$

2.7.3 Breast Milk Excretion of Radiopharmaceuticals

All women of lactating potential should be asked about breast-feeding practice prior to a nuclear medicine imaging procedure. If a woman is breast-feeding, two important considerations should be used in selecting an appropriate radiopharmaceutical for a specific procedure: (1) a radiopharmaceutical that is excreted less in breast milk and (2) the administered dose of a radiopharmaceutical that is the smallest amount possible to obtain a satisfactory imaging procedure. Following intravenous administration of radiopharmaceuticals, excretion of radioactivity into breast milk may be due to several different mechanisms, such as passive diffusion, active secretion by ions, or other transport pathways, or due to lipophilicity and protein binding of radiopharmaceuticals. In general, very small fractions of administered doses are excreted into milk. Specific radiopharmaceuticals (such as ^{99m}Tc pertechnetate, radioiodide, and ^{67}Ga-citrate) may show cumulative accumulations of > 10%.

For many radiopharmaceuticals, especially those with low excretion fractions into breast milk, interruption of breast-feeding is not necessary. However, in the literature, breast milk concentration of radiopharmaceuticals and half-times varied considerably between subjects. It is generally agreed that a reasonable ED criterion for interrupting breast-feeding is 0.1 rem (or 1.0 mSv) to the infant. A conservative recommendation is to discard the first milk produced within the first 4 hours following radiopharmaceutical administration. Certain radiopharmaceuticals, however, do require long periods of interruption or complete cessation as shown in ▶ Table 2.9.

2.7.4 Altered Biodistribution of Radiopharmaceuticals

One of the most common problems associated with radiopharmaceuticals is an unanticipated or altered biodistribution, which can have a significant clinical impact on scan interpretation and diagnostic imaging accuracy. While several factors may contribute to the altered biodistribution of radiopharmaceuticals, radiopharmaceutical preparation and formulation problems are mainly

Table 2.9 Recommended breast-feeding interruption schedule

Radiopharmaceutical	Interruption
^{99m}Tc Pertechnetate	12 h
^{99m}Tc-MAA	12 h
^{99m}Tc-RBC	12 h
^{99m}Tc-Complexes	4 h
^{123}I-Sodium iodide	> 3 wk
^{123}I-MIBG	> 3 wk
^{111}In-WBC	No
^{111}In-Octreotide	No
^{67}Ga-Citrate	> 3 wk
^{201}Tl-Chloride	48 h

associated with the increased production of radiochemical and chemical impurities. During preparation of radiopharmaceuticals, deviations from the official instructions (as described in the package insert), such as improper mixing or heating or incubation delays, whether purposeful or inadvertent, may result in suboptimal radiochemical impurities. With ^{99m}Tc radiopharmaceuticals the most common impurities are free ^{99m}TcO$_4^-$ and particulate impurities, such as ^{99m}Tc colloids or ^{99m}Tc-RH species. The predominant concern with radioiodinated radiopharmaceuticals is the radiolytic production of free radioiodide. In addition, problems associated with drug stability and delays before dispensing may also increase the relative amounts of radiochemical impurities. Since the biodistribution of radiochemical impurities may be significantly different compared to that of radiolabeled drug product of interest (▶ Table 2.10), the imaging studies may show altered biodistribution of the radiopharmaceuticals.

Faulty injection, such as dose infiltration or contamination with antiseptics and aluminum during dose administration, may cause significant artifacts. The patient's own medical problems, such as abnormalities in the regulation of hormone levels, failure in the function of excretory organs and systems (e.g., hepatobiliary and genitourinary systems), and even simple conditions (e.g., excessive talking) may contribute to altered biodistribution of radiopharmaceuticals. Previous medical procedures (chemotherapy, radiation therapy, dialysis) and drug interaction are some of the nontechnical factors responsible for unanticipated biodistribution of radiopharmaceuticals.

2.7.5 Adverse Reactions to Radiopharmaceuticals

An adverse reaction to radiopharmaceuticals is defined as any symptom or response that is unexpected, or unusual and undesirable. Most radiopharmaceuticals are used for diagnostic purposes and are administered in microdoses, that is, doses too low (a few micrograms) to cause pharmacological effects but high enough to allow the cellular response to be studied. Thus, significantly, unlike conventional drugs, there is no dose–response relationship for radiopharmaceuticals. Therefore, adverse reactions to radiopharmaceuticals are generally rare, mild, and reversible without medical treatment. Recently, a database software application Datinrad (datinrad@radiopharmacy.

Table 2.10 Expected in vivo distribution of radiochemical and chemical impurities in SPECT radiopharmaceuticals

Radiopharmaceuticals			
^{99m}Tc agents	Radiochemical impurities	Free ^{99m}TcO$_4^-$	Uptake in stomach, GI tract, thyroid, salivary glands
		^{99m}Tc-RH colloid, ^{99m}Tc-Sn(OH)$_n$ colloid	Phagocytized by the cells of RES located in liver, spleen, and bone marrow
		^{99m}Tc particles (> 10 μ)	Physically lodged in pulmonary capillaries
		Hydrophilic impurities	Uptake in kidney and bladder
		Lipophilic impurities	Uptake in liver and GI tract
	Chemical impurity (Al^{3+})	^{99m}Tc colloids and particles	Uptake in lung and RES
^{111}In agents	Radiochemical impurities	Free ^{111}In (as ^{111}In-DTPA)	Urinary excretion, bladder activity
		Free ^{111}In (as ^{111}In-transferrin or ^{111}In-RBCs	Increased blood pool and background activity
$^{123/131}$I agents	Radiochemical impurities	Free iodide (I$^-$)	Uptake in stomach, GI tract, thyroid, salivary glands

Abbreviations: GI, gastrointestinal; RES, reticuloendothelial system.

net), has been developed that contains all the information published to date about radiopharmaceutical drug interactions and adverse reactions.

Suggested Reading

[1] Andersson M, Johansson L, Minarik D, Leide-Svegborn S, Mattsson S. Effective dose to adult patients from 338 radiopharmaceuticals estimated using ICRP biokinetic data, ICRP/ICRU computational reference phantoms and ICRP 2007 tissue weighting factors. EJNMMI Phys. 2014;1(1):9

[2] Gómez Perales JL, Martínez AA. A portable database of adverse reactions and drug interactions with radiopharmaceuticals. J Nucl Med Technol. 2013;41(3):212–215

[3] ICRP Publication 106, a 3rd amendment to ICRP publication 53, vol. 38, nos. 1–2, 2008. Available at http://www.icrp.org/publication.asp?id=ICRP%20Publication%20106

[4] Kowalsky RJ, Falen SW. Radiopharmaceuticals in Nuclear Pharmacy and Nuclear Medicine. 3rd ed. Washington, DC: American Pharmacists Association; 2011

[5] Stabin MG, Breitz HB. Breast milk excretion of radiopharmaceuticals: mechanisms, findings, and radiation dosimetry. J Nucl Med. 2000;41(5):863–873

[6] Treves ST. Pediatric Nuclear Medicine/PET. New York, NY: Springer; 2007

[7] Vallabhajosula S. Molecular Imaging: Radiopharmaceuticals for PET and SPECT. Berlin, Heidelberg: Springer-Verlag; 2009

[8] Vallabhajosula S, Killeen RP, Osborne JR. Altered biodistribution of radiopharmaceuticals: role of radiochemical/pharmaceutical purity, physiological, and pharmacologic factors. Semin Nucl Med. 2010; 40(4):220–241

3 SPECT and SPECT/CT in Neuroscience

Tarun Singhal and Chun K. Kim

3.1 Radiopharmaceuticals for Brain SPECT Imaging

- *Brain perfusion agents:* for example, technetium-99 m (^{99m}Tc)-ethyl cysteinate dimer (ECD) and ^{99m}Tc-hexamethylpropyleneamine oxime (HMPAO).
- *Neurotransmitter agents:* for example, iodine-123 (^{123}I)-ioflupane.
- *Brain tumor agents:* for example, thallium-201 (^{201}Tl)-chloride.

3.2 Perfusion SPECT Imaging in Dementia

Dementia is a chronic, progressive neurodegenerative condition that affects multiple higher cognitive functional domains. There are several subtypes of dementia based on underlying pathology. Single-photon emission computed tomography (SPECT) demonstrates hypoperfusion patterns that differ among various dementia subtypes. These patterns are often analogous to patterns of hypometabolism seen on fluorodeoxyglucose positron emission tomography (FDG-PET).

3.2.1 Alzheimer's Disease

Posterior temporal and inferior parietal hypoperfusion generally precedes the onset of clinical symptoms (▶ Fig. 3.1 **a**). Precuneus hypoperfusion may be seen in some cases. A review of sagittal images is often helpful in diagnosis (▶ Fig. 3.1 **b**). Frontal hypoperfusion may be seen in advanced stages. There is usual sparing of the sensorimotor cortex and occipital lobes. Hypoperfusion may be asymmetric in the early stages and may extend to involve both hemispheres.[1]

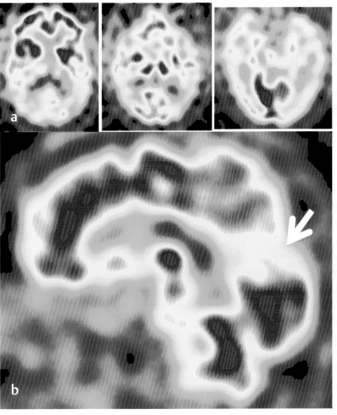

Fig. 3.1 Alzheimer's disease. **(a)** Three selected axial SPECT images show bilateral temporoparietal hypoperfusion with relative sparing of basal ganglia, frontal lobes, and occipital lobes. **(b)** A sagittal SPECT image shows precuneus hypoperfusion. Precuneus hypoperfusion (*arrow*) is an early sign of Alzheimer's disease.

3.2.2 Frontotemporal Dementia

Bilateral frontal and anterior temporal hypoperfusion is seen in patients with predominantly behavioral variant frontotemporal dementia (▶ Fig. 3.2). Frontal hypoperfusion may also be seen in depression and schizophrenia, and clinical correlation is necessary to interpret SPECT findings.

3.2.3 Vascular Dementia

Patchy areas of hypoperfusion involving the cortical hemispheres or subcortical structures may be seen in patients with vascular dementia (▶ Fig. 3.3).

3.2.4 Primary Progressive Aphasia

Left temporal hypoperfusion (particularly in right-handed individuals) is seen in the semantic dementia variant of primary progressive aphasia (▶ Fig. 3.4). Semantic dementia is clinically characterized by a fluent aphasia and is associated with frontotemporal dementia–type pathology. However, patients with a logopenic variant of primary progressive aphasia (clinically characterized by slow speech, word retrieval difficulty, and speech paucity and dysfluency) may show an asymmetric Alzheimer's disease pattern, often affecting the language-dominant left hemisphere (▶ Fig. 3.5).

3.2.5 Corticobasal Degeneration and Progressive Supranuclear Palsy

In addition to cerebral cortex involvement, these syndromes may present with hypoperfusion in the basal ganglia involving the caudate and putamen.

3.2.6 Diffuse Lewy Body Disease

The hypoperfusion pattern in Lewy body dementia is similar to that seen in Alzheimer's disease, except that there is prominent involvement of the occipital lobes.

3.3 Perfusion SPECT in Epilepsy

Chronic refractory epilepsy is defined as repeated, unprovoked seizures that do not respond to two or more antiepileptic drugs. Surgical resection of the epileptogenic zone in the cerebral cortex is warranted in such cases to improve clinical outcomes. Structural magnetic resonance imaging (MRI), interictal FDG-PET, and ictal and interictal perfusion SPECT images are obtained to identify the epileptogenic zone. The goal of the ictal SPECT study is to identify the epileptogenic zone by detecting localized hyperperfusion during an acute seizure episode. This technique is particularly helpful in MRI-negative temporal and extratemporal epilepsy.

3.3.1 Ictal Injection

For the most effective ictal study, the radiotracer should be injected immediately after seizure onset, ideally before completion of the acute seizure. The switch from ictal hyperperfusion to peri-ictal hypoperfusion ("postictal switch") has been estimated to occur 1 to 2 minutes after seizure completion in temporal-onset seizures. Similarly, in extratemporal seizures, the best performance is obtained when there is ongoing seizure activity for at least 10 to 15 seconds after tracer injection.[2]

3.3.2 Image Interpretation

Increased radiotracer activity in the epileptogenic zone is seen during the ictal scan (▶ Fig. 3.6).

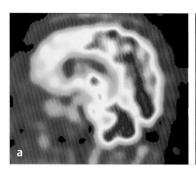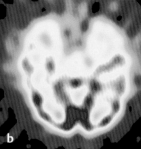

Fig. 3.2 Frontotemporal dementia. (**a**) Sagittal and (**b**) axial SPECT images show bilateral anterior temporal and frontal hypoperfusion with sparing of the posterior temporal, parietal, and occipital cortices.

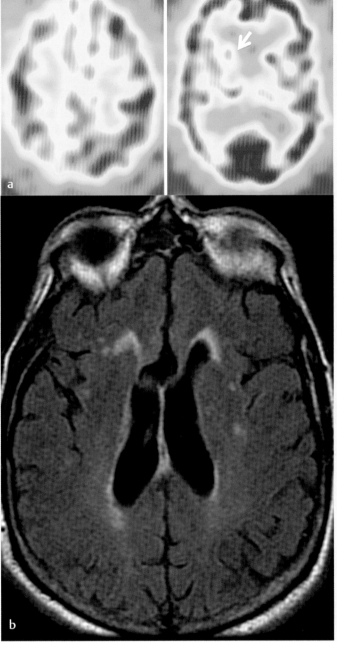

Fig. 3.3 Vascular dementia. (**a**) Axial SPECT images show heterogeneous radiotracer activity in the cerebral cortex with decreased activity in the right caudate (*arrow*) reflecting subcortical involvement. (**b**) Axial T2-weighted fluid attenuation inversion recovery MR image of the brain showing microangiopathic changes (periventricular hyperintensities).

Subtracting the interictal perfusion image from the ictal scan and coregistering the images with the patient's MRI (also known as subtraction ictal SPECT coregistered to MRI [SISCOM]) has been used to increase the sensitivity of the technique. Software-based image interpretation of subtraction images is superior to visual image analysis for detecting the epileptogenic zone (88% localization rate using SISCOM vs. 38% on visual analysis).[3]

3.3.3 Study Performance

The sensitivity and specificity of the study vary based on numerous factors, including injection technique and approaches to image interpretation. Delayed injections for ictal SPECT decrease the diagnostic yield and may also result in incorrect localization. Statistical analysis using SISCOM with lower threshold values increases sensitivity and decreases specificity, while higher threshold values increase specificity and decrease sensitivity.

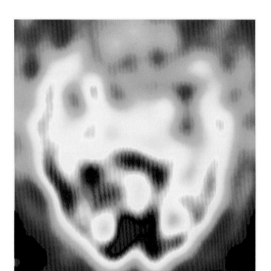

Fig. 3.4 Primary progressive aphasia (semantic dementia). An axial SPECT image shows asymmetric left temporal hypoperfusion.

3.4 Perfusion SPECT in Cerebrovascular Disease

Stenosis of extracranial or intracranial vessels leads to decreased brain perfusion and increased risk of transient ischemic attack (TIA) or stroke. Hypoperfusion or decreased regional cerebral blood flow may be demonstrated on SPECT in acute and chronic phases of stroke. Stenotic vessels also lead to a decreased regional cerebral vascular reserve (rCVR), which is defined by the ability of the vascular bed to increase blood flow in response to vasodilatory stimuli.[4]

3.4.1 Acetazolamide Challenge Perfusion Imaging

Administration of acetazolamide (a carbonic anhydrase inhibitor) leads to dilatation of cerebral vessels and increased cerebral perfusion. Stenosis of a major vessel leads to a blunting of the distal

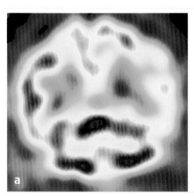
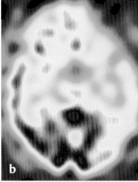

Fig. 3.5 Logopenic variant of primary progressive aphasia. (a) Coronal and (b) axial SPECT images show asymmetric left temporal and parietal hypoperfusion.

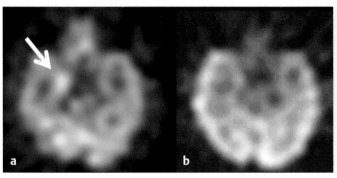

Fig. 3.6 Epilepsy. (a) Ictal SPECT shows hyperperfusion in the medial right temporal lobe (arrow), representing the epileptogenic focus. (b) Interictal SPECT.

vascular response to acetazolamide and a relative decrease in cerebral perfusion (in comparison to other cerebral regions) that is detectable on perfusion SPECT images as reduced radiotracer activity in the vascular bed of affected vessels.

- A brain perfusion SPECT study is performed after administration of 1,000 mg of acetazolamide intravenously.
- If acetazolamide challenge imaging is abnormal, a repeat baseline study is performed at least 24 hours later without acetazolamide.
- A relative decrease in tracer activity (on acetazolamide challenge imaging compared with baseline imaging) is seen in the vascular territory of the stenosed artery, suggesting a reduced rCVR (▶ Fig. 3.7).
- Demonstration of decreased rCVR is a predictor of significantly increased risk of subsequent development of TIA or stroke.

3.5 Dopamine Transporter SPECT in Parkinsonism

3.5.1 Parkinson's Disease and Other Parkinsonian Neurodegenerative Syndromes

Parkinson's disease is second only to Alzheimer's disease as a cause of neurodegenerative disease. Motor symptoms of Parkinson's disease result from a loss of dopaminergic neurons originating in the substantia nigra that project to the caudate and putamen. Dopamine transporter molecules expressed on the nerve terminals of these neurons in the caudate and putamen are reduced in patients with Parkinson's disease and other neurodegenerative parkinsonian syndromes.

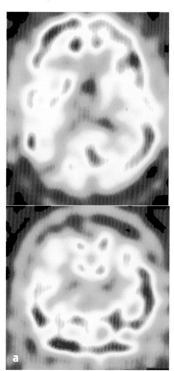
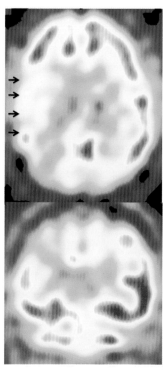
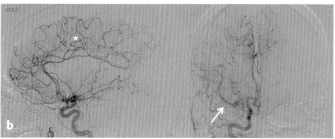

Fig. 3.7 Chronic ischemia. (a) Axial and coronal baseline SPECT (left) and axial and coronal postacetazolamide SPECT (right) show worsening of hypoperfusion in the right middle cerebral artery territory after administration of acetazolamide (*arrows*). (b) Angiograms demonstrate extensive collateral vessel development in the right cerebral hemisphere (*asterisk*) from chronic hypoperfusion due to right middle cerebral artery stenosis (*arrow*) leading to a "Moyamoya" pattern.

Common indications of the study include distinguishing essential, psychogenic or drug-induced tremors from tremor due to a neurodegenerative parkinsonian syndrome and distinguishing diffuse Lewy body dementia from Alzheimer's disease.[5,6]

3.5.2 ^{123}I-ioflupane

[123]I-ioflupane is an imaging analogue of cocaine that binds to dopamine transporters in the nerve terminals of the neurons arising from the substantia nigra. SPECT is typically performed 3 to 6 hours after a slow injection of 111 to 185 MBq of the tracer. Potassium perchlorate or Lugol's solution may be administered at least 1 hour before the tracer injection to prevent thyroid gland exposure to [123]I.

In Parkinson's disease, the pattern of reduced uptake is often asymmetric, with unilateral involvement contralateral to the side of clinical symptoms, particularly in early stages. Moreover, the posterior putamen is involved before the anterior putamen or caudate nucleus is involved. Hence a dot- or period-shaped abnormal appearance has been described as opposed to a comma-shaped normal appearance

(▶ Fig. 3.8). Atypical neurodegenerative parkinsonian syndromes tend to demonstrate bilateral and more prominent caudate involvement.

3.6 Brain Tumor Imaging

Distinguishing recurrent, viable brain tumor from radiation necrosis can be challenging as both conditions may present as contrast-enhancing, space-occupying lesions on conventional MRI scans.

3.6.1 ^{201}Tl-Chloride

[201]Tl is a potassium ion analogue that does not cross an intact blood–brain barrier. However, if there is blood–brain barrier breakdown, ^{201}Tl will be taken up by viable tumor cells but not by necrotic tissue. Hence an increased radiotracer activity is seen in viable brain tumor as compared to radiation necrosis[7] (▶ Fig. 3.9).

With the advent of several PET radiotracers aimed at distinguishing recurrent viable brain tumor from radiation necrosis, there has been a decline in use of ^{201}Tl for this indication, but it

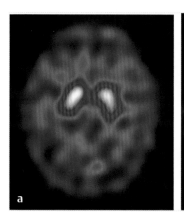
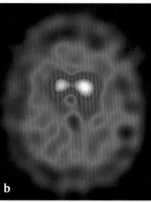

Fig. 3.8 Dopamine transporter scan. (a) Axial SPECT demonstrates homogeneous tracer activity in both the caudate and the putamen bilaterally (comma-shaped appearance, normal scan). (b) Axial SPECT demonstrates reduced activity in both putamina, worse on the right, and milder decreased activity in the right caudate (dot- or period-shaped appearance, abnormal scan).

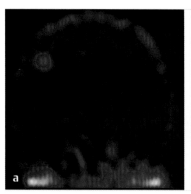
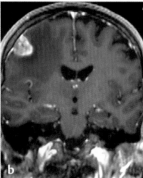

Fig. 3.9 ^{201}Tl SPECT. (a) Coronal SPECT shows increased radiotracer activity in the right parietal hemisphere corresponding to (b) a contrast-enhancing dural-based lesion on MRI. This lesion was confirmed to be viable melanoma metastasis on biopsy.

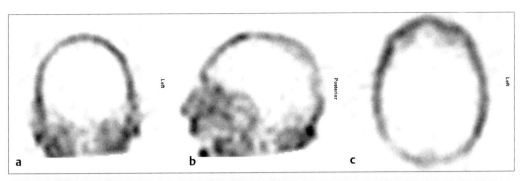

Fig. 3.10 Brain death. (**a**) Coronal, (**b**) sagittal, and (**c**) axial [99mTc-ECD] SPECT images show absent cerebral perfusion consistent with the clinical findings of brain death. Planar images (not shown) also demonstrated absent blood flow to the brain. Please note that brain death is a clinical diagnosis, with imaging used to provide supportive evidence.

may still be useful when PET is not readily available.

3.7 Brain Death

Brain scintigraphy, including perfusion SPECT, plays a supportive and confirmatory role in diagnosis of brain death in tandem with clinical findings and other investigations. In brain death, there is complete absence of blood flow to the brain.

3.7.1 [99mTc-ECD] or [99mTc-HMPAO]

With perfusion tracers, planar imaging may be sufficient if tracer activity is clearly present in the brain, which excludes brain death. If planar images are equivocal, SPECT may be performed in addition to dynamic flow and planar images (▶ Fig. 3.10) as it better portrays the intracranial perfusion and also provides a better view of the posterior fossa, including the brain stem.[8] However, SPECT may become logistically challenging, with unstable patients on life support.

References

[1] Herholz K. Perfusion SPECT and FDG-PET. Int Psychogeriatr. 2011;23 Suppl 2:S25–S31

[2] Van Paesschen W. Ictal SPECT. Epilepsia. 2004;45 Suppl 4:35–40

[3] O'Brien TJ, So EL, Mullan BP, et al. Subtraction ictal SPECT co-registered to MRI improves clinical usefulness of SPECT in localizing the surgical seizure focus. Neurology. 1998;50 (2):445–454

[4] Lewis DH, Toney LK, Baron JC. Nuclear medicine in cerebrovascular disease. Semin Nucl Med. 2012;42(6):387–405

[5] Bairactaris C, Demakopoulos N, Tripsianis G, et al. Impact of dopamine transporter single photon emission computed tomography imaging using I-123 ioflupane on diagnoses of patients with parkinsonian syndromes. J Clin Neurosci. 2009; 16(2):246–252

[6] Walker Z, Moreno E, Thomas A, et al. DaTSCAN DLB Phase 4 Study Group. Clinical usefulness of dopamine transporter SPECT imaging with 123I-FP-CIT in patients with possible dementia with Lewy bodies: randomised study. Br J Psychiatry. 2015;206(2):145–152

[7] Sun D, Liu Q, Liu W, Hu W. Clinical application of 201Tl SPECT imaging of brain tumors. J Nucl Med. 2000;41(1):5–10

[8] Donohoe KJ, Agrawal G, Frey KA, et al. SNM practice guideline for brain death scintigraphy 2.0. J Nucl Med Technol. 2012; 40(3):198–203

4 SPECT/CT for the Thyroid and Parathyroid Glands with Cases

Elisa Franquet-Elía and Kevin J. Donohoe

4.1 Introduction

Single-photon emission computed tomography/computed tomography (SPECT/CT) has substantially improved patient care in the management of several endocrine disorders previously managed with planar imaging or with planar imaging and SPECT together. Before the advent of hybrid imaging systems (positron emission tomography [PET]/CT and SPECT/CT), the CT images were collected separately from the planar or nuclear tomographic images, and the interpreting physician would look at the separate image sets and make a best guess at the "fusion" of the data sets. In some cases, the fusion was relatively easy to observe, such as when a solitary pulmonary nodule was found on CT and determined to be the same size and at the same location as a solitary focal concentration of tracer seen on fluorodeoxyglucose (FDG)-PET images. In many endocrine cases, however, lesions are small and often adjacent to structures that normally concentrate tracer, such as the gastrointestinal (GI) tract or salivary glands. Differentiating normal activity from abnormal activity then becomes a bigger challenge, particularly in postsurgical patients. As with FDG-PET/CT in patients with other malignant disease, SPECT/CT has drastically reduced the difficulty of fusing anatomical and physiological data sets obtained at different time points, improving the accuracy of tracer localization in many patients with thyroid and parathyroid neoplastic disease.

Pearls and pitfalls of SPECT/CT include the following:

- Tracer uptake may be faint and require additional time for SPECT data acquisition.
- Small focal sites of tracer uptake near the diaphragm may be subject to motion artifact, making localization more difficult or blurring the activity such that it cannot be seen at all.
- In the thyroid bed, artifact from intense iodine-131 (^{131}I) uptake following a therapeutic dose may render identification of adjacent nodal uptake difficult.
- If diffuse uptake of radioiodine is seen in the lung and the CT scan shows no anatomical signs of metastasis, the iodine uptake is still most likely secondary to metastatic thyroid disease.

- Posttherapy radioiodine imaging is more sensitive (and specific) for metastatic spread of thyroid cancer to the lungs than noncontrast chest CT and chest X-ray.[1,2,3,4]

4.2 For Benign Thyroid Disease

SPECT/CT is not often used for benign thyroid conditions, such as Graves' disease, thyroid nodules, or thyroiditis. If anatomical information is needed, a thyroid ultrasound is usually sufficient. Planar images with marker views of a palpable thyroid nodule can be correlated easily enough with ultrasound imaging. While SPECT/CT is not commonly used for benign thyroid disease, in some cases it can be helpful.

4.2.1 Case 1: Multinodular Goiter

History

A 76-year-old woman with known multinodular goiter and hyperthyroidism presented to her endocrinologist because a left thyroid nodule was increasing in size. Ultrasound showed multiple nodules bilaterally, with a cyst at the upper pole on the right. Because there was a question of the functional status of the enlarging nodule, a SPECT/CT was performed.

Physical Examination

Physical examination revealed a markedly enlarged, nontender, partially substernal multinodular thyroid gland.

Imaging Findings

The 24-hour uptake of radioiodine (iodine-123 [^{123}I]) was measured to be 40%. The planar images show an enlarged thyroid gland with heterogeneous iodine uptake (▶ Fig. 4.1). There are multiple areas with decreased tracer uptake and fewer areas with relatively increased tracer uptake. The biggest defect is noted in the left lower lobe (shown on the planar images).

On SPECT/CT (▶ Fig. 4.2), the low-resolution CT of the SPECT/CT shows that most of the thyroid nodules have no iodine uptake. Sites of increased tracer uptake in the posterior, medial, and upper poles of both lobes correspond to thyroid tissue with no nodule (▶ Fig. 4.2 c).

Discussion/Diagnosis

In this case, focal uptake in the thyroid gland on planar scintigraphy raised the concern of a hyper-functioning nodule, possibly contributing to the hyperthyroidism. SPECT/CT showed that the

nodules seen on ultrasound did not take up tracer, while the sites of increased tracer uptake were associated with nonnodular thyroid tissue, consistent with Graves' disease in a multinodular goiter.

Functioning nodules (showing iodine uptake) are so rarely associated with thyroid malignancy that they do not need biopsy. In addition, hyper-functioning nodules can show distorted follicular architecture and therefore can be difficult to distinguish from neoplastic tissue upon histological examination.[5,6,7]

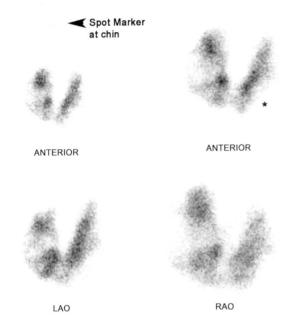

Fig. 4.1 Multinodular goiter with Graves' disease. Pinhole images of the neck obtained following administration of ^{123}I show an enlarged thyroid gland with heterogeneous uptake. The most prominent area of decreased uptake is located in the left lower pole (*asterisk*) and corresponded to a palpable nodule.

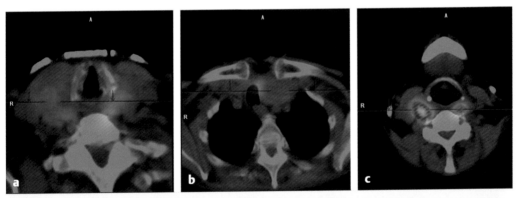

Fig. 4.2 Fused SPECT/CT images of the neck show two large nodules, **(a)** one in the lower pole of the right thyroid lobe and **(b)** another in the lower pole of the left thyroid lobe, which were relatively photopenic. **(c)** The thyroid parenchyma between the nodules (such as in the upper pole of the right thyroid lobe) shows homogeneous diffusely increased tracer uptake.

The dominant cold nodule was biopsied, but the results of the histological examination are not available.

4.2.2 Case 2: Hyperfunctioning and Hypofunctioning Nodules

History

A 53-year-old woman presented with three nodules seen on ultrasound of the right thyroid lobe. The functional status of the nodules is being pursued. The thyroid-stimulating hormone is suppressed.

Physical Examination

Thyroid examination was difficult secondary to body habitus; however, palpation of the right thyroid lobe revealed it to be prominent with an irregular surface.

Imaging Findings

The 24-hour uptake of radioiodine was measured to be 22%. Planar images show irregular uptake throughout the thyroid gland with relatively increased tracer uptake on the right compared to the left. The dominant nodule on palpation was marked using a cobalt-57 string marker, which, on imaging, appeared to be placed over the lower pole of the right thyroid lobe in a region of minimal iodine uptake. Because there was difficulty palpating the thyroid gland, the correct placement of the marker over the dominant nodule was questioned (▶ Fig. 4.3).

On SPECT/CT, the two sites of increased tracer uptake correspond to nodules in the upper pole and middle portion of the right thyroid lobe, and the inferior nodule shows no tracer uptake. The two relatively hyperfunctioning nodules are suppressing the function of the rest of the thyroid gland (▶ Fig. 4.4).

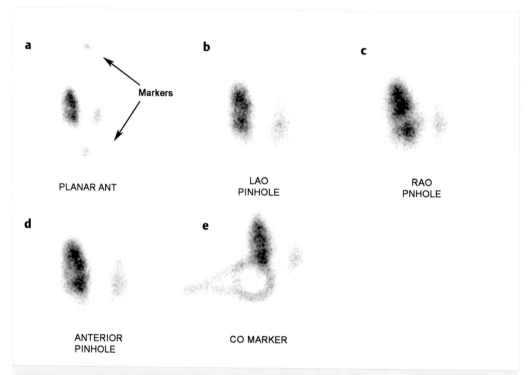

Fig. 4.3 Multinodular goiter. **(a–d)** Multiple pinhole views show tracer uptake in the right lobe. The left lobe has very little iodine uptake due to suppression of that portion of the gland. **(e)** A cobalt-57 string marker was placed on the palpated nodule.

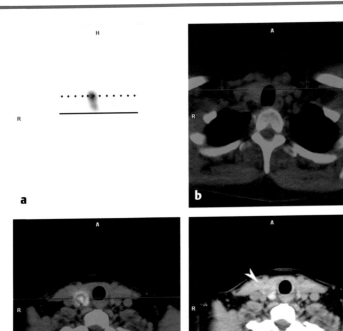

Fig. 4.4 Localization with SPECT/CT. (a) On the maximal intensity projection view, the right thyroid lobe functioning nodules stand out from the rest of the gland. The horizontal solid line is placed on the top of the cold nodule, which is marked in ▶ Fig. 4.3 with the Cobalt-57 string, and the dotted line on the upper functioning nodule. (b) The first axial fused image corresponds to the nodule at the solid line level and shows minimal tracer uptake at that site. (c) The fused SPECT/CT and (d) low-resolution CT images correspond to the dotted line level and show the functioning right upper lobe nodule (white arrow head).

Discussion/Diagnosis

While correlation of ultrasound findings with physical examination and planar images with marker views is often adequate to determine the functional status of thyroid nodules, when physical examination is difficult and reliable placement of the marker is questioned, SPECT/CT can be very helpful. SPECT/CT, in this case, confirmed that the dominant nodule in the lower pole of the right thyroid lobe was nonfunctioning, while the two nodules in the right middle and upper thyroid lobe corresponded to hyperfunctioning nodules. The lower pole nodule was biopsied and found to be benign. The relatively hyperfunctioning nodules higher in the right thyroid lobe were suppressing tracer uptake in the left thyroid lobe.

Pearls

Hyperthyroidism associated with Graves' disease usually results in an elevated 24-hour uptake of radioiodine in the thyroid gland; however, a hyperfunctioning nodule may not store as much iodine as the entire gland; therefore, whole-thyroid uptake measurements in glands with hyperfunctioning nodules can often be normal.

4.2.3 Case 3: Prominent Pyramidal Lobe

History

A 45-year-old woman presented with Graves' disease. The patient gave a history of hyperthyroidism for approximately 10 years, treated with methimazole for the past 8 years. A prior scan at another institution showed an unusual contour of the right upper pole/pyramidal lobe region and raised a question of a hypofunctioning nodule versus a large medial pyramidal lobe. Ultrasound showed heterogeneous iodine uptake throughout the gland, with several small nodular regions. The largest nodule in the left lower pole was 1 cm. Biopsy of that nodule was negative.

Physical Examination

Physical examination revealed an enlarged, soft, nontender thyroid gland that is slightly irregular without clear nodules. Palpated tissue near the midline, in the expected location of the pyramidal lobe, was more prominent than usual.

Imaging Findings

The 24-hour uptake of radioiodine was measured to be 95%. There was misregistration of SPECT and CT data, but the thyroid gland, including the pyramidal lobe, can be detected by increased attenuation on CT. There is no focal area of decreased tracer uptake that correlates with the expected location of the thyroid nodule. The pyramidal lobe shows tracer uptake (▶ Fig. 4.5).

Discussion/Diagnosis

This is an unusual case in which the pyramidal lobe of a hyperfunctioning gland made correlation of ultrasound, physical exam, and planar imaging difficult. SPECT/CT was helpful to show that the defect on the planar images did not correspond to the nodule seen on ultrasound. The final diagnosis was Graves' disease with a prominent pyramidal lobe.

Pearls

When viewing hybrid imaging studies (PET/CT and SPECT/CT), the possibility of misregistration between the CT and the scintigraphic data should always be considered, particularly when small structures are being evaluated. Determining if misregistration has occurred can be particularly difficult with thyroid imaging using radioiodine because of the lack of tracer uptake in adjacent landmarks.

4.2.4 Case 4: Ectopic Thyroid Tissue

History

A 27-year-old man presented with hypothyroidism. No thyroid tissue was seen on ultrasound.

Physical Examination

No thyroid tissue was palpated.

Imaging Findings

Planar images show no tracer uptake in the region of the thyroid bed; however, focal uptake is seen high in the neck (▶ Fig. 4.6). SPECT/CT showed that the site of tracer uptake was at the base of the tongue on the right (▶ Fig. 4.7). Visual examination of the base of the tongue showed evidence of a very small rest of lingual thyroid tissue on the right.

Discussion/Diagnosis

SPECT/CT is very useful for distinguishing functioning ectopic tissue from adjacent structures that can normally show iodine concentration, such as salivary glands, collections of saliva in the mouth, and swallowed saliva in the esophagus.

Pearls

Ectopic thyroid tissue typically does not function normally, nor is it the same size as a normal thyroid gland; therefore, measurement of 24-hour

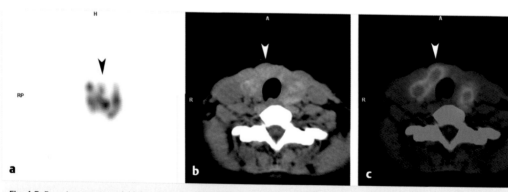

Fig. 4.5 Prominent pyramidal lobe. **(a)** Maximal intensity projection view shows heterogeneous increased tracer uptake throughout the gland, consistent with Graves' disease in a multinodular gland. The prominent pyramidal lobe (*black arrowhead*) corresponds to the palpated finding noticed by the patient (refer to text). **(b)** Low-resolution CT and fused **(c)** SPECT/CT show a multinodular thyroid gland and the functioning pyramidal lobe (*white arrowheads*), which corresponds to the palpated neck mass.

uptake of radioiodine cannot be compared to normal values and is not helpful for patient management.[8]

4.2.5 Case 5: Retrosternal Goiter

History

A 50-year-old woman presented with a mediastinal mass incidentally discovered on CT scan.

Physical Examination

Thyroid function tests were normal. The thyroid was normal on palpation except for evidence of fullness inferiorly.

Imaging Findings

The thyroid planar images (▶ Fig. 4.8) and SPECT/CT (▶ Fig. 4.9) demonstrated uptake of iodine within the mass, therefore confirming the presence of thyroid tissue. Histological sampling was

unsuccessful, and the mass was removed by partial thyroidectomy.

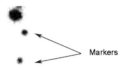

Fig. 4.6 Sublingual thyroid. Anterior planar ^{123}I thyroid scan. In the thyroid bed (between the two spot markers), there is no tracer concentration. Focal uptake is seen in the upper neck, with a second site of focal uptake just above it partially included in the field of view.

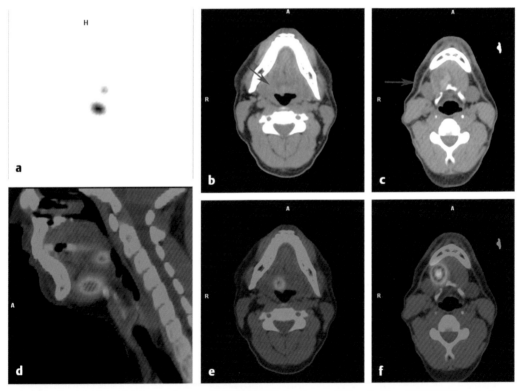

Fig. 4.7 Sublingual thyroid. **(a)** Sagittal maximal intensity projection view and **(d)** sagittal fused SPECT/CT images show two sites of focal uptake at the tongue base. **(b,c)** Low-resolution CT and **(e,f)** fused SPECT/CT images localize **(b,e)** the small site of uptake as well as **(c,f)** the larger site of uptake. The CT shows the increased attenuation of the iodine-rich thyroid tissue in the undescended portions of the gland (*red arrows*).

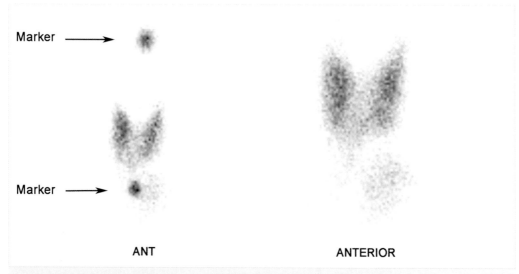

Marker ⟶

Marker ⟶

ANT

ANTERIOR

Fig. 4.8 Retrosternal goiter. [123]I thyroid scan shows a normally shaped thyroid gland located between the markers (*arrows*). A subtle and diffuse area of uptake is seen inferior to this.

Discussion/Diagnosis

Tissue masses just inferior to the thyroid gland in the anterior mediastinum may be suspected to be thyroid tissue; however, the differential diagnosis includes a number of neoplasms, and a tissue diagnosis is needed, particularly if the mass is causing symptoms such as shortness of breath or dysphagia due to airway or esophageal obstruction. Imaging with ^{123}I or ^{131}I can be helpful for confirming the presence of thyroid tissue. Substernal thyroid tissue often does not function normally, and iodine uptake may be diminished compared to uptake in normal thyroid tissue, as in this case. Pathology demonstrated the mass to be multinodular thyroid tissue.

Pearls

The four most common causes of anterior mediastinal masses can be remembered as the "four Ts":
• Teratoma/germ cell tumor.
• Thymoma.
• Thyroid tissue.
• Terrible lymphoma.

4.3 For Thyroid Cancer

According to the American Cancer Society, approximately 60,000 thyroid cancers occurred in the United States in 2014, yet in that same year there

were fewer than 2,000 deaths from thyroid cancer. The indolent nature of the disease is partly responsible for the low mortality; however, the incidence of thyroid cancer is increasing more rapidly than any other malignancy in the United States. Part of this increase in incidence may be attributable to the practice of head and neck irradiation, which occurred more commonly in the first half of the 20th century to treat skin diseases in children. More recently, much of the increase is thought to be secondary to the increased utilization of neck imaging, such as ultrasound, and the ease of histological sampling with fine-needle aspiration.[9,10,11,12]

While the indolent nature of the disease helps to keep the mortality low, proper staging of the disease remains important because patients with stage III and stage IV disease have increased mortality, albeit with evidence of prolonged life span following ^{131}I therapy.[13,14,15] Staging of thyroid cancer is usually based on the TNM (tumor, node, metastasis) system.[1,16] SPECT/CT can be an important tool for improving specificity over planar imaging for the diagnosis of metastatic disease, as well as improving sensitivity for nodal disease in the region of the thyroid bed.[13,17,18,19]

In the thyroid bed, SPECT/CT following thyroid surgery is helpful for separating local nodal uptake from remnant thyroid tissue. Local nodal disease, particularly outside the thyroid bed, may be treated more aggressively than remnant thyroid

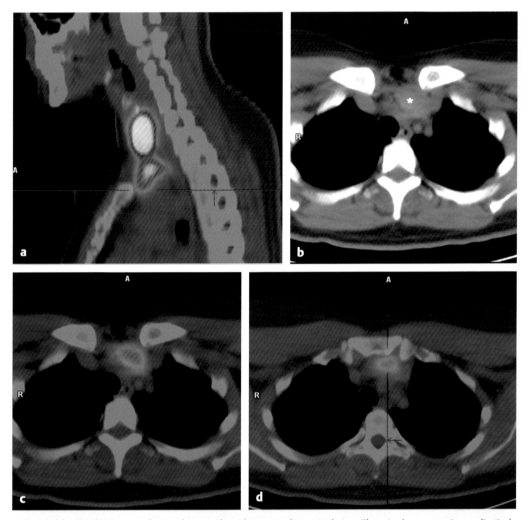

Fig. 4.9 (a) SPECT/CT images show orthotopic thyroid tissue in the sagittal view. There is also an anterior mediastinal mass (b, *asterisk*) with ^{123}I uptake (c,d). This ectopic thyroid tissue extends into the superior mediastinum just behind the manubrium.

tissue alone.[20,21] Focal tracer uptake at a distant site of disease in the chest, abdomen, or pelvis may also be more easily found using SPECT/CT. Sites of metastatic tracer uptake distant to the thyroid gland can be confused with normal structures, such as tracer normally found in the urinary collecting system or GI tract. In some cases, uptake in the region of the diaphragm seen on planar images can be either in the lungs or normal tracer concentration in the bowel or kidneys.

Identification of the cause and location of focal tracer uptake can be helpful in the initial staging of patients with thyroid cancer and at the time of subsequent visits as well.

4.3.1 Case 6: Thyroid Bed Uptake

History

A 74-year-old man presented with follicular variant papillary thyroid cancer.

Physical Examination

Physical examination was not performed.

Imaging Findings

[123]I planar images (▶ Fig. 4.10) show sites of tracer uptake in the base of the neck. There was a question as to the exact location of the uptake, and

SPECT/CT was performed. SPECT/CT images show focal uptake in the left thyroid bed (▸ Fig. 4.11 a) and anterior to the trachea (▸ Fig. 4.11 b, c), consistent with a thyroglossal duct remnant.

Discussion/Diagnosis

SPECT/CT is not always needed for postthyroidectomy imaging, particularly during routine posttherapy scans when tracer uptake is noted in the

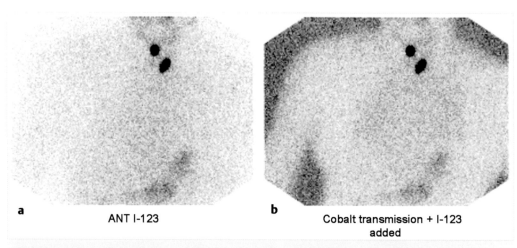

a ANT I-123

b Cobalt transmission + I-123 added

Fig. 4.10 (a,b) Planar ^{123}I images show two foci of tracer uptake in the neck following thyroidectomy. Planar images do not localize the sites of uptake well, and there was a question as to whether or not any of the sites of uptake were outside the thyroid bed.

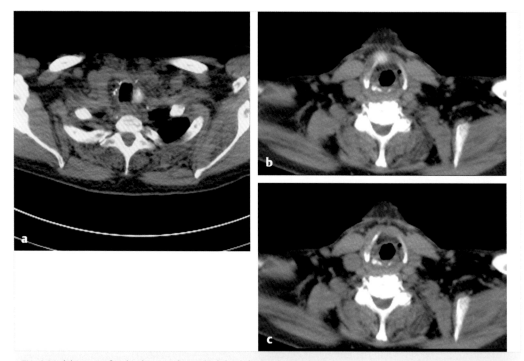

Fig. 4.11 (a) Intense focal iodine uptake to the left of the trachea and inferior to the thyroid cartilage corresponded to remnant thyroid tissue. (b) SPECT/CT fused images and (c) nonfused low-resolution CT better localize the uptake to confirm it is remnant tissue in the thyroid bed and thyroglossal duct.

region of the thyroid bed. However, the location of tracer uptake can sometimes be difficult to determine on planar images.

On this patient, a cobalt flood source was placed behind the patient to provide a body contour outline to better localize the sites of tracer uptake. In patients with exaggerated kyphosis or scoliosis of the cervical spine, remnant tissue in the thyroid bed may appear to be in an atypical location. Documentation of tracer uptake in local nodes or in tissue outside the thyroid bed may alter management. The SPECT/CT in this patient confirmed tracer uptake was confined to the thyroid bed.

Pearls

We often think of the thyroid gland as being at the base of the neck, and we think that the neck stops at the level of the shoulders. The body outline shown by the cobalt source in this patient reminds us that the thyroid bed actually lies below the top of the shoulders.

Variations in the location of remnant thyroid tissue can be substantial. If there is any question about local nodal uptake, SPECT/CT is much more helpful than oblique views or SPECT alone in determining the exact site of tracer uptake.

4.3.2 Case 7: Metastases

History

A 66-year-old man presented with thyroid cancer.

Physical Examination

Physical examination was not performed.

Imaging Findings

Following ^{131}I therapy, multiple sites of tracer uptake are seen in the lungs and bones. Although several sites of osseous uptake show correlating CT changes, others, such as in the sternum, show only subtle CT abnormalities, and one site (fourth left rib) shows no CT abnormalities at all (▶ Fig. 4.12).

Discussion/Diagnosis

Thyroid metastases can be discovered with either ^{123}I or ^{131}I. ^{123}I has a photon energy that is better suited to imaging with standard gamma cameras (159 keV), but ^{131}I has a longer half-life allowing more time for concentration of tracer in metastatic deposits and longer time for clearance of tracer from the soft tissue background. In addition, ^{131}I therapy doses allow for higher photon flux. Both isotopes have their advantages.

Some of the sites of radioiodine uptake in this patient are seen at sites with correlating CT abnormalities, while others are not. In addition, several abnormalities seen on CT (lung nodules—images not shown) show no radioiodine uptake. If the radioiodine images are negative and there is no other evidence for metastatic disease, including negative thyroglobulin and thyroglobulin antibody, further diagnostic imaging may not be

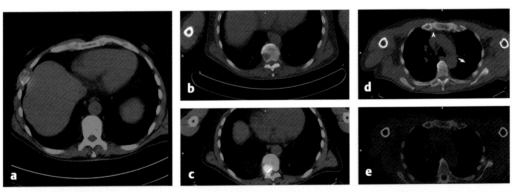

Fig. 4.12 ^{131}I posttherapy SPECT/CT shows multiple bone metastases that could not be confidently localized to bone on planar images (not shown). Some lesions are easily identifiable on CT because of the lytic bone lesion and soft tissue component (such as the sixth right rib lesion in **a**) or just the lytic bone lesion (T8 vertebral body in **b,c**). In other cases, the morphological appearance of the lesions can be more subtle, such as the lytic lesion within the manubrium (*arrowhead* in **d**), where the iodine uptake directed our attention to the CT finding. There can also be absent anatomical abnormalities, but clear iodine uptake (fourth left rib lesion in **e**, *white arrow* in **d**).

necessary. If there is a clinical suggestion of disease, such as a positive or rising thyroglobulin level, additional imaging might begin with an ultrasound of the neck. Whole-body imaging with CT or PET/CT may be considered if the ultrasound is negative.

The patient in this case developed widespread metastatic disease that no longer concentrated iodine. Fluoro-2-deoxy-D-glucose (FDG) PET/CT showed the progression of disease, and the patient succumbed to his disease several years after the iodine imaging study was obtained.

Pearls

Some literature suggests that if thyroid metastases are iodine-avid, they are not FDG-avid, and if they are FDG-avid, they do not concentrate iodine. While this has been demonstrated in some patients, other patients show avidity to both tracers or to neither, and some patients with a number of metastases show lesions that exclusively take up iodine, while other lesions only take up FDG and still others concentrate both iodine and FDG.[22]

Depending on the location of the metastatic disease and patient preparation, iodine imaging is the most accurate study (sensitive and specific) for identifying differentiated thyroid cancer metastatic deposits. However, as with other tests, it is not 100% accurate, and sometimes other testing is needed.

Medullary thyroid cancer does not concentrate iodine, but it may be localized with somatostatin receptor agents, such as pentetreotide labeled with indium-111.

4.3.3 Case 8: Pleural Effusion

History

A 68-year-old woman presented with a history of thyroid cancer resected several years earlier, now with rising thyroglobulin.

Imaging Findings

Planar images with ^{123}I prior to therapy show a normal distribution of tracer uptake with no uptake in the thyroid bed, consistent with prior thyroidectomy and ^{131}I ablation. A normal pattern of tracer uptake is also seen in the bowel (▶ Fig. 4.13).

A therapy dose of 175 mCi ^{131}I was administered. The dose was chosen based on a second

neck exploration, which revealed 4/10 nodes positive for thyroid cancer, as well as several small nodules in the lungs.

Following ^{131}I therapy, whole-body images were obtained approximately 1 week posttherapy. These images showed intense tracer uptake in the region of the stomach as well as diffuse liver uptake (▶ Fig. 4.13). In addition, there were two sites of faint uptake in the right anterior upper chest that were considered possible metastases (arrows in ▶ Fig. 4.13).

SPECT/CT was obtained (1) to assess the intense uptake in the epigastric region because intense gastric uptake was unexpected 1 week following therapy, and its appearance was different from that seen on the ^{123}I scan, and (2) because the diffuse liver uptake suggested functioning iodine-avid tissue somewhere in the body, and two sites of faint uptake in the right upper chest were considered possible sources.

Discussion/Diagnosis

SPECT/CT images show that the uptake in the region of the stomach is actually a loculated pleural effusion (▶ Fig. 4.14 a, b). Of the two right chest lesions, the lateral one (arrow in ▶ Fig. 4.13) was a second site of loculated pleural fluid (▶ Fig. 4.14 c). A possible cause of the pleural tracer uptake is passive diffusion into an exudative effusion. The mild midline uptake seen in the whole-body ^{131}I scan (arrowhead in ▶ Fig. 4.13) corresponded to mediastinal lymph nodes on the SPECT/CT (▶ Fig. 4.14 d).

Images approximately 1 week following ^{131}I therapy will occasionally show sites of tracer uptake in metastatic disease that were missed on the pretherapy imaging.[23] A second therapy dose cannot be administered at this time, but the information obtained is important for future management. Surgical resection of the metastatic disease may be possible if the site of tracer uptake on ^{131}I imaging is solitary and in a location amenable to surgery. Otherwise, uptake seen on ^{131}I imaging may help with decisions regarding future ^{131}I therapy. The fact that the metastatic deposit is iodine-avid suggests that ^{131}I therapy is still a treatment option, and the distribution of metastatic disease may also suggest the dose of ^{131}I for future treatment.

Pearls

Diffuse liver uptake suggests functioning iodine-avid thyroid tissue somewhere in the body, likely

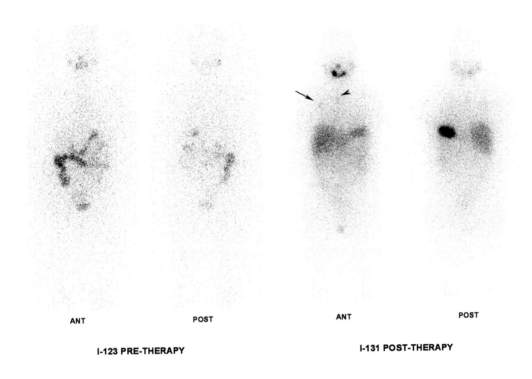

ANT   POST   ANT   POST

I-123 PRE-THERAPY   I-131 POST-THERAPY

Fig. 4.13 Whole-body scans performed before and after radioiodine therapy. The ^{123}I scan shows a normal distribution of uptake, with bowel uptake also noted. [131]I whole-body scan shows intense focal uptake in the region of the stomach. This amount of gastric uptake is unusual 1 week following therapy. Also, there is diffuse uptake in the liver, suggesting radioiodine labeling of thyroglobulin, which is metabolized in the liver, and two foci of mild uptake are noted in the right upper chest (*arrow* and *arrowhead*).

being the metastatic mediastinal lymph nodes in this case. The radioiodine is incorporated into thyroid hormone that is metabolized in the liver. While liver metastatic disease can (rarely) occur, it does not occur diffusely throughout the liver.

There is some debate about the need for ^{123}I whole-body imaging prior to ^{131}I therapy.[24] At our institution, we frequently use information obtained with ^{123}I images to alter management and the ^{131}I therapy dose.

4.3.4 Case 9: Contamination

History

A 74-year-old man presented with thyroid cancer. A scan of the ^{131}I treatment dose was obtained approximately 1 week following ^{131}I administration.

Imaging Findings

Planar ^{131}I whole-body images show tracer uptake in the region of the thyroid bed (▶ Fig. 4.15) as well as several sites of focal uptake scattered over the lower chest and abdomen on the anterior view. SPECT/CT images after removal of clothing demonstrate that the activity over the chest is superficial (▶ Fig. 4.16). Repeat imaging at other sites following removal of the clothing showed resolution of the focal tracer uptake and no evidence of metastatic disease.

Discussion/Diagnosis

SPECT/CT was definitive in showing that the sites of uptake distant to the thyroid bed were located outside the body and secondary to contamination. Another clue to the location of the tracer uptake is

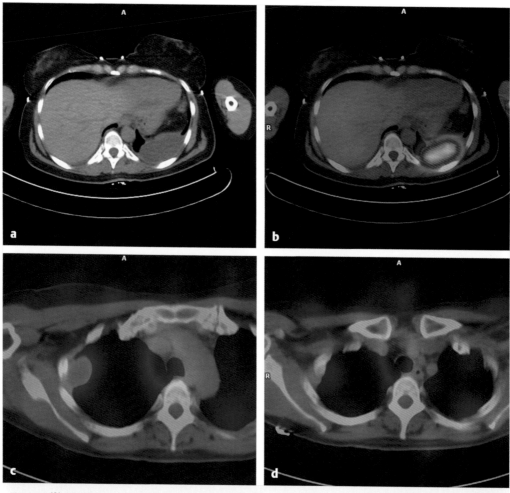

Fig. 4.14 ^{131}I SPECT/CT demonstrates two loculated pleural effusions: **(a,b)** a 7.5-cm pleural effusion in the left lower hemithorax with intense iodine uptake and **(c)** a 2.7-cm loculated pleural effusion in the right apex with low uptake. This right-sided pleural lesion was faintly present on the ^{131}I planar images in ▶ Fig. 4.13 (*arrow*). **(d)** The lesion located in the midline of the chest corresponds in the SPECT/CT to subcentimeter paratracheal lymph nodes. Lung windows (not shown) showed multiple noniodine-avid nodules.

that the uptake is seen on the anterior images but not the posterior images, suggesting an anterior location.

SPECT/CT may not be needed to diagnose contamination if contamination is always considered for sites of tracer accumulation. Inconsistent movement of sites of tracer uptake between different views suggests the sites are contamination of clothing, gowns, or other objects external to the body. Simple removal of clothing or using a damp cloth to wipe the suspected area is often sufficient to remove or at least relocate the contamination.

Tracer is excreted in the GI tract, genitourinary tract, and sweat and can easily contaminate handkerchiefs, tissues, undergarments, and outer clothing.

4.3.5 Case 10: Bochdalek's Hernia

History

A 63-year-old woman had thyroidectomy recently for papillary thyroid cancer.

Imaging Findings

Planar images show uptake in the thyroid bed as well as uptake at the base of the lungs (▶ Fig. 4.17).

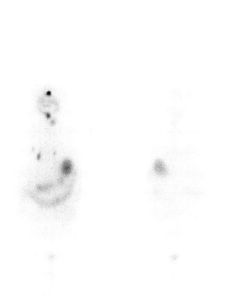

Fig. 4.15 ^{131}I posttherapy whole-body scan. There are foci of radioiodine uptake in the neck corresponding to remnant thyroid tissue. There are also three foci of uptake in the chest on the anterior view, not visible on the posterior view. There is normal uptake of iodine throughout the GI tract.

ANT   POST

I-131 POST-THERAPY

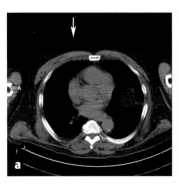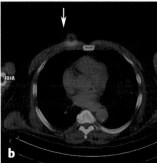

Fig. 4.16 ^{131}I posttherapy SPECT/CT. **(a)** The fused image shows focal uptake on the skin. **(b)** The CT image shows no evidence of a lesion in this area. This patient changed her clothes before the SPECT/CT, removing the other two sites of focal uptake seen on the anterior view (▶ Fig. 4.15). The SPECT/CT helped to confirm these sites were contamination, not metastatic disease.

SPECT/CT shows the tracer uptake to be in the stomach that has herniated through the diaphragm (▶ Fig. 4.18).

Discussion/Diagnosis

SPECT/CT proved very important in the staging of this patient, showing that the uptake in the chest was secondary to physiological accumulation of tracer in the GI tract. At our institution, we routinely image with ^{123}I prior to ^{131}I treatment to help determine the distribution of metastatic disease. Only patients with suspected tracer uptake outside the thyroid bed are imaged with SPECT/CT. We have found several patients with histologically indolent disease to have unexpected distant metastases. Findings on SPECT/CT not uncommonly alter our ^{131}I therapeutic dose.

61

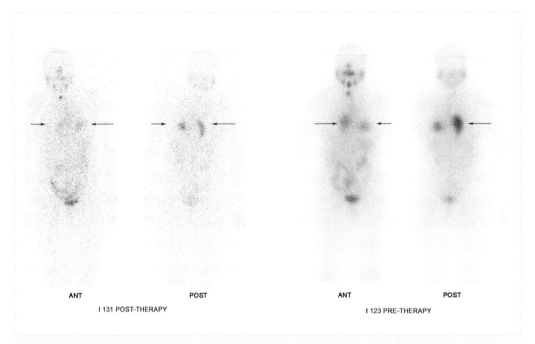

| ANT | POST | ANT | POST |

I 131 POST-THERAPY   I 123 PRE-THERAPY

Fig. 4.17 Post-therapy ^{131}I whole-body scan shows focal increase of uptake in the neck corresponding to remnant tissue. There are two areas of increased iodine uptake in the thorax, better seen on the posterior image (*arrows*). Otherwise, normal biodistribution of ^{131}I is seen in the salivary glands, intestines, and bladder.

Pearls

There are several benefits of ^{123}I imaging prior to ^{131}I therapy: to document iodine avidity in metastatic tissue, to localize metastatic deposits for staging, to help determine ^{131}I therapy dose, and, if appropriate, to localize metastatic disease prior to resection. Occasionally, the ^{123}I uptake and scan following surgery shows substantial residual thyroid tissue in the thyroid bed (uptake > 5%). In these patients, lowering the initial ^{131}I therapy dose can help to avoid local radiation injury beyond the intended remnant ablation.

If the thyroglobulin is elevated and there is no evidence of iodine-avid disease on ^{123}I imaging, FDG may be helpful for staging and localization of metastases prior to possible surgical removal.

4.4 For Parathyroid Disease

There are typically four parathyroid glands: two just posterior to the upper poles of the thyroid gland and two just posterior to the lower poles. The inferior parathyroid glands may more commonly be found at ectopic sites, from the carotid bifurcation to the mediastinum.[25] Five parathyroid glands are not uncommon, but three glands are rare.[26]

Primary hyperparathyroidism most commonly presents as asymptomatic hypercalcemia caused by a solitary hyperfunctioning adenoma almost 90% of the time. Other causes of hyperparathyroidism include multiple adenomas, parathyroid hyperplasia, and rarely parathyroid carcinoma.

There is debate about the need for surgical treatment of asymptomatic hyperparathyroidism with hypercalcemia of 1 to 1.5 mg/dL above normal levels. Many patients with asymptomatic hyperparathyroidism will not have progression of disease; therefore, surgery may not be necessary. Others argue that symptoms are often subtle and that the costs of monitoring these patients for progression of disease and the relative ease of localized surgery favor surgical intervention in most patients with primary hyperparathyroidism. If surgery is not considered, there is little need for parathyroid imaging.

Approximately 80% of solitary parathyroid adenomas should be detected on Tc-99 m methoxyisobutylisonitrile (MIBI) imaging. The sensitivity decreases substantially with multiple adenomas and parathyroid hyperplasia.[27]

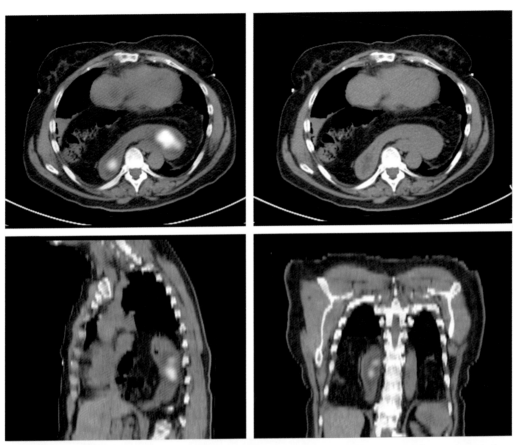

Fig. 4.18 Thoracoabdominal ¹³¹I posttherapy SPECT/CT shows the tracer uptake to be in a herniated stomach, not in the lungs, substantially changing staging and management.

Normally functioning parathyroid glands are too small and too metabolically quiescent to localize with radiotracers. However, hyperplastic, hyperfunctioning parathyroid glands can be detected with nuclear medicine techniques. The most common tracer now used for localization of hypertrophic parathyroid glands is Tc-99 m MIBI, an agent also used for myocardial perfusion SPECT and scintimammography.[28,29] MIBI is a lipophilic cationic compound that can easily transit cell membranes and then associate with negatively charged regions inside the cell, often around active mitochondria.

4.4.1 Case 11: Parathyroid Adenoma

History

An 83-year-old woman presented to the emergency room with altered mental status. Serum calcium was elevated at 12 mg/dL. The serum parathyroid hormone (PTH) levels were elevated at 446 pg/mL.

Imaging Findings

The parathyroid scan with 10 mCi Tc-99 m MIBI at 20 minutes shows focal tracer uptake inferior to the right thyroid lobe. At 2 hours, there is partial washout of the tracer from the thyroid gland and at the site of focal uptake below the right lobe of the thyroid gland (▶ Fig. 4.19 a). SPECT/CT performed following the planar images obtained at 20 minutes demonstrates the presence of a hyperfunctioning 2-cm nodule located behind the brachiocephalic artery (▶ Fig. 4.19 b–d).

Discussion/Diagnosis

Following removal of the parathyroid gland, intraoperative PTH levels dropped to 10 pg/mL from more than 300 mg/mL prior to removal. The

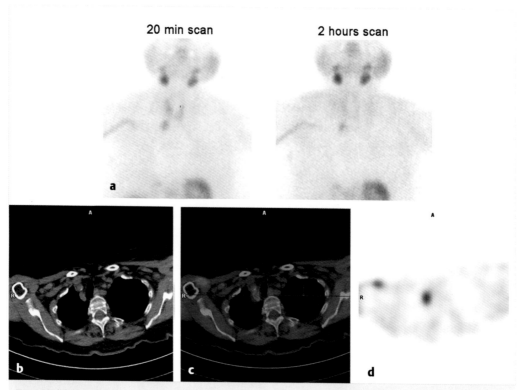

20 min scan   2 hours scan

Fig. 4.19 (a) Planar Tc-99 m MIBI images show a single focus of radiotracer uptake below the right thyroid lobe at 20 minutes and 2 hours. **(b–d)** SPECT/CT images show that this focus of uptake correlates with a 2-cm nodule located behind the brachiocephalic artery. A successful parathyroidectomy was planned based on the SPECT/CT.

histology confirmed the lesion was a parathyroid adenoma. This case shows a parathyroid adenoma below the right thyroid lobe, a typical location for adenomas on planar imaging. SPECT/CT, however, provides more accurate anatomical detail, allowing the surgeon to quickly locate the adenoma with less blind exploration. The incision can be more directed to the expected location of the lesion and surgical time is decreased.[30,31,32]

Pearls

Parathyroid scintigraphy is the procedure of choice for localization of parathyroid adenomas. While ultrasound is good, scintigraphy is more sensitive for ectopic lesions and more specific for the pathology.

Although textbooks describe the classical imaging pattern of a parathyroid adenoma as tracer uptake in both the parathyroid adenoma and the thyroid gland on early images, with washout of the tracer from the thyroid gland and retention of the tracer in the adenoma on delayed (2 hour)

images, it is not uncommon for parathyroid adenomas to show partial or complete washout on delayed imaging or for the thyroid gland to show incomplete washout on delayed imaging. Don't rely on persistence of tracer uptake to distinguish a parathyroid adenoma from normal structures.

4.4.2 Case 12: Parathyroid Adenoma

History

A 54-year-old woman presented with pneumonia and was found to be hypercalcemic. The PTH level was 131 pg/mL. A bone density study showed the patient was osteopenic.

Imaging Findings

Planar images (▶ Fig. 4.20 a) show a large, irregular area of tracer uptake at the level of the sternal notch. SPECT/CT shows the extension of the mass into the mediastinum (▶ Fig. 4.20 b–d).

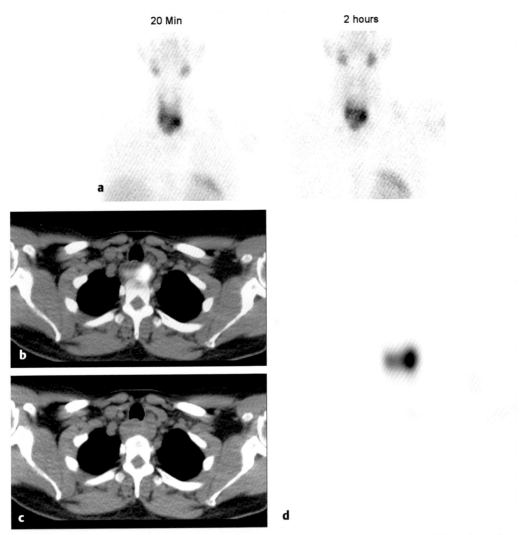

Fig. 4.20 **(a)** Planar Tc-99 m MIBI study at 20 minutes and 2 hours. A large area of irregular Tc-99 m MIBI uptake overlies the inferior lobes of the thyroid gland on both the early and the delayed planar images. **(b–d)** SPECT/CT better demonstrates the size of the lesion and that it is separate from the thyroid gland, extending into the superior mediastinum. Imaging changed the surgical approach to this lesion.

Discussion

At surgery, a large 22-g parathyroid adenoma was resected. SPECT/CT demonstrated the size and extent of the lesion to better assist in surgical planning. Following ultrasonographic correlation of the size and location of the mass, a limited surgical approach was no longer considered.

Pearls

The serum PTH level is not an indicator of the size of the parathyroid adenoma. Large adenomas can be accompanied by relatively low PTH levels, whereas smaller lesions (such as the first case) can have higher PTH levels.

MIBI is a perfusion agent that is not specific to parathyroid adenomas. Focal uptake of the tracer can be seen in hypervascular, metabolically active tissues other than parathyroid adenomas.

4.4.3 Case 13: Parathyroid Adenoma

History

A 74-year-old woman presented with documented hypercalcemia for several years as well as an elevated PTH.

Imaging Findings

The initial planar parathyroid images show focal uptake in the midline at the level of the sternal notch on both initial and delayed images (▶ Fig. 4.21 a). Claustrophobia prevented the patient from tolerating SPECT/CT. An ultrasound did not show a parathyroid adenoma. A second parathyroid scan 2 years later showed the midline focal tracer uptake. The patient was able to tolerate SPECT/CT, allowing the focal uptake to be discovered behind the trachea (▶ Fig. 4.21 b–d).

Discussion/Diagnosis

If the SPECT/CT shows a possible parathyroid adenoma and ultrasound does not detect the lesion, there is usually a reason for the discrepancy. The conflicting results should be communicated to the referring physician along with the reason as to why the lesion is not seen on one modality or the other, so that the referring physician is helped by the imaging results rather than confused by them.

Lesions seen on ultrasound but not with scintigraphy may have been missed secondary to small size, lack of sufficient metabolic activity, rapid washout of the tracer, or location adjacent to a multinodular thyroid gland. Lesions seen on scintigraphy but missed on ultrasound may have been

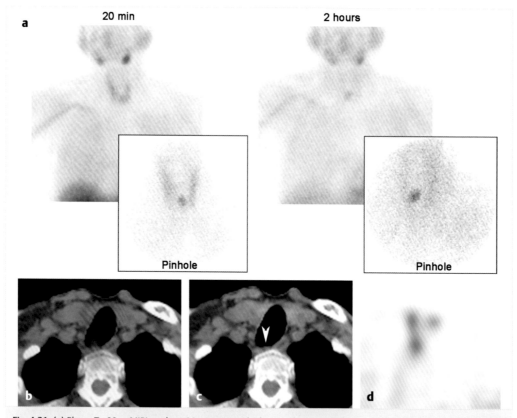

Fig. 4.21 (a) Planar Tc-99 m MIBI study at 20 minutes and 2 hours. The 20-minute large field-of-view planar image does not clearly show an abnormality; however, the pinhole image is more helpful. At 2 hours, the focal radiotracer uptake in the midline is more evident following washout of radiotracer from the thyroid gland. (b–d) SPECT/CT shows the site of focal uptake corresponds to a very small nodule seen on CT (*arrowhead*). This was a confirmed retrotracheal parathyroid adenoma.

mistaken for lymph nodes or may be ectopic lesions distant to the thyroid bed or behind bone or trachea.

At surgery, a retrotracheal parathyroid adenoma was found. The PTH and serum calcium levels reverted to normal following surgery.

Pearls

While it may seem to make sense to perform SPECT/CT at the 2-hour time point rather than the 20-minute time point, a study by Lavely et al[33] suggests the optimal time to perform a SPECT/CT in parathyroid scintigraphy is at 20 minutes. This is probably because some parathyroid adenomas washout by 2 hours and may not be visible on SPECT/CT at that time point. Also, at 20 minutes, the problem of separating parathyroid activity from adjacent thyroid activity on planar images is not as much of an issue with SPECT/CT.

4.4.4 Case 14: Ectopic Adenoma

History

A 72-year-old woman presented with chronic renal failure, diabetes, coronary artery disease, renal osteodystrophy, and osteoporosis and showed markedly elevated PTH levels of more than 1,800 pg/mL. She underwent a subtotal parathyroidectomy with three full, and three quarters of the fourth, glands removed (one-fourth of the lower left gland was not removed). The specimens showed parathyroid hyperplasia. Seven years after surgery, the patient presented with PTH rising again to more than 1,700 pg/mL. A parathyroid scan was requested.

Imaging Findings

Planar images at 20 minutes and 2 hours show two sites of focal tracer uptake (▶ Fig. 4.22 a) located inferior to the lower pole of the left thyroid lobe and in the mediastinum.

SPECT/CT (▶ Fig. 4.22 b–d) shows that the focal tracer uptake in the neck corresponds to a CT hypodense nodule close to the surgical bed (*white arrow*) that is consistent with a hyperplasia of the remnant gland. The second site of focal uptake was located in the anterior mediastinum (ectopic gland) and is clearly seen on the CT (*arrowhead* in ▶ Fig. 4.22 c, f). SPECT/CT helped localize the two lesions.

Discussion/Diagnosis

Parathyroid scanning is approximately 80 to 90% sensitive for solitary adenomas.[34] The sensitivity of the procedure drops substantially for multiple adenomas and parathyroid hyperplasia.[27] In this patient with end-stage renal disease and a subtotal parathyroidectomy in the past showing parathyroid hyperplasia, a parathyroid scan is not as likely to show parathyroid disease; however, the study is noninvasive and may be able to assist in the management of complicated patients such as this. The findings are consistent with tertiary hyperparathyroidism.[35,36]

4.4.5 Case 15: Intrathyroidal Parathyroid Adenoma

History

A 41-year-old woman presented with a 1-year history of hyperparathyroidism. The serum calcium level is 11.1 mg/dL and the PTH level is 96 pg/mL. She has no symptomatic manifestations of hyperparathyroidism.

Imaging Findings

Planar images at 20 minutes and 2 hours show focal tracer uptake in the region of the thyroid isthmus, just to the left of midline (▶ Fig. 4.23 a). SPECT/CT images show no extrathyroidal tissue correlating to the site of focal tracer uptake; however, relatively hypodense soft tissue that appears to be inside the thyroid gland does correlate to the location of the tracer uptake (▶ Fig. 4.23 b).

Discussion/Diagnosis

Focal tracer uptake in the region of the lower thyroid bed on planar scintigraphy localized to soft tissue within the thyroid gland on SPECT/CT. Because Tc-99 m MIBI uptake is not specific to parathyroid tissue, other causes for the uptake should be considered. However, in a patient with primary hyperparathyroidism, parathyroid adenoma remains high on the differential diagnosis.

At surgery, an intrathyroidal parathyroid adenoma was discovered. A left hemithyroidectomy was performed. PTH and serum calcium levels returned to normal following the left hemithyroidectomy.

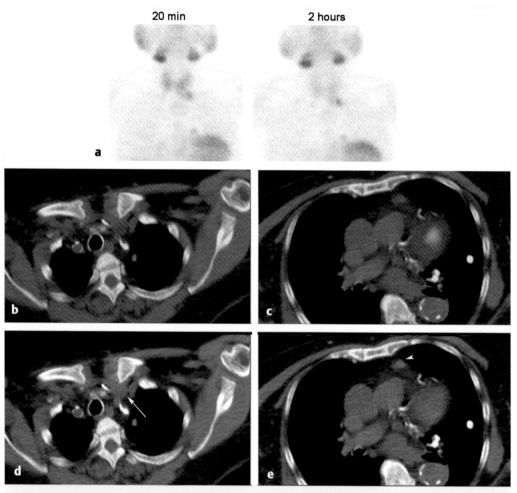

Fig. 4.22 **(a)** Planar Tc-99 m MIBI images at 20 minutes and 2 hours are shown. There are two foci of increased radiotracer uptake on the planar images: one is located just below the lower pole of the left thyroid lobe, and the other is located just above the normal cardiac uptake. **(b,d)** SPECT/CT images show a parathyroid adenoma located just below the left thyroid lobe (*white arrow*). **(c,e)** Images show the second parathyroid adenoma in the pericardial fat (*arrowhead*).

4.4.6 Case 16: Fifth Parathyroid Gland

History

A 37-year-old woman presented with elevated calcium and PTH levels. She initially had a blind neck exploration with four parathyroid glands seen, all appearing normal. Three of the four glands were removed, but there was no change in calcium or PTH level. Following this unsuccessful parathyroidectomy, a parathyroid scan was obtained with SPECT/CT.

Imaging Findings

Planar images (▶ Fig. 4.24 a) show focal tracer uptake below the sternal notch, just to the left of midline. SPECT/CT (▶ Fig. 4.24 b–d) shows that the focal uptake localizes behind the sternum to the left of midline.

Discussion

While parathyroid surgery can be successful without presurgical imaging, presurgical imaging localization of parathyroid adenomas allows minimally

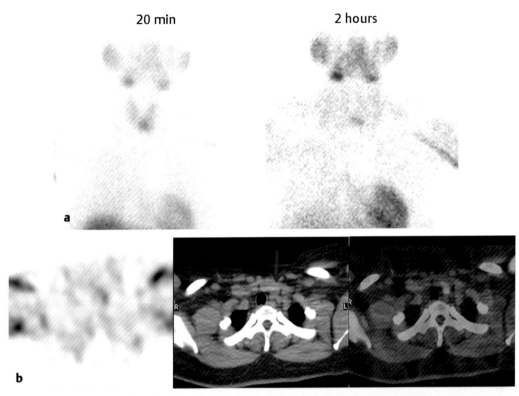

Fig. 4.23 **(a)** Planar images show focal tracer uptake in the lower pole of the left thyroid lobe. **(b)** SPECT/CT images show a low-attenuation nodule in the left thyroid lobe that corresponds to the site of focal tracer uptake (*red arrow*). This lesion was confirmed surgically to be an intrathyroid parathyroid adenoma.

invasive surgery with decreased operative morbidity (such as scarring and recurrent laryngeal nerve damage).[37,38] In this case, continued hypercalcemia was due to an ectopic fifth parathyroid gland seen on SPECT/CT.

Pearls

As mentioned previously, four parathyroid glands are most common, but five parathyroid glands occur. Three parathyroid glands are rare.[26,39]

4.4.7 Case 17: Brown Fat

History

A 57-year-old woman presented with osteoporosis, hypercalcemia, and PTH level at the upper limits of normal for several years.

Imaging Findings

Planar images at 20 minutes and 2 hours show irregular tracer uptake in the neck, supraclavicular region, and axillae (▶ Fig. 4.25 a). The thyroid gland has an abnormal contour on pinhole images at 20 minutes, with prominent activity medially in the region of the left upper pole. At 2 hours, tracer uptake in the thyroid gland washes out with focal uptake remaining in the region of the left upper pole. SPECT/CT shows focal activity in the left upper pole as well as irregular uptake within adipose tissue in the neck, supraclavicular region, and axillae (▶ Fig. 4.25 b, c).

Discussion/Diagnosis

This case illustrates that not all sites of MIBI uptake are related to a parathyroid adenoma. The focal

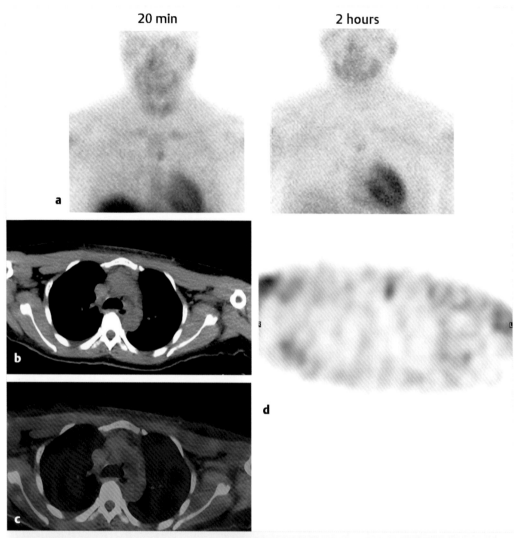

Fig. 4.24 **(a)** Planar Tc-99 m MIBI images at 20 minutes and 2 hours show focal tracer uptake at the level of the sternomanubrial junction. **(b–d)** SPECT/CT images localize the focal tracer uptake on the planar images just posterior to the sternum. At surgery, this was confirmed to be a parathyroid adenoma in an ectopic fifth parathyroid gland.

uptake adjacent to the thyroid gland correlated to a soft tissue nodule on ultrasound that eventually proved to be a parathyroid adenoma at the time of surgical removal. The uptake in the neck, supraclavicular region, and axillae was secondary to uptake in metabolically active brown adipose tissue. SPECT/CT localization of tracer uptake helps to distinguish brown fat uptake in parathyroid adenoma.

4.5 Acknowledgment

Dr. Franquet-Elía was supported by a grant from Fundación Alfonso Martín Escudero.

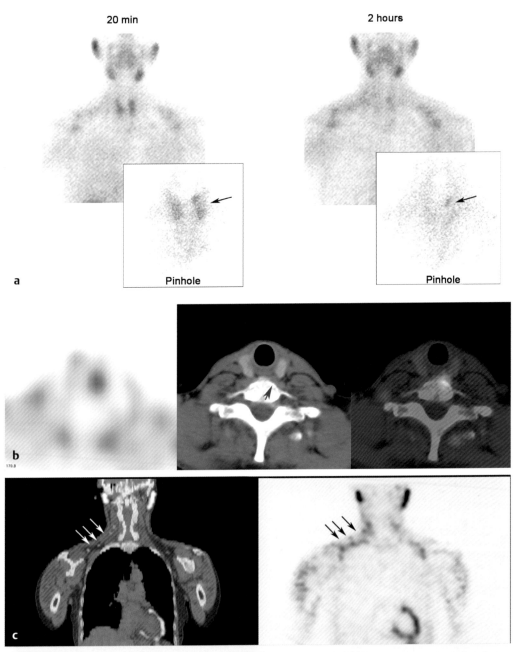

Fig. 4.25 **(a)** Planar images at 20 minutes and 2 hours with pinhole images show a focus of persistent tracer uptake in the medial aspect of the upper pole of the left thyroid lobe (*black arrow*). **(b)** Axial SPECT/CT images show that this site of uptake corresponds to a hypoattenuating prevertebral nodule (*red arrow*). **(c)** Metabolically active brown adipose tissue is seen in the supraclavicular regions bilaterally on both the planar images and the fused coronal SPECT/CT images (*triple arrows*).

References

[1] American Thyroid Association (ATA) Guidelines Taskforce on Thyroid Nodules and Differentiated Thyroid Cancer, Cooper DS, Doherty GM, Haugen BR, et al. Revised American Thyroid Association management guidelines for patients with thyroid nodules and differentiated thyroid cancer. Thyroid. 2009;19 (11):1167–1214

[2] Küçük ON, Gültekin SS, Aras G, Ibiş E. Radioiodine whole-body scans, thyroglobulin levels, 99mTc-MIBI scans and computed tomography: results in patients with lung metastases from differentiated thyroid cancer. Nucl Med Commun. 2006; 27(3):261–266

[3] Lorenzen J, Beese M, Mester J, Brumma K, Beyer W, Clausen M. Chest X ray: routine indication in the follow-up of differentiated thyroid cancer? [in German]. Nucl Med (Stuttg). 1998;37(6):208–212

[4] Ronga G, Filesi M, Montesano T, et al. Lung metastases from differentiated thyroid carcinoma. A 40 years' experience. Q J Nucl Med Mol Imaging. 2004;48(1):12–19

[5] Kresnik E, Gallowitsch HJ, Mikosch P, Unterweger O, Gomez I, Lind P. Scintigraphic and ultrasonographic appearance in different tumor stages of thyroid carcinoma. Acta Med Austriaca. 2000;27(1):32–35

[6] Kusić Z, Becker DV, Saenger EL, et al. Comparison of technetium-99 m and iodine-123 imaging of thyroid nodules: correlation with pathologic findings. J Nucl Med. 1990;31(4):393–399

[7] Beierwaltes WH. Comparison of technetium-99 m and iodine-123 nodules: correlation with pathologic findings. J Nucl Med. 1990;31(4):400–402

[8] Noussios G, Anagnostis P, Goulis DG, Lappas D, Natsis K. Ectopic thyroid tissue: anatomical, clinical, and surgical implications of a rare entity. Eur J Endocrinol. 2011;165 (3):375–382

[9] Morris LG, Sikora AG, Tosteson TD, Davies L. The increasing incidence of thyroid cancer: the influence of access to care. Thyroid. 2013;23(7):885–891

[10] Vigneri R, Malandrino P, Vigneri P. The changing epidemiology of thyroid cancer: why is incidence increasing? Curr Opin Oncol. 2015;27(1):1–7

[11] Pellegriti G, Frasca F, Regalbuto C, Squatrito S, Vigneri R. Worldwide increasing incidence of thyroid cancer: update on epidemiology and risk factors. J Cancer Epidemiol. 2013; 2013:965212

[12] Joyce JM, Swihart A. Thyroid: nuclear medicine update. Radiol Clin North Am. 2011;49(3):425–434, v

[13] Avram AM. Radioiodine scintigraphy with SPECT/CT: an important diagnostic tool for thyroid cancer staging and risk stratification. J Nucl Med. 2012;53(5):754–764

[14] de Melo TG, Zantut-Wittmann DE, Ficher E, da Assumpção LV. Factors related to mortality in patients with papillary and follicular thyroid cancer in long-term follow-up. J Endocrinol Invest. 2014;37(12):1195–1200

[15] Jonklaas J, Sarlis NJ, Litofsky D, et al. Outcomes of patients with differentiated thyroid carcinoma following initial therapy. Thyroid. 2006;16(12):1229–1242

[16] Edge SBBD, Compton CC, Fritz AG, Greene FL, Trotti A, eds. AJCC Cancer Staging Manual. 7th ed. New York, NY: Springer; 2010

[17] Mariani G, Bruselli L, Kuwert T, et al. A review on the clinical uses of SPECT/CT. Eur J Nucl Med Mol Imaging. 2010;37 (10):1959–1985

[18] Xue YL, Qiu ZL, Song HJ, Luo QY. Value of 131I SPECT/CT for the evaluation of differentiated thyroid cancer: a systematic review of the literature. Eur J Nucl Med Mol Imaging. 2013; 40(5):768–778

[19] Schmidt D, Szikszai A, Linke R, Bautz W, Kuwert T. Impact of 131I SPECT/spiral CT on nodal staging of differentiated thyroid carcinoma at the first radioablation. J Nucl Med. 2009; 50(1):18–23

[20] Grewal RK, Tuttle RM, Fox J, et al. The effect of posttherapy 131I SPECT/CT on risk classification and management of patients with differentiated thyroid cancer. J Nucl Med. 2010; 51(9):1361–1367

[21] Maruoka Y, Abe K, Baba S, et al. Incremental diagnostic value of SPECT/CT with 131I scintigraphy after radioiodine therapy in patients with well-differentiated thyroid carcinoma. Radiology. 2012;265(3):902–909

[22] Iwano S, Kato K, Ito S, Tsuchiya K, Naganawa S. FDG-PET performed concurrently with initial I-131 ablation for differentiated thyroid cancer. Ann Nucl Med. 2012;26(3):207–213

[23] Bravo PEGB, Goudarzi B, Rana U, et al. Clinical significance of discordant findings between pre-therapy (123)I and post-therapy (131)I whole body scan in patients with thyroid cancer. Int J Clin Exp Med. 2013;6(5):320–333

[24] Van Nostrand D, Aiken M, Atkins F, et al. The utility of radioiodine scans prior to iodine 131 ablation in patients with well-differentiated thyroid cancer. Thyroid. 2009;19(8):849–855

[25] Noussios G, Anagnostis P, Natsis K. Ectopic parathyroid glands and their anatomical, clinical and surgical implications. Exp Clin Endocrinol Diabetes. 2012;120(10):604–610

[26] Eslamy HK, Ziessman HA. Parathyroid scintigraphy in patients with primary hyperparathyroidism: 99mTc sestamibi SPECT and SPECT/CT. Radiographics. 2008;28(5):1461–1476

[27] Caldarella C, Treglia G, Pontecorvi A, Giordano A. Diagnostic performance of planar scintigraphy using 99mTc-MIBI in patients with secondary hyperparathyroidism: a meta-analysis. Ann Nucl Med. 2012;26(10):794–803

[28] Greenspan BS, Dillehay G, Intenzo C, et al. SNM practice guideline for parathyroid scintigraphy 4.0. J Nucl Med Technol. 2012;40(2):111–118

[29] Rauth JD, Sessions RB, Shupe SC, Ziessman HA. Comparison of Tc-99 m MIBI and Tl-201/Tc-99 m pertechnetate for diagnosis of primary hyperparathyroidism. Clin Nucl Med. 1996; 21(8):602–608

[30] Noda S, Onoda N, Kashiwagi S, et al. Strategy of operative treatment of hyperparathyroidism using US scan and (99m) Tc-MIBI SPECT/CT. Endocr J. 2014;61(3):225–230

[31] Lorberboym M, Minski I, Macadziob S, Nikolov G, Schachter P. Incremental diagnostic value of preoperative 99mTc-MIBI SPECT in patients with a parathyroid adenoma. J Nucl Med. 2003;44(6):904–908

[32] Hindié E, Mellière D, Perlemuter L, Jeanguillaume C, Galle P. Primary hyperparathyroidism: higher success rate of first surgery after preoperative Tc-99 m sestamibi-I-123 subtraction scanning. Radiology. 1997;204(1):221–228

[33] Lavely WC, Goetze S, Friedman KP, et al. Comparison of SPECT/CT, SPECT, and planar imaging with single- and dual-phase (99m)Tc-sestamibi parathyroid scintigraphy. J Nucl Med. 2007;48(7):1084–1089

[34] Ruda JM, Hollenbeak CS, Stack BC, Jr. A systematic review of the diagnosis and treatment of primary hyperparathyroidism from 1995 to 2003. Otolaryngol Head Neck Surg. 2005;132 (3):359–372

[35] Madorin C, Owen RP, Fraser WD, et al. The surgical management of renal hyperparathyroidism. Eur Arch Otorhinolaryngol. 2012;269(6):1565–1576

[36] Lorenz K, Sekulla C, Dralle H. Surgical management of renal hyperparathyroidism [in German]. Zentralbl Chir. 2013;138 Suppl 2:e47–e54

[37] Gasparri G, Camandona M, Bertoldo U, et al. The usefulness of preoperative dual-phase 99mTc MIBI-scintigraphy and IO-PTH assay in the treatment of secondary and tertiary hyperparathyroidism. Ann Surg. 2009;250(6):868–871

[38] Fuster D, Ybarra J, Ortin J, et al. Role of pre-operative imaging using 99mTc-MIBI and neck ultrasound in patients with secondary hyperparathyroidism who are candidates for subtotal parathyroidectomy. Eur J Nucl Med Mol Imaging. 2006;33 (4):467–473

[39] Smith JR, Oates ME. Radionuclide imaging of the parathyroid glands: patterns, pearls, and pitfalls. Radiographics. 2004;24 (4):1101–1115

5 SPECT and SPECT/CT for the Cardiovascular System

Stephen J. Horgan and Sharmila Dorbala

5.1 Introduction

Cardiac single-photon emission computed tomography (SPECT) is widely used for the evaluation of myocardial ischemia, infarction, viability, and function. Scintigraphic images identify selective uptake of a radiotracer by functioning myocardial tissue. Thallium-201 chloride (^{201}Tl) was the original myocardial perfusion tracer used initially with planar imaging and later in dual-isotope protocols with SPECT. Despite excellent first-pass myocardial extraction characteristics, ^{201}Tl provided limited image quality, due to the low-energy photons associated with this radioisotope; in addition, with a half-life of 73 hours, it is associated with the risk of excessive radiation exposure to the patient.[1] Technetium-99 m (^{99m}Tc)-sestamibi and ^{99m}Tc-tetrofosmin are the most commonly used radiotracers today because of the relatively short half-life of ^{99m}Tc (6 hours), easy availability, and high-quality myocardial perfusion and gated images.[2] In this chapter, we will provide a brief overview of ^{99m}Tc SPECT myocardial perfusion imaging (MPI) followed by a problem-oriented approach to MPI using SPECT, SPECT/computed tomography (CT), novel semiconductor detector scanner platforms, and software, emphasizing their potential advantages and pitfalls.[3,4,5,6]

5.2 Stress Testing and Myocardial Perfusion Imaging

Flow-dependent uptake of the radioactive tracer reveals relative blood flow to the different regions of the myocardium. As myocardial blood flow at rest may remain normal, even with high-grade coronary stenosis,[7] a stress test prior to injection of the radiotracer is needed to produce flow heterogeneity between the normal and the diseased myocardial segments and to noninvasively identify hemodynamically significant coronary artery disease (CAD). Radionuclide MPI is therefore typically performed at rest and during maximal hyperemic stress.

5.3 Stress Testing Protocols

Myocardial stress is achieved either by exercise (preferred) or pharmacologically with regadenoson,

adenosine, or dipyridamole (as an alternate to exercise) using standard protocols.[8] Treadmill exercise with the standard Bruce protocol (3-minute stages) is most widely used in the United States, while bicycle exercise is more common in the European Union. Symptom-limited exercise testing, rather than exercise termination due to attainment of age-predicted maximal heart rate (APMHR; 85% of 220 – age), is critical. At least 1-mm horizontal or downsloping ST depression or 1-mm ST elevation (in non-Q-wave leads) in a single lead for three consecutive beats is considered an ischemic response. Exercise-induced ischemic changes typically resolve with termination of exercise. If not, sublingual nitroglycerin 0.4 mg may be administered after ascertaining that there are no contraindications (systolic blood pressure < 90 mm Hg or use of phosphodiesterase inhibitors). If symptoms persist and blood pressure remains stable, then intravenous beta blockers (Lopressor, 5 mg, slow intravenous push) can be used to decrease the heart rate and reduce ischemia.

Regadenoson is administered as a nonweight-based slow bolus injection of 0.4 mg over 10 seconds, whereas adenosine (140 µg/kg/min to a maximum of 60 mg) and dipyridamole (142 µg/kg/min to a maximum of 60 mg) are weight-based injections administered over 4 minutes. Adenosine is short acting and typically the effects wear off when infusion is terminated. If wheezing occurs with any of the agents or in patients who are symptomatic or demonstrate ischemic changes, the effects of regadenoson or dipyridamole can be reversed with intravenous aminophylline, 1.0 to 1.5 mg/kg, slow IV push over 2 minutes.[8] Dobutamine is occasionally required when there is a contraindication to the previously mentioned vasodilators, including active wheezing, high-grade atrioventricular block without a pacemaker, or hypotension (systolic blood pressure < 90 mm Hg).[8] Intravenous beta blockers as described previously can be used to alleviate tachycardia or adverse effects from dobutamine infusion.

5.4 Myocardial Perfusion Imaging Protocols

Typically, both rest imaging and stress imaging are performed on the same day, with the stress portion of the test performed after the rest imaging has been completed, although stress-first imaging is gaining popularity.[9] A 2-day study is preferred in obese patients (typically men > 250 lb, women > 225 lb).[9] For single-day protocols, the radiotracer dose is administered three times for the second scan. If the stress perfusion is normal, the rest scan can be avoided with cost, radiotracer, radiation, and time savings, with excellent outcomes for a normal stress–only MPI.[10,11]

In the figures of this chapter, stress and rest myocardial perfusion images are displayed in alternate rows. The short-axis images (SA, top two rows) are displayed from apex to base (left to right), the horizontal long-axis imaging (HLA, middle two rows) are displayed from the inferior to the anterior wall (left to right), and the vertical long-axis imaging (VLA, bottom two rows) are displayed from septum to the lateral wall (left to right). The polar plots show raw polar plots (left column), polar plots compared to a normal limits database (middle column), and percent peak activity (right column). The top row is stress, the middle row is rest, and the bottom row the difference polar plot. All SPECT scans in this chapter are conventional Anger SPECT (A-SPECT) images, unless otherwise specified. All the cadmium zinc telluride (CZT) SPECT images were acquired using a D-SPECT scanner (Spectrum Dynamics).

Myocardial perfusion may be normal with relative homogeneous perfusion throughout the left ventricle (LV) or abnormal with fixed or reversible perfusion defects. ▶ Fig. 5.1 demonstrates an example of a reversible defect in the left circumflex artery territory indicating myocardial ischemia. Fixed defects can be associated with normal wall motion (suggesting artifact) or abnormal wall motion (suggesting scar or hibernating myocardium). Identifying and troubleshooting potential artifacts on cardiac SPECT are necessary for accurate image interpretation.

SPECT MPI is highly accurate (83%; sensitivity: 85%; specificity: 72%) and is comparable with (or better than) other noninvasive tests for the evaluation of ischemic heart disease.[12] Indeed, the major advantage of SPECT MPI is that perfusion defect size, severity, location,

and reversibility not only guide coronary revascularization (▶ Fig. 5.1) but also provide powerful prognostic information about risk of future cardiac death or myocardial infarction (MI).[12] However, the high diagnostic and prognostic value of SPECT MPI relies on accurate scan interpretation; false-positive rate remains problematic, particularly in women and in obese patients, and the optimal specificity of MPI depends on accurate identification of artifacts.[13] The advent of ^{99m}Tc radiotracers and electrocardiographic (ECG) gated SPECT MPI in the late 1990s allowed for accurate measurements of ventricular wall motion and thickening, ejection fraction, and ventricular volumes, and was a major step forward in distinguishing real defects from attenuation artifact.[14,15] Repeat image acquisition and motion correction software (for minor simple motion) help with motion artifacts.[9]

Also, after several decades of using the robust conventional A-SPECT scanners, with limited count sensitivity from the collimators, there have been several major recent advances in SPECT technology. High-sensitivity semiconductor detectors with cardiofocal collimation (D-SPECT, Spectrum Dynamics [all CZT SPECT figures in this chapter]; Alcyone, GE; or Cardius, Digirad), attenuation-corrected SPECT (radionuclide or CT), and novel software advances (fully iterative reconstruction with resolution recovery and scatter correction) have improved quality of images obtained with low and very low radiation dose SPECT MPI.[3,4,5,6] As with conventional SPECT technology, this new technology poses specific imaging challenges that will be discussed in this chapter.

5.5 Troubleshooting Traditional and Novel SPECT MPI

Rest and stress MPI should be interpreted systematically, starting with a review of the rotating projection images and followed by a review of the static perfusion images, polar plots, and gated images. A perfusion defect seen at rest and at stress is called a fixed defect, whereas a perfusion defect seen at stress but not at rest is called a reversible perfusion defect. The differential diagnosis of fixed and reversible perfusion defects is listed in ▶ Table 5.1.

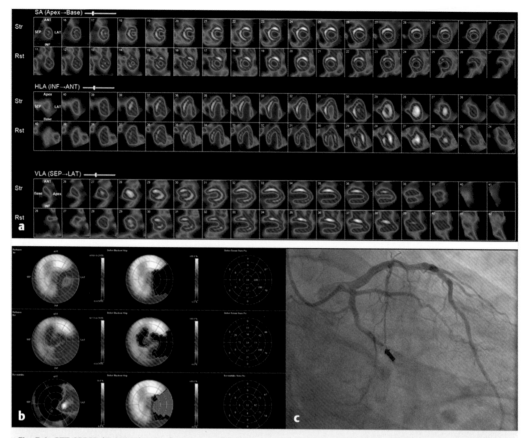

Fig. 5.1 CZT SPECT (D-SPECT) MPI of a 50-year-old man with atypical chest pain. His coronary risk factors include hypertension, dyslipidemia, a positive family history for CAD, tobacco use, and obesity. The patient exercised according to the Bruce protocol (9:30 minutes, 10.8 metabolic equivalents, maximal heart rate of 151 beats per minute [bpm], 89% of APMHR), with chest discomfort at 8 minutes into the test (heart rate of 145 bpm) that resolved 3 minutes into recovery. Blood pressure response to exercise was normal. There were 1 mm horizontal ST depressions in leads of V3–V5, which started 2 minutes into recovery and resolved at 7 minutes. He received 6.6 mCi and 22.3 mCi of ^{99m}Tc-sestamibi at rest and at peak exercise, respectively.
The left ventricle (LV) appears mildly dilated with no transient ischemic dilatation. The right ventricle is normal in size with normal radiotracer uptake. (a) The stress and rest MPI demonstrates a large, severe perfusion defect involving the mid and basal anterolateral and inferolateral walls and the apical lateral walls, showing significant but not complete reversibility. (b) Semiquantitative assessment of perfusion on the polar plots confirms that the mean regional counts in each of these segments are ≥ 50%, suggesting preserved viability. Gated SPECT MPI demonstrates akinesis of the entire lateral wall with reduced regional wall thickening (**Video 1**). The left ventricular ejection fraction (LVEF) was 57% and the LV end-diastolic volume index (LVEDVI) was 37 mL/m². These findings are consistent with a large region of nontransmural scar/hibernation with significant peri-infarct ischemia in the distribution of the left circumflex coronary artery. (c) Based on the scan results, an invasive coronary angiogram was performed (left anterior oblique caudal projection showing the left main, left anterior descending coronary artery and the left circumflex coronary artery with occlusion, red arrow), and the left circumflex coronary artery was revascularized percutaneously with a stent.

5.6 Fixed Anterior Wall Abnormalities

The differential diagnosis of fixed defects in the anterior wall includes breast attenuation artifact in female or obese male patients, or infarction or hibernating myocardium in the territory of the left anterior descending (LAD) artery. It is vital to exclude breast tissue attenuation artifact in order to make an accurate diagnosis of LAD pathology. Of note, sometimes breast tissue attenuation may coexist with LAD pathology.

5.6.1 Breast Attenuation

Breast attenuation is a frequently encountered artifact[9] (▶ Fig. 5.2) in A-SPECT and is less apparent with D-SPECT. This artifact typically presents as a fixed perfusion defect in the mid and apical anterior wall and/or anteroseptum on A-SPECT and may appear as a photopenic defect in the middle of the sinogram on D-SPECT (▶ Fig. 5.3). The main reason a fixed anterior wall perfusion defect is less apparent with D-SPECT may be upright imaging (wherein the breast tissue is located lower down as a result of gravity), high count sensitivity, or a combination of both.

Table 5.1 Differential diagnosis for fixed and reversible defects

Perfusion pattern	Differential diagnosis
Fixed defect	Attenuation
	Scar
	Hibernation
Reversible defect	Motion
	Misregistration
	Scanner failure
	Ischemia

Pearls

- Review the rotating projection images on A-SPECT to observe for attenuation from breast tissue.[9]
- When using D-SPECT, breast tissue attenuation is identified by reviewing the rotating projection images as well as the sinograms. Typically,

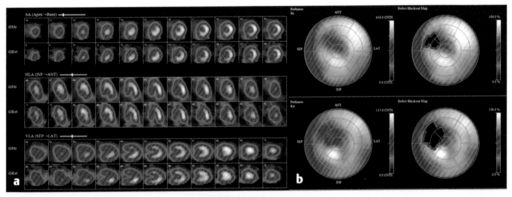

Fig. 5.2 Breast attenuation artifact. A 70-year-old woman with dyslipidemia and obesity was referred for evaluation of chest pain. She underwent a vasodilator stress test with regadenoson and there were no significant symptoms or ECG changes. She received 8 and 29 mCi of ^{99m}Tc-tetrofosmin at rest and during maximal vasodilator stress, respectively, and was imaged on a SPECT scanner. A breast shadow is identified on the rotating projection images (Video 2a). The LV and RV are normal in size with normal RV radiotracer uptake. (a) The stress and rest MPI demonstrates a fixed defect in the mid and apical anteroseptum. The gated SPECT MPI demonstrated normal wall motion and thickening, confirming breast tissue attenuation (Video 2b; LVEF 65% and LVEDVI 36 mL/m^2). (b) The polar plots demonstrate mildly reduced perfusion in the mid and apical anteroseptal walls but no abnormality when compared with a normal female database.

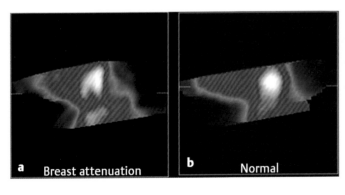

Fig. 5.3 On a D-SPECT scanner, review of the sinogram images may indicate (a) breast attenuation typically identified as a photopenic region in the midportion of the sinogram compared to (b) a normal sinogram without breast tissue attenuation.

counts are reduced in the midportion of the sinogram (▶ Fig. 5.3).

- Review regional wall motion and wall thickening; if normal, breast attenuation artifact is confirmed. In a prospective study of 99mTc SPECT (and 201Tl SPECT), Taillefer et al showed that concomitant analysis of gated images in female patients improved specificity for CAD detection from 84 to 92%.[16]
- Most SPECT software packages include quantitative programs that compare patient scans with a normal database, allowing (to some degree) for typical breast attenuation artifact in women.
- The optimal solution for attenuation artifact is attenuation correction using a radionuclide source or CT transmission scan. If a SPECT MPI study is equivocal due to suspected attenuation on SPECT, a positron emission tomography (PET) MPI study should be considered for further evaluation (▶ Fig. 5.4).[15,17,18]

Pitfalls

- Lack of recognition of breast attenuation artifact may result in an incorrect diagnosis of an infarct in the location of the perfusion defect.
- Depending on body habitus and the position of the breast, the lateral wall can also be involved.
- If the breast position shifts between rest and stress acquisitions, as identified on the rotating projection images, there may be an apparent reversible perfusion defect mimicking LAD ischemia. Gated SPECT cannot help in this situation. Attenuation-correct MPI is recommended when shifting breast tissue attenuation is suspected.
- Small or nontransmural scars (< 50% scar on cardiac magnetic resonance imaging [CMR]) may have preserved wall motion on gated SPECT and may not be identified by SPECT MPI. In one study, 13% of patients with nontransmural scar on CMR had normal rest 201Tl SPECT MPI.[19] In

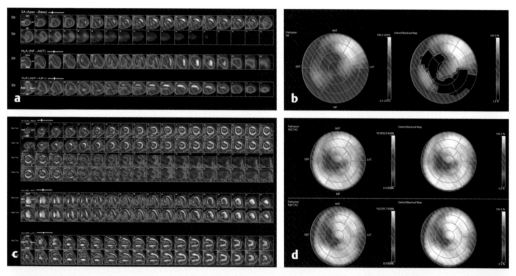

Fig. 5.4 Soft tissue attenuation in an obese patient. An obese 70-year-old woman (61 inches height, 290 lb weight) with hypertension, dyslipidemia, and diabetes was referred for a SPECT MPI to evaluate atypical chest pain. A 2-day stress-first 99mTc-tetrofosmin imaging (28 mCi) was performed due to her high BMI of 54.8 (rotating projection images, **Video 3a**). She underwent a vasodilator stress test with regadenoson, with no significant symptoms or ECG changes. **(a)** Stress perfusion images with **(b)** corresponding polar plots. The LV and RV are normal in size and RV radiotracer uptake is normal. There are medium-sized moderate-intensity perfusion defects in the apical anterior wall and the basal to mid inferior and inferolateral walls. **(c,d)** Due to her high BMI and concern for attenuation artifacts, 13N-ammonia PET MPI was recommended, which showed normal myocardial perfusion and normal LV function (**Video 3b**; LVEF 64% and LVEDVI 59 mL/m²).

animal models of MI, with histological gold standard comparison, both cardiac SPECT and CMR identified all segments with transmural scar (> 75%); however, small and nontransmural scar (< 50%) was better identified by CMR (92 vs. 28% of the segments).[19]

- Prone imaging aggravates anterior wall attenuation artifact and is not recommended when troubleshooting possible breast attenuation.

5.6.2 Myocardial Scar and Hibernating Myocardium

Fixed defects in the anterior wall with associated impairment of regional wall motion and thickening typically represent a true abnormality, such as myocardial scar (▶ Fig. 5.5) or hibernating myocardium (▶ Fig. 5.6).

Both of these entities are characterized by abnormal wall motion and wall thickening. Myocardial metabolic imaging with fluorine-18 fluorodeoxyglucose (^{18}F-FDG) PET, however, can differentiate them: the metabolically active hypoperfused region (mismatch between perfusion and metabolic activity) is hibernating, while the metabolically inactive hypoperfused region (matched reduced in perfusion and metabolic activity) is scar. The mismatch pattern is the hallmark of hibernating myocardium and portends an excellent likelihood of recovery of regional function following successful revascularization. Indeed, ^{18}F-FDG PET is the gold standard test to identify myocardial hibernation[20] and can be considered when the percent peak radiotracer uptake is between 40 and 60%[21] and the patient is a potential candidate for coronary revascularization.[22] A detailed description of myocardial viability assessment with ^{18}F-FDG PET is beyond the scope of this chapter, and readers are referred to other excellent reviews on this topic.[22] When ^{18}F-FDG cardiac PET is not available, ^{201}Tl SPECT may be used to assess myocardial viability (see Case 2 in Chapter 11), although it is less accurate than PET.

Pearls

- Defect size and severity are similar at rest and stress.
- Hibernation or scar may coexist with peri-infarct ischemia in the same or in another coronary distribution.
- The gated images demonstrate a regional wall abnormality in both infarcted and hibernating territories.

Pitfalls

- A small or nontransmural scar with no obvious regional wall motion abnormality may be interpreted as an artifact.
- Attenuation correction may improve an apparent perfusion defect when coexistent attenuation artifact is present.
- In regions of dense scar with minimal or absent radiotracer uptake, the SPECT software may incorrectly track the area of the infarct, resulting in a spurious increase or decrease in ejection fraction.

5.7 Fixed Inferior Wall Abnormalities

A fixed defect in the inferior wall may be due to infarction or hibernating myocardium in the right coronary artery (RCA) territory (▶ Fig. 5.7). More commonly, however, an apparent inferior wall perfusion defect represents an artifact resulting from diaphragmatic attenuation (▶ Fig. 5.8 and ▶ Fig. 5.9). This artifact is typically seen in men or in women with larger body mass index (BMI).

There are several reasons for artifacts in the inferior wall. First, a fixed inferior wall defect with normal wall motion may represent diaphragmatic attenuation. Next, with the use of filtered back projection for image reconstruction, fixed or reversible (if only stress images are affected) inferior wall defects may be a result of a ramp filter artifact.[6,23] This is particularly evident when there is prominent activity in subdiaphragmatic organs adjacent to the heart. Typically, this activity interferes with evaluation of the adjacent inferior wall, but, rarely, in the setting of a hiatal hernia, the lateral wall can be affected.[13] Lastly, Compton scatter from intense radiotracer activity in the subdiaphragmatic region may mask true inferior wall perfusion defects.[6,23,24]

5.7.1 Diaphragmatic Attenuation

Pearls

- Regional wall motion abnormality is normal on the gated images.
- Most SPECT software programs include quantitative programs that compare patient scans with normal databases, allowing for the typical inferior wall artifact in men.
- Prone images may minimize diaphragmatic attenuation.

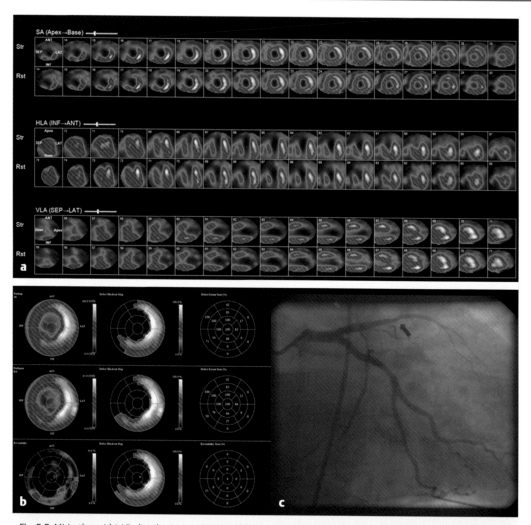

Fig. 5.5 MI in the mid-LAD distribution. A 64-year-old man with a known history of MI, dyslipidemia, diabetes, and hypertension was referred for chest pain evaluation. He underwent a vasodilator stress test with regadenoson and there were no significant symptoms or ECG changes. He received 8.5 and 30 mCi of ^{99m}Tc-tetrofosmin at rest and during maximal vasodilator stress, respectively, and underwent SPECT imaging. The LV appears mildly dilated with no transient ischemic dilatation. The RV is normal in size with normal radiotracer uptake. **(a)** The stress and rest MPI demonstrates a large and severe perfusion defect involving the mid and basal anterior and anteroseptal walls, and all four apical segments and LV apex without reversibility. **(b)** The polar plots confirm a large fixed defect in the typical territory of the mid-LAD coronary artery (a mid-LAD defect involves the midventricular anterior and anteroseptal walls, as well as the apical segments). Gated SPECT MPI demonstrates akinesis of the affected segments with absent wall thickening (**Video 4**). The LVEF is 39% and the LVEDVI is 109 mL/m². **(c)** The invasive coronary angiogram is an LAO caudal projection showing normal left main coronary artery, normal left circumflex coronary artery, and an occluded LAD coronary artery (*red arrow*). The severity of the perfusion defect (percent peak activity 30%) suggests a transmural scar rather than hibernating myocardium. As this was a known remote MI, an ^{18}F-FDG PET scan to identify hibernating myocardium was not performed.

- However, the optimal solution for attenuation artifacts is attenuation-corrected imaging with radionuclide source or CT-based transmission imaging.

Pitfalls

- Lack of recognition of an inferior wall diaphragmatic attenuation artifact may result in an incorrect diagnosis of inferior wall infarct.[13]

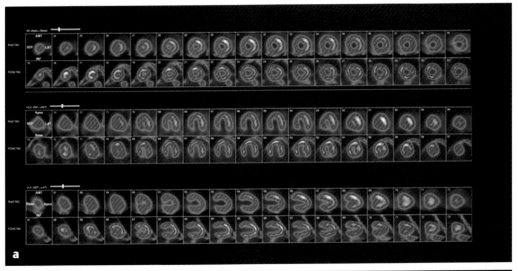

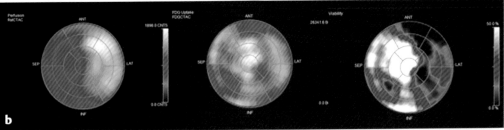

Fig. 5.6 Viability study. A 63-year-old woman with known CAD was referred for evaluation of myocardial viability for potential coronary revascularization. She underwent a gated rest ^{99m}Tc-sestamibi SPECT/CT (20 mCi) scan followed by ^{18}F-FDG PET scan. To maximize glucose utilization by the myocardium, an oral glucose load was provided followed by intravenous injection of regular insulin (2-unit increments to a total of 10 units) prior to administration of 10 mCi of ^{18}F-FDG and PET imaging 60 minutes later. **(a)** Rest perfusion and ^{18}F-FDG images are displayed in alternate rows. The perfusion images demonstrate medium-sized severe-intensity perfusion defects in the mid and apical anterior walls, septum, and apex, with mismatch on the ^{18}F-FDG images (reduced perfusion with preserved glucose utilization). In addition, there is a moderate perfusion defect in the basal and mid inferior and inferoseptal walls with a mismatch. The gated SPECT images demonstrate an LVEF of 36% (**Video 5**) with dilated volumes (LVEDVI of 93.5 mL/m²). **(b)** The polar plots demonstrate a perfusion (left) to metabolism (middle row) mismatch (right). These findings are consistent with hibernating myocardium in the LAD and RCA territories.

- Prone imaging can result in apparent perfusion defects in other myocardial regions, particularly the anterior wall. Hence, in cases of rest inferior wall defects, it is recommended to acquire both supine (for interpreting the anterior wall) and prone (for interpreting the inferior wall) stress images.[13]
- Attenuation correction increases the specificity to diagnose obstructive epicardial CAD but may reduce sensitivity, particularly for inferior wall defects in the RCA distribution.[17]

5.7.2 Excessive Subdiaphragmatic Activity

Pearls

- A drink of water or fatty foods (milk) may clear radiotracer activity from the bowel.[25,26]
- Repeating the scan after a delay may improve subdiaphragmatic activity.
- Exercising the patient (even if undergoing pharmacological stress) reduces splanchnic blood

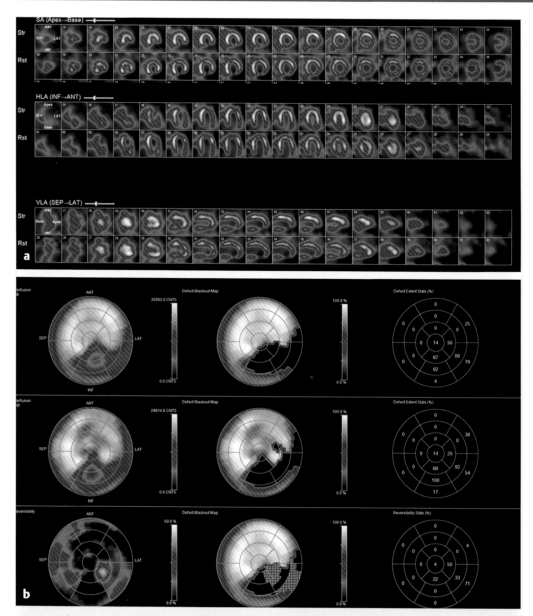

Fig. 5.7 Inferior wall MI. A 66-year-old man with a history of MI and coronary artery bypass grafting was referred for evaluation of dyspnea. His coronary risk factors included hypertension, dyslipidemia, diabetes, a positive family history for CAD, and obesity. He exercised on a Bruce protocol for 2:52 minutes, with a maximal heart rate of 104 bpm (68% of APMHR) and normal blood pressure response. He was limited by dyspnea. As APMHR was not achieved, the test was terminated and a regadenoson stress study was performed. He received 7.1 mCi and 21 mCi of ^{99m}Tc-sestamibi at rest and at peak hyperemia, respectively, and gated CZT SPECT imaging was performed. LV is normal with no transient ischemic dilatation. The RV is normal in size with normal radiotracer uptake. The LVEF is 58% and the LVEDVI is 37.8 mL/m^2 (**Video 6**). (**a,b**) The stress and rest myocardial perfusion images demonstrate a medium-sized perfusion defect of severe intensity in the mid and apical inferior and the mid and basal inferolateral walls that was minimally reversible in inferolateral segments. The gated images (**Video 6**) demonstrate reduced wall motion and thickening in the corresponding region, indicating infarction or hibernating myocardium in the RCA territory. Abnormal septal motion (paradoxical motion) is likely from prior coronary artery bypass grafting.

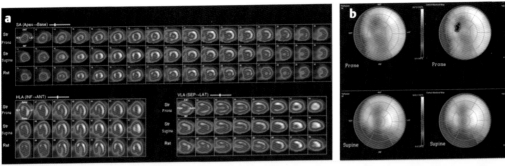

Fig. 5.8 Inferior wall attenuation artifact. (a) A 69-year-old man (BMI = 26.5) with hypertension, dyslipidemia, and no known CAD was referred for chest pain evaluation. He underwent a vasodilator stress test with regadenoson and there were no significant symptoms or ECG changes. Gated SPECT imaging was performed with ^{99m}Tc-sestamibi at rest (7 mCi) and poststress (31 mCi), respectively. The rotating projection images demonstrate patient motion that improved with prone imaging (**Video 7a**). The LV and RV are normal in size with normal RV radiotracer uptake. There is an apparent basal to mid inferior wall defect seen on the supine stress and rest images. Prone imaging has eliminated the defect and improved the perfusion (top row). (b) A stress polar plot representation of the perfusion in the prone and supine positions. Gated images show preserved wall motion and wall thickening (**Video 7b**; the LVEF is 65% and the LVEDVI is 68 mL/m^2).

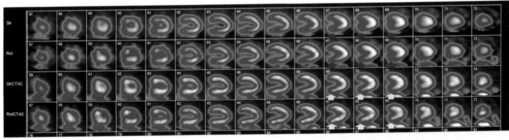

Fig. 5.9 An example from a different patient with a similar inferior wall attenuation artifact (*red arrows*, top two rows) that resolved with CT-based attenuation correction (*green arrows*, bottom two rows).

flow by increasing skeletal muscle blood flow, hence reducing bowel uptake of the radiopharmaceutical.[27] This is particularly important for patients scheduled for vasodilator stress testing.

- Reconstruction of the images with iterative reconstruction methods (ordered subset expectation maximization) will help in cases where ramp filter artifact is suspected.
- Lastly, if all measures fail, repeat imaging with [201]Tl (typically on another day) may help improve subdiaphragmatic activity.

Pitfalls

- If the subdiaphragmatic activity is variable at rest and at stress, apparent reversibility may be seen in the inferior wall leading to erroneous diagnosis of ischemia.

- If the subdiaphragmatic activity is intense and overlies the inferior wall, the images may be uninterpretable.

5.7.3 Myocardial Infarction in the RCA Territory

Pearls

- Defect size and severity are similar at rest and at stress.
- The defect may be larger or more intense at stress due to peri-infarct ischemia.
- The defect may involve the basal inferoseptal wall and/or the basal inferolateral wall.
- The gated images demonstrate abnormal wall motion and thickening, confirming pathology: MI or hibernating myocardium.

Pitfalls

- A true infarct could be misinterpreted as an artifact as a result of diaphragmatic attenuation.

5.8 Reversible Perfusion Defects

Most reversible perfusion defects are real and represent ischemia. However, it is important to recognize causes of artifactual reversible perfusion defects and exclude them prior to interpretation of the scans as ischemia. Patient motion, especially if noted only on the stress images, variable breast tissue position, misregistration of the emission and transmission images, and detector failure may result in artifactual reversible perfusion defects.

5.8.1 Patient Motion

Due to the scan acquisition over 8 to 15 minutes, a very important source of error with MPI is patient motion.[9,13,23] This may result in a false-positive study with defects in the anterior, inferior, lateral, or septal walls (► Fig. 5.10). One study demonstrated that patient motion was present in as many as 36% of clinical studies.[28] Detection of patient motion can be challenging with CZT SPECT or PET wherein imaging is not in a multiframe mode.

Pearls

- Patient motion is identified by a review of the rotating projection images.[9]
- The rotating projection images and the sinogram detect z-axis motion, whereas the linogram identifies horizontal x–y-axis or complex motion (► Fig. 5.11).[9]

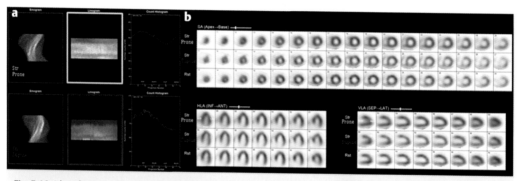

Fig. 5.10 Identification of motion artifacts. (**a**) The stress supine linogram (red box) demonstrates a very irregular jagged line indicating patient motion in the x–y-axis. An irregular breathing pattern can cause this artifact. (**b**) On the perfusion images, the LV and RV are normal in size with normal RV radiotracer uptake. The supine images (middle row) show defects in the anterior and inferior walls. Due to motion artifact, imaging was repeated in the prone position. The linogram (**a**, green box) of the patient in the prone position shows a much smoother line, and the corresponding prone perfusion images are normal (**b**, top row); see **Video 8**.

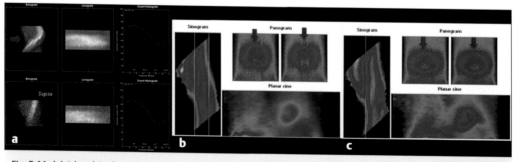

Fig. 5.11 (**a**) A break in the contour of the sinogram (*red arrow*) indicates patient motion in the z-axis or complex patient motion (**Video 9**). (**b**) (CZT SPECT images) shows an irregular panogram indicating patient motion contrasted with (**c**) a normal (smooth) panogram.

- With a D-SPECT scanner, there is a striped appearance of the sinogram images or a difference or shift in the two panogram images (▶ Fig. 5.11).
- When motion is identified, the solution is to repeat image acquisition, sometimes in the prone position. Imaging the patient in the prone position will reduce motion artifact. Motion correction software algorithms appear to work well when there is only simple one-time motion.[29] For this reason, it is always recommended to repeat image acquisition in cases of complex motion. The best solution is to prevent patient motion by careful patient instruction and positioning.
- If the myocardial perfusion scan is totally normal, there may be no need to repeat image acquisition.

Pitfalls

- There could be misinterpretation of a fixed or reversible defect in the anterior or inferior wall.

5.8.2 Misregistration

Attenuation of photons within the body is a recognized limitation reducing the specificity of SPECT for the detection of perfusion defects. Attenuation correction with dedicated radionuclide source transmission imaging or hybrid SPECT/CT systems has enhanced image quality and improved the specificity of MPI.[17,18,30] While CT transmission–based attenuation correction represents a major advancement compared to traditional line source transmission attenuation correction, due to the differences in image resolution between CT and radionuclide methods, artifacts may arise (▶ Fig. 5.12 and ▶ Fig. 5.13).

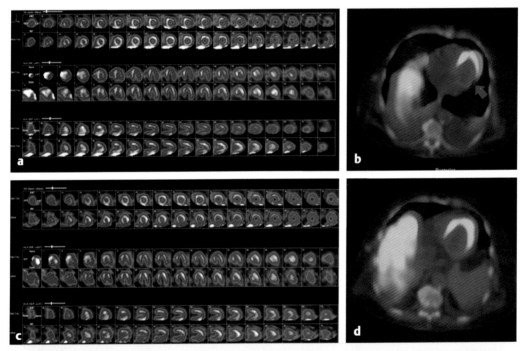

Fig. 5.12 Misregistration artifact. A 66-year-old woman with dyslipidemia and a family history of CAD was referred for evaluation of nonanginal chest pain. She exercised for 4:30 minutes (Bruce protocol), reaching 6.3 METS, and achieved a maximal heart rate of 136 bpm (88% of APMHR). The test was terminated due to dyspnea and fatigue. The blood pressure response to exercise was normal and there were no ECG changes. Gated SPECT/CT imaging was performed with ^{99m}Tc-sestamibi at rest (11.8 mCi) and poststress (32.6 mCi), respectively (**Video 10**). The LV and RV are normal in size with normal radiotracer uptake. The LVEF is 51% and the LVEDVI is 58.3 mL/m².
(**a**) There is an apparent medium-sized perfusion defect of moderate intensity in the entire lateral wall that was reversible. (**b**) However, on inspection of the overlay of the stress emission and the CT transmission images, misregistration is evident, with the emission scan overlying the lung fields (*red arrow*). (**c**) On the newly reconstructed images, the stress perfusion is normal, following appropriate registration of (**d**) the transmission and emission images using specific software for correction of misregistration.

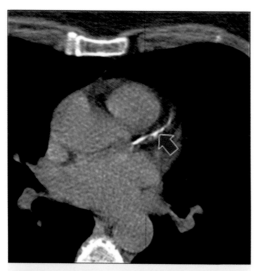

Fig. 5.13 A calcium score scan (prospectively triggered gated noncontrast CT scan) on this patient shows extensive LAD calcification (*red arrow*). Despite having a normal SPECT MPI scan, the patient was commenced on preventive therapy as her Agatston coronary calcium score was 180.

Pearls

- Close attention to quality assurance is required by viewing the fused emission and transmission images in all three projections (axial, sagittal, and coronal) to ensure accurate coregistration.
- A registration error of just 7 mm can result in a substantial reduction in quality of the attenuation-corrected images.[31]
- Superimposition of myocardial radiotracer activity on the lung, due to undercorrection of attenuation (as attenuation coefficients of air are applied to the myocardium), can produce artifacts simulating significant perfusion defects in the lateral wall.
- When misregistration is identified, the transmission and emission images must be coregistered, a new attenuation map (mu map) produced, and the perfusion images reconstructed by applying this new mu map.

Pitfalls

- There could be misinterpretation of an apparent perfusion defect as a result of misregistration artifact.
- Care must be taken when reading the low-dose (10–15 mA) free-breathing CT for incidental findings.

- Moving the emission and transmission images to coregister them using fusion software does not change the myocardial perfusion images.
- If misregistration is due to physical patient motion during the emission or the transmission images, coregistration and new reconstructions may not help. The images have to be repeated.

5.8.3 Scanner Failure

Scanner failure is an uncommon source of error. Regular scanner maintenance and quality control are critical.[9] Detector head misalignment, with dual-detector systems, is a frequent source of error, which can appear as patient motion on the rotating projection images. Another error includes imaging a ^{99m}Tc MPI study using a ^{201}Tl photopeak (dual-isotope imaging or during periods of ^{99m}Tc shortage). When identified, the scan should be repeated with the correct photopeak. A cause of scanner malfunction with the novel dedicated SPECT scanner (D-SPECT) is failure of electronics of one of the nine collimators. This is identified by a review of the sinogram when a slab of data (pertaining to the malfunctioning detector) is absent (► Fig. 5.14). The missing data may result in a false perfusion defect. When this is identified, the acquisition should be repeated.

Pearls

- Quality control should always include a review of the raw data.

Pitfalls

- There could be misinterpretation of a defect.

5.9 Balanced Ischemia

Once all sources of artifact have been evaluated and excluded, the MPI may be interpreted and reported. Despite excellent quality imaging, balanced ischemia (globally reduced tracer uptake without any relative difference between different coronary territories) may result in a negative SPECT MPI study (► Fig. 5.15 and ► Fig. 5.16). Indeed, in patients with ≥ 50% left main CAD, perfusion defects (visual or quantitative) were only present in only 56 to 59% of the patients, leading to significant underestimation of ischemia.[32] The addition of gated SPECT, as well as the identification of increased radiotracer activity in the lung, and particularly transient ischemic dilation (TID)

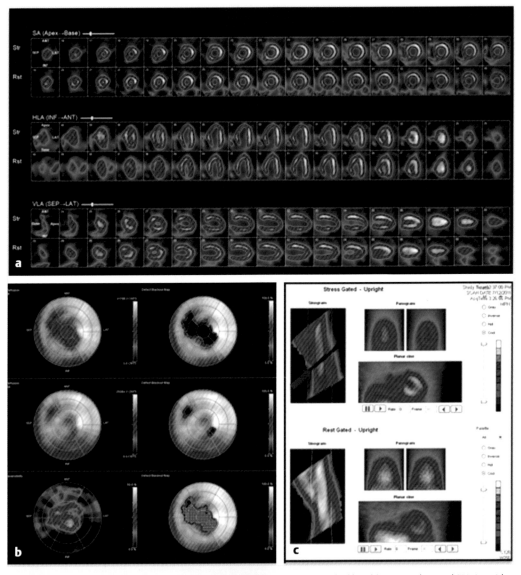

Fig. 5.14 Detector failure. **(a,b)** The perfusion images demonstrate transiently dilated LV size and normal RV size with normal RV radiotracer uptake. There is an apparent reversible defect in the mid and apical anterior and anteroseptal walls and apex. **(c)** However, review of the raw data shows a slab of missing information (*red arrow*) on the stress sinogram. This appearance is a classic example of malfunction of the electronics of a novel CZT scanner. As it is possible that this defect is an artifact caused by detector failure, the scan was repeated and was normal.

of the LV, increased the detection rate of left main disease.[32] In order to identify balanced ischemia, it is critical to look for high-risk features on stress testing and on SPECT MPI.

Exercise is the preferred stress modality in patients who are able to achieve at least 85% of age-adjusted maximal predicted heart rate and five metabolic equivalents (METS) of workload. Exercise stress testing is a powerful risk stratification tool and is useful in assessing symptoms in patients with known or suspected CAD. High-risk markers on exercise testing include low exercise capacity, angina at low workloads, ST-segment depression (≥1 mm of horizontal or downsloping depression) occurring early in exercise and lasting long into recovery, or ≥3 mm ST segment depression, ST segment evaluation (>1 mm) in leads without diagnostic Q waves except for leads

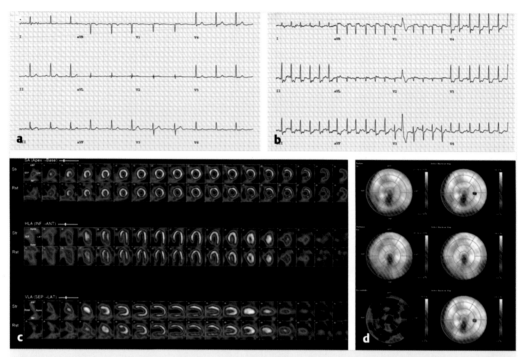

Fig. 5.15 Balanced ischemia. A 73-year-old man with hypertension, dyslipidemia, and diabetes was referred for a SPECT MPI to evaluate chest pain, dyspnea, and syncope. The patient exercised for 3:27 minutes (5.1 METS) on a standard Bruce protocol, reaching a maximal heart rate of 148 bpm (101% of APMHR). He did not have any symptoms, and the blood pressure response was normal. Exercise was terminated due to ischemic ECG changes. (a) While the ECG at rest was normal, (b) the peak exercise ECG was strongly positive, with 3 mm of horizontal ST depression in leads II, III, aVF, and V4–V6. CZT gated SPECT imaging was performed with ^{99m}Tc-sestamibi at rest (5.8 mCi) and poststress (17 mCi), respectively. Left and right ventricular sizes are normal, there is no TID, and RV radiotracer uptake is normal (a). The gated SPECT images show normal function with an LVEF of 67% and an LVEDVI of 54.8 mL/m^2 (**Video 11**). (c,d) The rest and stress perfusion images are also normal. However, reduced exercise capacity and ischemic ECG changes at low workload are high-risk features.

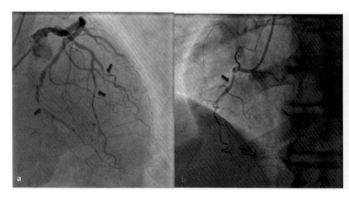

Fig. 5.16 Despite normal MPI, the patient was referred for left heart catheterization that demonstrated severe stenoses in the mid-LAD artery and the first diagonal and left circumflex arteries *(red arrows)* . (a) RAO caudal projection. (b) Mid-RCA (LAO cranial).

V1 and a VR, sustained ventricular tachycardia, development of left bundle branch block or intraventricular conduction delay that cannot be distinguished from ventricular tachycardia and a drop in systolic blood pressure of greater than 10 mm Hg from baseline, despite an increase in workload, when accompanied by other evidence of ischemia.[33] Most of these high-risk markers are not evident or do not occur during vasodilator stress, making exercise stress particularly important in individuals with known or suspected three-vessel obstructive CAD.

High-risk imaging features include increased radiotracer uptake in the lungs (lung uptake), a reduction in LV function at stress compared to that at rest (postischemic stunning), transiently increased right ventricular tracer uptake, and TID of the LV.[34,35,36,37,38,39] Of note, TID without perfusion defects has a poor predictive accuracy as a marker of high-risk CAD.[40,41]

5.9.1 Pearls

- Look for high-risk markers on the exercise treadmill test. This is particularly important when the SPECT study is normal or only mildly abnormal.
- Look for high-risk markers on SPECT imaging.
- If balanced ischemia is suspected based on high-risk exercise features, an invasive coronary angiogram is frequently recommended. However, if the high-risk exercise features are not definitive, or a pharmacological (instead of exercise) stress was performed, or the patient prefers a noninvasive evaluation, then a CT coronary angiogram, a vasodilator PET with flow quantitation, or, in some cases, dobutamine or exercise echocardiogram may be considered for further evaluation. With the novel CZT SPECT scanners, dynamic imaging with quantitation of radiotracer retention is feasible[42] and may, in future, enable better detection of underlying multivessel CAD.
- Evaluate the coronary calcium score when SPECT/CT is performed.[43] This can help identify underlying calcified atherosclerosis independent of perfusion imaging. The CT scan can be used to detect significant coronary calcifications and make a qualitative assessment of coronary calcification (despite being low dose, free breathing, and 5-mm slice thickness).[43,44]
- Most hybrid SPECT/CT scanners have calcium-scoring capabilities, and even in those that do not, coronary artery calcium can also be identified on the low-dose CT scan. A dedicated gated, high-dose, noncontrast coronary CT for calcium score can be performed with the MPI study when feasible; it can be helpful for patient management, especially when the MPI is normal (▶ Fig. 5.13), and is also effective for further risk stratification in patients who are asymptomatic.[45] A normal MPI portends an excellent short-term prognosis,[46] while a high calcium score portends a worse long-term prognosis.[47] In

fact, substantial coronary artery calcium is associated with an increase of almost 10 times in adverse coronary events after multivariable adjustment and may be associated with superior CAD risk factor modification.[48] Indeed, in one study, 88% of the ischemic scans were observed in patients with calcium score ≥ 100, and about half of the patients with normal MPI have underlying coronary artery calcification.[49] Currently, a calcium score of more than 400, or 100-400 in diabetics, is considered an appropriate referral for stress and rest MPI.[50]

5.9.2 Pitfalls

- TID alone in the absence of myocardial perfusion defects is unreliable as a high-risk marker.
- TID may be seen in patients with left ventricular hypertrophy. However, patients with left ventricular hypertrophy frequently have high-risk coronary disease as well.

5.10 Conclusion

SPECT MPI is a highly accurate imaging modality for evaluating patients with known or suspected CAD. However, a sound knowledge of the pitfalls of SPECT is integral to maintaining and improving diagnostic accuracy. The pearls described in this chapter will provide the reader with insights and useful techniques to troubleshoot potential artifacts.

Menu of Accompanying Videos

Video 1: Left circumflex ischemia
Video 2a: Breast attenuation: projection rotating images
Video 2b: Breast attenuation: function
Video 3a: High BMI SPECT
Video 3b: High BMI PET
Video 4: Left anterior descending infarction
Video 5: Hibernating myocardium
Video 6: Right coronary artery infarction
Video 7a: Inferior wall defect
Video 7b: Inferior wall defect on A-SPECT
Video 8: Motion
Video 9: Complex motion
Video 10: Misregistration artifact
Video 11: Balanced ischemia

References

[1] Cerqueira MD, Allman KC, Ficaro EP, et al. Recommendations for reducing radiation exposure in myocardial perfusion imaging. J Nucl Cardiol. 2010;17(4):709–718

[2] Dilsizian V, Taillefer R. Journey in evolution of nuclear cardiology: will there be another quantum leap with the F-18-labeled myocardial perfusion tracers? JACC Cardiovasc Imaging. 2012;5(12):1269–1284

[3] Garcia EV, Faber TL, Esteves FP. Cardiac dedicated ultrafast SPECT cameras: new designs and clinical implications. J Nucl Med. 2011;52(2):210–217

[4] Madsen MT. Recent advances in SPECT imaging. J Nucl Med. 2007;48(4):661–673

[5] Slomka PJ, Berman DS, Germano G. New cardiac cameras: single-photon emission CT and PET. Semin Nucl Med. 2014; 44(4):232–251

[6] DePuey EG. Advances in SPECT camera software and hardware: currently available and new on the horizon. J Nucl Cardiol. 2012;19(3):551–581, quiz 585

[7] Gould KL, Lipscomb K, Hamilton GW. Physiologic basis for assessing critical coronary stenosis. Instantaneous flow response and regional distribution during coronary hyperemia as measures of coronary flow reserve. Am J Cardiol. 1974;33 (1):87–94

[8] Henzlova MJ, Cerqueira MD, Hansen CL, Taillefer R, Yao S. ASNC Imaging Guidelines for Nuclear Cardiology Procedures: stress protocols and tracers. 2009. http://www.asnc.org/files/Stress%20Protocols%20and%20Tracers%202009.pdf

[9] Holly TA, Abbott BG, Al-Mallah M, et al. ASNC Imaging Guidelines for Nuclear Cardiology Procedures: single photon-emission computed tomography. 2010. http://www.asnc.org/files/SPECT%202010.pdf

[10] Mahmarian JJ. Stress only myocardial perfusion imaging: is it time for a change? J Nucl Cardiol. 2010;17(4):529–535

[11] Chang SM, Nabi F, Xu J, Raza U, Mahmarian JJ. Normal stress-only versus standard stress/rest myocardial perfusion imaging: similar patient mortality with reduced radiation exposure. J Am Coll Cardiol. 2010;55(3):221–230

[12] Shaw LJ, Hage FG, Berman DS, Hachamovitch R, Iskandrian A. Prognosis in the era of comparative effectiveness research: where is nuclear cardiology now and where should it be? J Nucl Cardiol. 2012;19(5):1026–1043

[13] DePuey EG, Garcia EV. Optimal specificity of thallium-201 SPECT through recognition of imaging artifacts. J Nucl Med. 1989;30(4):441–449

[14] DePuey EG, Rozanski A. Using gated technetium-99m-sestamibi SPECT to characterize fixed myocardial defects as infarct or artifact. J Nucl Med. 1995; 36(6):952–955

[15] Links JM, DePuey EG, Taillefer R, Becker LC. Attenuation correction and gating synergistically improve the diagnostic accuracy of myocardial perfusion SPECT. J Nucl Cardiol. 2002; 9(2):183–187

[16] Taillefer R, DePuey EG, Udelson JE, Beller GA, Latour Y, Reeves F. Comparative diagnostic accuracy of Tl-201 and Tc-99 m sestamibi SPECT imaging (perfusion and ECG-gated SPECT) in detecting coronary artery disease in women. J Am Coll Cardiol. 1997;29(1):69–77

[17] Hendel RC, Berman DS, Cullom SJ, et al. Multicenter clinical trial to evaluate the efficacy of correction for photon attenuation and scatter in SPECT myocardial perfusion imaging. Circulation. 1999;99(21):2742–2749

[18] Hendel RC, Corbett JR, Cullom SJ, DePuey EG, Garcia EV, Bateman TM. The value and practice of attenuation correction for myocardial perfusion SPECT imaging: a joint position statement from the American Society of Nuclear Cardiology and the Society of Nuclear Medicine. J Nucl Cardiol. 2002;9 (1):135–143

[19] Wagner A, Mahrholdt H, Holly TA, et al. Contrast-enhanced MRI and routine single photon emission computed tomography (SPECT) perfusion imaging for detection of subendocardial myocardial infarcts: an imaging study. Lancet. 2003;361 (9355):374–379

[20] Partington SL, Kwong RY, Dorbala S. Multimodality imaging in the assessment of myocardial viability. Heart Fail Rev. 2011;16(4):381–395

[21] Udelson JE, Coleman PS, Metherall J, et al. Predicting recovery of severe regional ventricular dysfunction. Comparison of resting scintigraphy with 201Tl and 99mTc-sestamibi. Circulation. 1994;89(6):2552–2561

[22] Klocke FJ, Baird MG, Lorell BH, et al. American College of Cardiology, American Heart Association Task Force on Practice Guidelines, American Society for Nuclear Cardiology. ACC/AHA/ASNC guidelines for the clinical use of cardiac radionuclide imaging—executive summary: a report of the American College of Cardiology/American Heart Association Task Force on Practice Guidelines (ACC/AHA/ASNC Committee to Revise the 1995 Guidelines for the Clinical Use of Cardiac Radionuclide Imaging). Circulation. 2003;108(11):1404–1418

[23] Burrell S, MacDonald A. Artifacts and pitfalls in myocardial perfusion imaging. J Nucl Med Technol. 2006;34(4):193–211, quiz 212–214

[24] Garcia EV, Cooke CD, Van Train KF, et al. Technical aspects of myocardial SPECT imaging with technetium-99 m sestamibi. Am J Cardiol. 1990;66(13):23E–31E

[25] van Dongen AJ, van Rijk PP. Minimizing liver, bowel, and gastric activity in myocardial perfusion SPECT. J Nucl Med. 2000; 41(8):1315–1317

[26] Hurwitz GA, Clark EM, Slomka PJ, Siddiq SK. Investigation of measures to reduce interfering abdominal activity on rest myocardial images with Tc-99 m sestamibi. Clin Nucl Med. 1993;18(9):735–741

[27] Vitola JV, Brambatti JC, Caligaris F, et al. Exercise supplementation to dipyridamole prevents hypotension, improves electrocardiogram sensitivity, and increases heart-to-liver activity ratio on Tc-99 m sestamibi imaging. J Nucl Cardiol. 2001;8(6):652–659

[28] Wheat JM, Currie GM. Incidence and characterization of patient motion in myocardial perfusion SPECT: part 1. J Nucl Med Technol. 2004;32(2):60–65

[29] Leslie WD, Dupont JO, McDonald D, Peterdy AE. Comparison of motion correction algorithms for cardiac SPECT. J Nucl Med. 1997;38(5):785–790

[30] Dvorak RA, Brown RK, Corbett JR. Interpretation of SPECT/CT myocardial perfusion images: common artifacts and quality control techniques. Radiographics. 2011;31(7):2041–2057

[31] Kennedy JA, Israel O, Frenkel A. Directions and magnitudes of misregistration of CT attenuation-corrected myocardial perfusion studies: incidence, impact on image quality, and guidance for reregistration. J Nucl Med. 2009;50(9):1471–1478

[32] Berman DS, Kang X, Slomka PJ, et al. Underestimation of extent of ischemia by gated SPECT myocardial perfusion imaging in patients with left main coronary artery disease. J Nucl Cardiol. 2007;14(4):521–528

[33] Gibbons RJ, Balady GJ, Bricker JT, et al. American College of Cardiology/American Heart Association Task Force on Practice Guidelines (Committee to Update the 1997 Exercise Testing Guidelines). ACC/AHA 2002 guideline update for exercise testing: summary article: a report of the American College of Cardiology/American Heart Association Task Force on

Practice Guidelines (Committee to Update the 1997 Exercise Testing Guidelines). Circulation. 2002;106(14):1883–1892

[34] Leslie WD, Tully SA, Yogendran MS, Ward LM, Nour KA, Metge CJ. Prognostic value of lung sestamibi uptake in myocardial perfusion imaging of patients with known or suspected coronary artery disease. J Am Coll Cardiol. 2005;45 (10):1676–1682

[35] Borges-Neto S, Javaid A, Shaw LK, et al. Poststress measurements of left ventricular function with gated perfusion SPECT: comparison with resting measurements by using a same-day perfusion-function protocol. Radiology. 2000;215 (2):529–533

[36] Emmett L, Iwanochko RM, Freeman MR, Barolet A, Lee DS, Husain M. Reversible regional wall motion abnormalities on exercise technetium-99m-gated cardiac single photon emission computed tomography predict high-grade angiographic stenoses. J Am Coll Cardiol. 2002;39(6):991–998

[37] Mannting F, Zabrodina YV, Dass C. Significance of increased right ventricular uptake on 99mTc-sestamibi SPECT in patients with coronary artery disease. J Nucl Med. 1999;40 (6):889–894

[38] McClellan JR, Travin MI, Herman SD, et al. Prognostic importance of scintigraphic left ventricular cavity dilation during intravenous dipyridamole technetium-99 m sestamibi myocardial tomographic imaging in predicting coronary events. Am J Cardiol. 1997;79(5):600–605

[39] McLaughlin MG, Danias PG. Transient ischemic dilation: a powerful diagnostic and prognostic finding of stress myocardial perfusion imaging. J Nucl Cardiol. 2002;9(6):663–667

[40] Mandour Ali MA, Bourque JM, Allam AH, Beller GA, Watson DD. The prevalence and predictive accuracy of quantitatively defined transient ischemic dilation of the left ventricle on otherwise normal SPECT myocardial perfusion imaging studies. J Nucl Cardiol. 2011;18(6):1036–1043

[41] Halligan WT, Morris PB, Schoepf UJ, et al. Transient ischemic dilation of the left ventricle on SPECT: correlation with findings at coronary CT angiography. J Nucl Med. 2014;55 (6):917–922

[42] Ben-Haim S, Murthy VL, Breault C, et al. Quantification of myocardial perfusion reserve using dynamic SPECT imaging in humans: a feasibility study. J Nucl Med. 2013;54(6):873–879

[43] Dorbala S, Di Carli MF, Delbeke D, et al. SNMMI/ASNC/SCCT guideline for cardiac SPECT/CT and PET/CT 1.0. J Nucl Med. 2013;54(8):1485–1507

[44] Einstein AJ, Johnson LL, Bokhari S, et al. Agreement of visual estimation of coronary artery calcium from low-dose CT attenuation correction scans in hybrid PET/CT and SPECT/CT

with standard Agatston score. J Am Coll Cardiol. 2010;56 (23):1914–1921

[45] Budoff MJ, Achenbach S, Blumenthal RS, et al. American Heart Association Committee on Cardiovascular Imaging and Intervention, American Heart Association Council on Cardiovascular Radiology and Intervention, American Heart Association Committee on Cardiac Imaging, Council on Clinical Cardiology. Assessment of coronary artery disease by cardiac computed tomography: a scientific statement from the American Heart Association Committee on Cardiovascular Imaging and Intervention, Council on Cardiovascular Radiology and Intervention, and Committee on Cardiac Imaging, Council on Clinical Cardiology. Circulation. 2006;114 (16):1761–1791

[46] Rozanski A, Gransar H, Wong ND, et al. Clinical outcomes after both coronary calcium scanning and exercise myocardial perfusion scintigraphy. J Am Coll Cardiol. 2007;49 (12):1352–1361

[47] Chang SM, Nabi F, Xu J, et al. The coronary artery calcium score and stress myocardial perfusion imaging provide independent and complementary prediction of cardiac risk. J Am Coll Cardiol. 2009;54(20):1872–1882

[48] Rozanski A, Gransar H, Shaw LJ, et al. Impact of coronary artery calcium scanning on coronary risk factors and downstream testing the EISNER (Early Identification of Subclinical Atherosclerosis by Noninvasive Imaging Research) prospective randomized trial. J Am Coll Cardiol. 2011;57(15):1622–1632

[49] Berman DS, Wong ND, Gransar H, et al. Relationship between stress-induced myocardial ischemia and atherosclerosis measured by coronary calcium tomography. J Am Coll Cardiol. 2004;44(4):923–930

[50] Hendel RC, Berman DS, Di Carli MF, et al. American College of Cardiology Foundation Appropriate Use Criteria Task Force, American Society of Nuclear Cardiology, American College of Radiology, American Heart Association, American Society of Echocardiology, Society of Cardiovascular Computed Tomography, Society for Cardiovascular Magnetic Resonance, Society of Nuclear Medicine. ACCF/ASNC/ACR/AHA/ASE/SCCT/ SCMR/SNM 2009 Appropriate Use Criteria for Cardiac Radionuclide Imaging: A Report of the American College of Cardiology Foundation Appropriate Use Criteria Task Force, the American Society of Nuclear Cardiology, the American College of Radiology, the American Heart Association, the American Society of Echocardiography, the Society of Cardiovascular Computed Tomography, the Society for Cardiovascular Magnetic Resonance, and the Society of Nuclear Medicine. J Am Coll Cardiol. 2009;53(23):2201–2229

6 SPECT and SPECT/CT for the Respiratory System

Paul J. Roach and Geoffrey P. Schembri

6.1 Introduction

Since its first description by Wagner et al in 1964,[1] the planar lung scan has been one of the most commonly performed studies in nuclear medicine. While it can be used to investigate various respiratory disorders, its primary role is in the diagnosis and evaluation of pulmonary embolism (PE). However, planar ventilation–perfusion (V/Q) scanning, a two-dimensional technique, has well-recognized limitations, particularly related to overlap of anatomical segments. Embolic defects may not be detected if there is "shine-through" occurring from underlying lung segments with normal perfusion, thus resulting in an underestimation of the extent of perfusion loss.[2] Furthermore, the medial basal segment of the right lower lobe is often not visualized on planar scans. Assigning defects to specific lung segments on planar imaging is often difficult due to the variability in segment size and shape between patients.[3] Single-photon emission computed tomography (SPECT) overcomes this limitation through its ability to generate three-dimensional (3D) imaging data. V/Q SPECT is increasingly being used in many imaging centers and has been shown to have a higher sensitivity, specificity, and accuracy, as well as a lower indeterminate rate, than planar imaging.[4] Hybrid SPECT/computed tomography (CT) scanners can now perform combined V/Q SPECT with CT (generally using low-dose CT protocols) to further enhance diagnostic accuracy of V/Q SPECT. This chapter will summarize how V/Q SPECT and SPECT/CT are performed, outline strengths and weaknesses compared to planar lung scans and CT pulmonary angiography (CTPA), describe typical patterns, normal variants, and caveats relevant to image interpretation, and outline applications in areas other than the evaluation of PE.

6.2 Performing V/Q SPECT

As with planar imaging, the usual approach with SPECT is to perform a ventilation study followed by the perfusion study when technetium-99 m (^{99m}Tc)-based agents are used.

6.2.1 Ventilation

- For ventilation imaging, several alternatives exist.[5] These include the following:
  ○ Inert radioactive gases such as krypton-81 m (^{81m}Kr) and xenon-133 (^{133}Xe).
  ○ Radiolabeled aerosols, most commonly ^{99m}Tc-diethylenetriaminepentaacetic acid (^{99m}Tc-DTPA) but occasionally sulfur colloid or albumen.
  ○ Technegas (^{99m}Tc ultrafine carbon suspension) (Cyclopharm, Sydney, Australia).
- Each has its advantages and disadvantages (▶ Table 6.1); however, most centers performing SPECT would use either Technegas (preferable, especially if underlying airways disease[6]) or ^{99m}Tc-DTPA aerosol. ^{81m}Kr is also an ideal ventilation agent for SPECT; however, it is expensive, requires continuous administration, it is no longer available in the United States, and its use is limited to some European centers. Although still used in the United States for planar imaging, ^{133}Xe is unsuitable for SPECT due to its low-energy photons leading to poor resolution and high scatter.

6.2.2 Perfusion

- ^{99m}Tc-macroaggregated albumin (^{99m}Tc-MAA) is generally used to assess perfusion.[7]
- The dose of ^{99m}Tc-MAA used is dependent on the ventilation agent used.
- If a radioactive gas is used, the dose of perfusion agent is typically lower than if a technetium-based ventilation agent is used as the signal from the radioactive gas can be separated from that of the perfusion agent based on the energy level of the emitted photons.
- If a technetium-based agent is used for both ventilation and perfusion imaging, a greater dose of perfusion agent (resulting in a perfusion–ventilation dose ratio of at least 4:1) is required to "drown out" the underlying ventilation signal.[7]
- The administered activity of ^{99m}Tc-MAA is typically 2.5 to 6 mCi (100–250 MBq).[5,7]

Table 6.1 Comparison of different ventilation agents

	^{133}Xe	^{81m}Kr	^{99m}Tc-Aerosols (e.g., ^{99m}Tc-DTPA)	Technegas
Physical half-life	5.3 d	13 s	6 h	6 h
Gamma photon energy	80 keV (low)	193 keV (ideal)	140 keV (ideal)	140 keV (ideal)
Alveolar penetration	Excellent	Excellent	Good, unless COPD	Excellent
Image quality	Poor	Excellent (▶ Fig. 6.1)	Good, unless COPD (▶ Fig. 6.2)	Very good (▶ Fig. 6.3)
Continuous administration required during image acquisition	Yes, due to recirculation[7]	Yes	No, but alveolar absorption accelerated in inflammatory conditions and smokers	No
Availability	Limited (but still used in the United States)	Limited (mainly used in Europe)	Widespread	Widespread (but not FDA-approved in the United States)
Cost	Varies	High	Very low	Low
SPECT imaging capability	No	Yes	Yes	Yes

Abbreviations: COPD, chronic obstructive pulmonary disease; SPECT, single-photon emission computed tomography.

- For pregnant patients, dose reduction is usually implemented. This can be achieved by reducing the administered dose of both the ventilation and perfusion agents, usually by half.[8] This will necessitate a longer acquisition time to maintain images of good quality. Some centers advocate omitting the ventilation scan; however, the radiation savings from this approach are minimal, and diagnostic accuracy may be adversely impacted.[9] In centers performing SPECT/CT imaging, consideration can be given to omitting the CT scan to reduce breast radiation exposure.

6.2.3 Image Acquisition and Processing

- Multihead gamma cameras (either dual or triple head) are required for SPECT imaging.[5] Acquisition times become prohibitive for standard clinical practice if a single-head camera is used.
- A typical protocol that uses a multihead camera requires 15 to 25 minutes of total acquisition time for a V/Q data set.[5,10] This is faster than traditional six- or eight-view planar imaging.[10,11]
- If V/Q can be performed simultaneously (e.g., when ^{81m}Kr is used for ventilation), the acquisition time is halved.[12]

Table 6.2 Typical acquisition and processing parameters for V/Q SPECT (protocol from Royal North Shore Hospital, Sydney, Australia)

SPECT acquisition	Three-degree steps over 360 degrees
Acquisition time per projection	12 s (ventilation) 8 s (perfusion)
Collimator	Low energy, high resolution
Matrix size	128 × 128 (64 × 64 can also be used)
Reconstruction	OSEM (eight iterations, four subsets)
Postreconstruction filter	3D Butterworth, cutoff 0.8 cycles/cm, order 9

Abbreviations: OSEM, ordered subset expectation maximization; SPECT, single-photon emission computed tomography.

- Representative acquisition and processing parameters are shown in ▶ Table 6.2. Note that if ^{81m}Kr is used for ventilation, a medium energy collimator is typically used.
- SPECT/CT imaging is acquired on a hybrid SPECT/CT scanner.

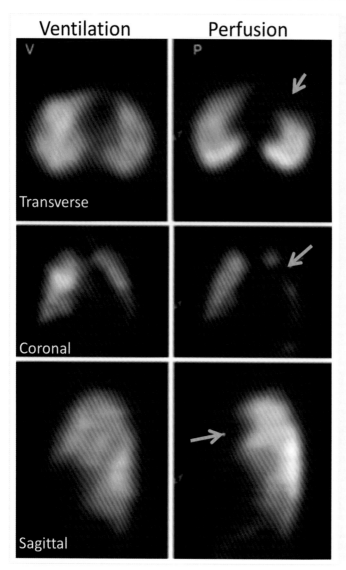

Ventilation   **Perfusion**

Transverse

Coronal

Sagittal

Fig. 6.1 [81mKr] ventilation SPECT (left) and [99mTc]-MAA perfusion SPECT images in patient with left upper lobe PE (*arrow*). [81mKr] produces SPECT ventilation images of good quality.

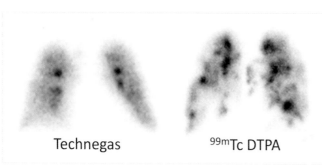

Technegas   [99mTc] DTPA

Fig. 6.2 COPD. Ventilation images (anterior planar) acquired in the same patient using Technegas (left) and [99mTc]-DTPA aerosol (right) show better peripheral penetration, a more uniform pattern, and less central clumping with Technegas. In patients with COPD, central clumping and poor peripheral penetration are often seen with [99mTc]-DTPA aerosol.

- While most hybrid scanners can perform diagnostic quality CT, they can also be operated solely for attenuation correction and anatomical localization using "low-dose" parameters.[13]

- For lung scanning, the CT acquisition is typically acquired immediately after the perfusion SPECT. Intravenous contrast is not required, and a reduced beam current of the order of 20 to 80 mA will suffice.[4] This results in an absorbed dose of the order of 1 to 2 mSv.[7,9,12,14] This compares favorably with the 2 to 2.5 mSv from the V/Q scan itself and is well below the levels received from a diagnostic CTPA.[9,15,16]
- Due to the duration of acquisition time for SPECT imaging, breath holding is not feasible, and these are therefore performed during free breathing. To better match the CT images to SPECT acquisitions, it has been suggested that they be performed using a mid inspiratory breath hold, or during shallow breathing, rather than at maximal inspiration.[17]
- The CT acquisition time is rapid (< 1 minute), and combined with the setup time, the procedure adds only 1 to 2 minutes to a V/Q SPECT study.

6.2.4 Image Display and Reviewing

- Image review should occur following coregistration of the V/Q SPECT data sets (as well as the CT data sets in the case of SPECT/CT).
- Images are best viewed simultaneously in transverse, coronal, and sagittal planes on a workstation (▶ Fig. 6.3). This allows the reporter to interactively examine and triangulate the linked V/Q SPECT studies as well as the CT in each of the three orthogonal imaging planes and to adjust the relative image intensities, especially of fused images (▶ Fig. 6.4).
- Review of images on a workstation also facilitates the viewing of CT data in different windows so that lungs, soft tissue, and bones can all be reviewed, as appropriate.

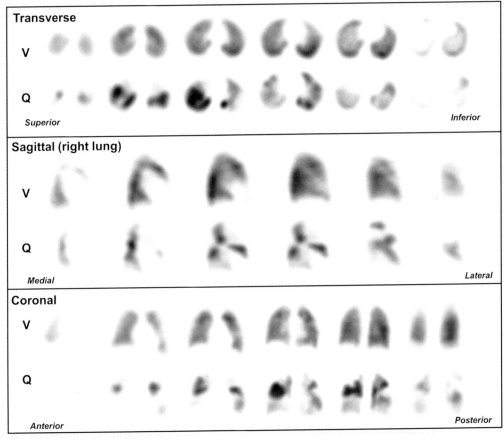

Fig. 6.3 Representative ventilation (V) and perfusion (Q) SPECT slices in a patient with multiple mismatched defects secondary to PE displayed in each of the three orthogonal planes.

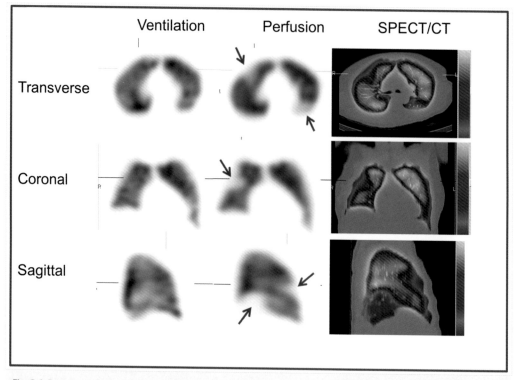

Fig. 6.4 Representative ventilation, perfusion, and fused SPECT/CT images in a patient with multiple PEs (*arrows*). Workstation review should include triangulation of any defects to determine if there is V/Q mismatch and if there is any underlying structure or abnormality on the CT.

- Segmental lung anatomy charts may be of help for reporting specialists, particularly for reporters who are inexperienced (▶ Fig. 6.5).[8]
- V/Q SPECT studies are usually reported using the European Association of Nuclear Medicine (EANM) reporting guidelines. These guidelines recommend that studies be reported as positive for PE if there is V/Q mismatch of at least one segment or two subsegments that conform to pulmonary vascular anatomy (▶ Table 6.3).[7] Probabilistic reporting (as used for planar scanning) is not recommended, and has not been validated, for V/Q SPECT.[11,18] While the EANM reporting guidelines do not specifically address hybrid imaging, these guidelines are also generally used to report V/Q SPECT/CT studies. Indeed, the addition of the CT component is likely to help classify the V/Q SPECT pattern more appropriately. The CT will provide patient-specific anatomical information, including the lung and segment borders, fissures, and the location of major vessels, as well as the presence of parenchymal disease (▶ Fig. 6.6).

- Further demonstration of V/Q abnormalities can be made by creating a quotient or ratio image. In these images, the ratio of counts is usually derived by the formula $\frac{V_1}{(Q - V_2)}$, where V_1 are counts at time of ventilation acquisition and V_2 decay corrected counts at time of perfusion acquisition. There are novel ways of displaying $V:Q$ quotient data to assist image reporting. Palmer et al have described a technique where these images can be presented as either 3D surface-shaded images or as tomographic sections in each of the orthogonal planes.[19] These "quotient images" can be helpful in facilitating image reporting and are a useful way of demonstrating the location and extent of mismatched defects (▶ Fig. 6.7).
- Planar-like images can be generated from SPECT data using several approaches. While Bailey et al have described a technique using reprojection,[20] many of the commercial vendors offer a simpler approach using an "angular summing" technique.[11] With this approach, images are generated by summing several consecutive projections from the SPECT

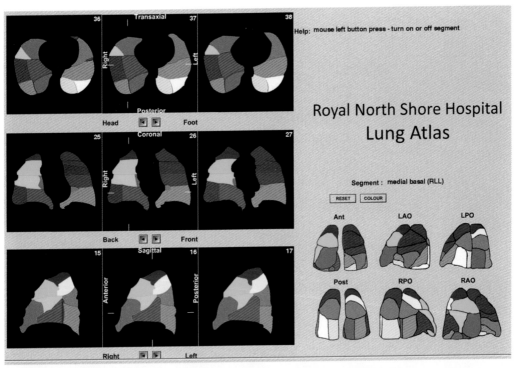

Fig. 6.5 Example of a computer-based lung segmental atlas. Using this program, individual lung segments are color coded on both planar and SPECT slices. Such an atlas is of particular value during the transition from planar to SPECT imaging or for inexperienced readers.

Table 6.3 EANM reporting guidelines for V/Q SPECT

No PE	• Normal perfusion pattern conforming to the anatomical boundaries of the lungs • Matched or reversed mismatch V/Q defects of any size, shape, or number in the absence of mismatch • Mismatch that does not have a lobar, segmental, or subsegmental pattern
Nondiagnostic	Multiple V/Q abnormalities not typical of specific diseases
PE positive	V/Q mismatch of at least one segment or two subsegments that conforms to the pulmonary vascular anatomy

Abbreviations: EANM, European Association of Nuclear Medicine; PE, pulmonary embolism; V/Q, ventilation–perfusion.
Source: Data from Bajc et al.[7]

acquisition. This can blur small defects as data are acquired over an arc; however, the images produced approximate true planar images (▶ Fig. 6.8).[21] These "pseudoplanar" images give a familiar and rapid view of the lungs for quick evaluation and may be of particular value during the transition phase from planar imaging to SPECT imaging.[8] As the images are generated from the SPECT data, no additional image acquisition time is required.

6.3 Clinical Indications

The main clinical roles of V/Q SPECT (and SPECT/CT) include the following:
• Diagnosis of patients with suspected PE.
• Monitoring of patients diagnosed with PE:
  ○ To assess for the development of interval PE.
  ○ To monitor defect reperfusion.
• To quantify regional lung V/Q, for example, in patients undergoing (or being considered for) lung cancer reduction surgery or to assist in radiotherapy planning.

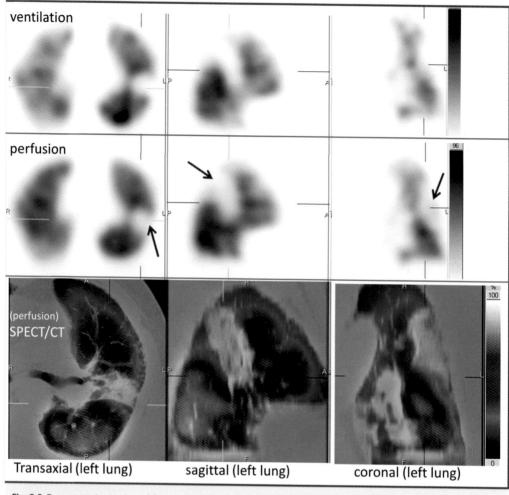

Fig. 6.6 Representative V, Q, and fused SPECT/CT images in an elderly male with dyspnea. A large matched defect is evident on SPECT in the left upper and midzone (*arrow*). SPECT/CT shows this to correspond with extensive consolidation.

6.4 Accuracy

- Based on pooled literature, V/Q SPECT has sensitivities ranging from 80 to 100% and specificities ranging from 93 to 100%.[4,7,18] Bajc et al, citing experience from more than 3,000 patients, quote negative predictive values for V/Q SPECT of 97 to 99%, sensitivities of 96 to 99%, and specificities of 91 to 98% for PE diagnosis.[7]
- V/Q SPECT imaging has also been consistently shown to have an indeterminate rate of less than 5%, typically in the 1 to 3% range.[5,7,10,22,23]

6.5 Comparison with Planar Imaging

Studies comparing planar and SPECT lung scanning have consistently demonstrated the superiority of SPECT over planar imaging.

- Animal studies done using dogs[24] and pigs[25] as well as studies using Monte Carlo simulation[26] have all shown a higher sensitivity for the detection of PE with SPECT compared with planar imaging.
- In humans, Bajc et al found SPECT to be more sensitive than planar imaging (100 vs. 85%) in

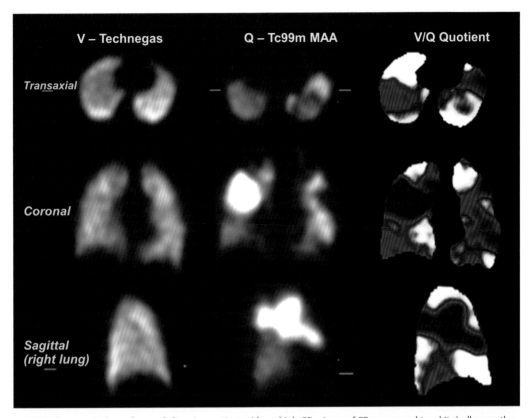

V – Technegas	Q – Tc99m MAA	V/Q Quotient
Transaxial		
Coronal		
Sagittal (right lung)		

Fig. 6.7 Representative orthogonal slices in a patient with multiple PEs. Areas of PE correspond to white/yellow on the V:Q quotient images, indicating areas with a high V:Q ratio value (normal V but reduced Q).

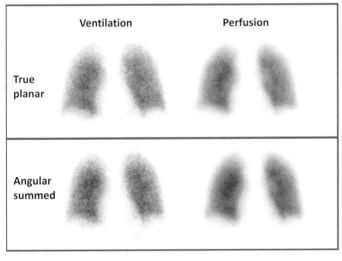

	Ventilation	Perfusion
True planar		
Angular summed		

Fig. 6.8 Anterior planar V and Q images in a patient without PE (top row). "Pseudoplanar" images have been generated from the SPECT data acquired in the same patient (bottom row). Note that they appear nearly identical to the true planar images. Planar-like images can be derived from the SPECT data using several approaches and can be of use to reporters and referrers by giving a general overview of V and Q, particularly for those familiar with planar imaging.

the detection of PE.[22] They showed that SPECT had less interobserver variation and better delineation of mismatched defects compared with planar imaging.

• Collart et al demonstrated that SPECT was also more specific than planar imaging (96 vs. 78%) and had better reproducibility, both intraobserver (94 vs. 91%) and interobserver (88 vs. 79%).[27]

- In a study of 83 patients, Reinartz et al demonstrated that, compared with planar imaging, SPECT had a higher sensitivity (97 vs. 76%), specificity (91 vs. 85%), and accuracy (94 vs. 81%).[11] In this series, SPECT increased the detection of segmental defects by 13% and subsegmental defects by more than 80%.
- Leblanc et al demonstrated that SPECT has a very high negative predictive value (98.5%) for PE.[10] Le Roux et al have shown that a negative V/Q SPECT based on EANM reporting criteria carries a 3-month thromboembolic event rate of less than 0.5%.[28]
- Multiple studies have demonstrated nondiagnostic rates of less than 5% for V/Q SPECT.[10,22,23] This is much lower than that reported for planar imaging. In the landmark PIOPED study (which used ^{133}Xe as the ventilation agent), the indeterminate rate was 39%.[29]

In summary, published literature has consistently demonstrated that SPECT has a greater sensitivity and specificity, improved reproducibility, and a lower indeterminate rate than planar lung scintigraphy, and it has a high negative predictive value.

6.6 Comparison with CTPA

Multidetector CTPA has evolved to the point where it is frequently used as the primary imaging investigation in patients with potential PE. This is certainly the case in the United States, where it has supplanted the V/Q scan as the initial imaging test for the assessment of PE in many institutions.[30]

6.6.1 Advantages of CTPA over V/Q SPECT

- Better availability in many centers (especially after hours).[15,31]
- Much faster acquisition times.[30,31]
- Relatively high interobserver agreement.[30]
- The ability to diagnose pathologies other than PE that could be accounting for the patient's symptoms, such as pneumonia and aortic dissection.[15,30,31]
- Referrer preference for binary reporting.[30]

6.6.2 Disadvantages of CTPA Compared with V/Q SPECT

Lower Sensitivity

Several studies have shown that CTPA is less sensitive than V/Q SPECT.

- In the large PIOPED II study, the sensitivity of CTPA was 83% (78% when technically suboptimal studies were included).[32] Accuracy was particularly suboptimal if there was discordance between scan results and clinical likelihood (as was the case with planar V/Q scanning in the original PIOPED study[29]).
- In a study of 81 patients, Gutte et al report a sensitivity of 68% for CTPA (16 slice).[12] In the same series, SPECT had a sensitivity of 97%.

Technical Artifacts

- Artifacts can adversely impact image quality of CTPA.
- These artifacts are primarily related to
  - poor contrast opacification of the pulmonary arteries.
  - motion artifacts.
  - image noise related to the body habitus of some patients.[33]
- Indeterminate rates due to technical factors have been estimated at 5 to 11%.[34]
- SPECT is rarely impacted by technical factors.[9]

Contrast Complications

- In the PIOPED II study, 22% of patients were excluded due to contrast allergy and impaired renal function.[32] It has been reported that CTPA is complicated by some type of immediate contrast reaction in 3%[35] and contrast-induced nephropathy in 1 to 3% of patients.[36] Adverse reactions to the radiopharmaceuticals used in V/Q SPECT (or V/Q SPECT/CT) are practically nonexistent.[9]

Higher Radiation Dose

- The radiation dose to the breast from CTPA has been estimated at 10 to 70 mGy, a particular concern in younger women.[16,37] By comparison, the breast radiation dose from the V/Q scan is on the order of 0.3 to 1 mGy.[38]

- CTPA has overall radiation effective doses on the order of 8 to 20 mSv, compared with approximately 2.5 mSv with V/Q SPECT.[9] Lower doses are possible with modern CT systems using dose modulation software and iterative reconstruction, but in standard clinical practice, the effective dose continues to be significantly higher for CTPA than for V/Q SPECT.[39]

Overdiagnosis

- There is increasing concern related to the detection of incidental and/or unrelated findings.[40] While CTPA may diagnose alternate pathologies in many patients (up to 33% in one series), these may not be the cause of patient symptoms.[41]
- Investigation of these incidental findings can be expensive and results in additional radiation/contrast exposure and performance of invasive procedures for uncertain return.[42]
- One study showed that only 3.2% of CTPAs in patients with low or intermediate pretest probability had a relevant alternate diagnosis that was not evident on the chest radiograph.[43]

Limitations in Pregnancy

- The accuracy of CTPA is lower in pregnant patients. As many as one-third of CTPA procedures, even with 64-slice CT scanners, are deemed to be indeterminate.[44,45] This is thought to be attributable to increased pressure in the inferior vena cava during pregnancy.[45] SPECT is preferable in pregnant patients due to its high accuracy, comparable fetal radiation dose, and much lower breast radiation dose than CTPA, which, despite dose reduction techniques on modern scanners, has recently been shown to still exceed 10 mSv.[39]

6.6.3 Accuracy of CTPA versus V/Q SPECT

Overall, relatively few studies have directly compared SPECT V/Q and CTPA.

- Reinartz et al showed that SPECT was more sensitive (97 vs. 86%) but less specific (91 vs. 98%) than CTPA (4 slice).[11]
- In a study of 100 patients using 16-slice CTPA, Miles et al also found the accuracy of each to be comparable. They noted that SPECT had fewer contraindications, a lower patient radiation dose, and fewer nondiagnostic findings.[46]

- In a study of 81 patients, Gutte et al found that V/Q SPECT had a higher sensitivity (97% compared with 68%) but a lower specificity (88% compared with 100%) than CTPA (16 slice).[12]
- These head-to-head studies consistently demonstrate that SPECT has a higher sensitivity and CTPA has a higher specificity and that the overall accuracy of each modality is comparable. The negative predictive value of CTPA, V/Q SPECT, and planar V/Q imaging is consistently reported as being very high.[31,47]
- With each modality having its strengths and weaknesses (▶ Table 6.4), the test selected for any individual patient should take into account patient factors (including age, gender, renal function, diabetes, and the presence of coexisting lung disease) as well as institutional factors (e.g., availability and local expertise).

6.7 Comparison of V/Q SPECT and V/Q SPECT/CT

6.7.1 Advantages of V/Q SPECT/CT over SPECT Alone

- While V/Q SPECT has a higher sensitivity than both planar scintigraphy and CTPA, the literature suggests a higher specificity for CTPA.[11,12,46]
- While lung scanning is based on the demonstration of V/Q mismatch, the hallmark of PE, other conditions can cause this appearance.[7] Furthermore, not all patients with PE have the classic V/Q "mismatch" pattern; some develop pulmonary infarction, resulting in matched defects.[7] For these reasons, many consider the chest X-ray appearances to be pivotal for interpreting the V/Q scan, and the findings are often used to improve the accuracy and specificity of V/Q reporting.[7,29,48]
- The development of SPECT/CT scanners has allowed the easy acquisition of a CT scan with the V/Q SPECT. This CT, even when a "low dose" study to minimize patient radiation exposure, allows many of the benefits of this modality to be obtained in the one combined study.
- V/Q mismatch due to conditions other than PE (e.g., radiation therapy-induced changes, emphysema, and extrinsic vascular compression from conditions such as neoplasm or mediastinal adenopathy) can be detected by SPECT/CT imaging (▶ Fig. 6.9).[7] Patients with cardiac failure have a characteristic antigravitational redistribution of perfusion that can cause a nonsegmental

Table 6.4 Comparison of strengths and weaknesses of CTPA, V/Q SPECT, and V/Q SPECT/CT

	CTPA	V/Q SPECT	V/Q SPECT/CT
Sensitivity	Moderate–high	Very high	Very high
Specificity	Very high	High	Very high
Accuracy with abnormal radiograph	Unaffected	Sometimes affected	Sometimes affected
Provides other diagnoses	Frequent	Rare	Relatively frequent
Incidental findings require follow-up	Frequent	Rare	Less frequent
Radiation dose	High	Low	Low–moderate
Possible allergic reaction	Yes	No	No
Risk of contrast nephropathy	Yes	No	No
Technical failure rate	Higher	Rare	Rare
Availability (especially out of routine hours)	High	Usually lower	Usually lower
Accuracy in pregnancy	Lower	High	High
Accuracy in chronic PE	Lower	High	High
Performance in obstructive lung disease	Unaffected	May be affected	May be affected
Role and accuracy in follow-up	Limited	Very good	Very good
Negative predictive value	Very high	Very high	Very high

Abbreviations: CTPA, computed tomography pulmonary angiography; PE, pulmonary embolism; V/Q SPECT, ventilation–perfusion single-photon emission computed tomography; V/Q SPECT/CT, ventilation–perfusion single-photon emission computed tomography/computed tomography.

mismatch on SPECT.[7,49] SPECT/CT can be useful in these patients by demonstrating interstitial edema in the area of reduced perfusion (▶ Fig. 6.10).

- SPECT/CT can help to characterize matched changes due to nonembolic etiologies, such as pneumonia (▶ Fig. 6.6), abscess, pleural or pericardial effusions, malignancy, and pulmonary infarction (▶ Fig. 6.11).[30,31,41] Hybrid SPECT/CT imaging therefore has the potential to increase the specificity of V/Q scanning by characterizing the causes of underlying perfusion defects.[12,13]

V/Q SPECT/CT offers the potential for a single imaging procedure yielding a high sensitivity and specificity for the detection of PE, with the added benefit of being able to identify various other pathologies that can account for chest pain and dyspnea.[4]

6.7.2 Accuracy of V/Q SPECT/CT

Several studies have shown that combined V/Q SPECT/CT imaging can further improve the specificity and overall diagnostic accuracy of V/Q SPECT.

- In a series of 48 patients, Herald et al showed that the addition of a low-dose (30–50 mAs) CT scan reduced the number of false-positive V/Q SPECT scans by 50% (from six patients to three).[50] In particular, it was noted that low-dose CT could characterize pulmonary vessels and fissures that can result in defects on perfusion scintigraphy (▶ Fig. 6.12). In this series, the addition of the low-dose CT did not improve the sensitivity of SPECT.
- In a larger prospective study of 81 consecutive patients (with ^{81m}Kr gas used as the ventilation agent), Gutte et al found that the sensitivities of V/Q SPECT alone and V/Q SPECT combined with low-dose CT were identical at 97%.[12] However,

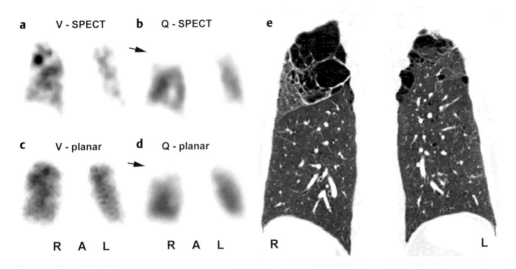

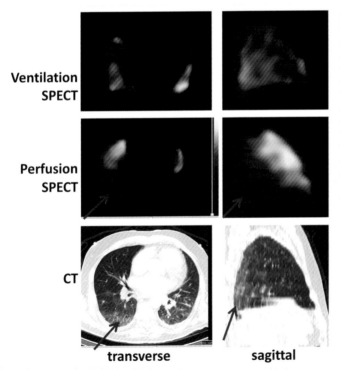

Fig. 6.9 (a–d) V and Q CT images in a patient with severe chronic obstructive pulmonary disease (COPD) and emphysema. **(e)** The right upper lobe mismatch demonstrated in the planar and SPECT images (*arrows*) was interpreted as positive for PE. However, the CT study reveals that the ventilation image appearance is due to Technegas ventilating emphysematous bullae in the right upper lobe. The CT study avoids a false-positive diagnosis for PE, thus improving specificity. (R, right; A, anterior; L, left). (Reproduced with permission from Reinartz et al.[11])

Fig. 6.10 Representative slices from a V/Q SPECT/CT scan in a patient with cardiac failure. While ventilation is normal, there is reduced perfusion in the posterior and inferior aspects of the lungs (*red arrows* in middle row). This causes V/Q mismatch, but the appearance is not segmental. Note cardiomegaly. In patients with cardiac failure, a craniocaudal shift (antigravitational) in perfusion is often demonstrated. This nonsegmental mismatch should not be confused with PE. Interstitial edema is demonstrated on the CT (*red arrows* in bottom row).

the addition of low-dose CT increased the specificity of SPECT from 88 to 100%. The addition of anatomical data demonstrated that mismatched perfusion defects could be attributed to structures, such as fissures, as well as pathological conditions, such as emphysema, pneumonia, atelectasis, and pleural fluid. The inconclusive rate for V/Q SPECT alone was only 5%, and this fell to zero when SPECT was combined with low-dose CT. While CTPA had a high specificity (100%,

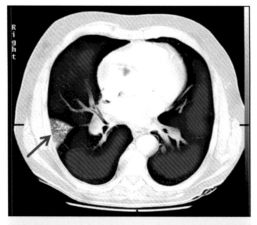

Fig. 6.11 Tranaxial perfusion SPECT/CT shows a perfusion defect in the right midzone, associated with a wedge-shaped peripheral area of consolidation (*arrow*), secondary to pulmonary infarction. SPECT/CT can help to characterize the cause of perfusion reductions due to consolidation, mass lesions, as well as pleural or pericardial effusions.

identical to that reported for V/Q SPECT/CT), it had a sensitivity much lower than either SPECT or SPECT/CT (68% compared with 97%).

- In a study of 106 patients, Ling et al showed that SPECT/CT had 93% sensitivity, 100% specificity, 97% accuracy, 1% inconclusive rate, and 97% negative predictive value.[14] The low-dose CT revealed abnormalities in 41% of patients, of which 27% were thought to account for the patient's clinical symptoms.

- Another benefit of SPECT/CT imaging is the ability to more accurately localize perfusion defects to the correct segments in each individual patient. Segmental reference lung maps, which are used to guide SPECT reporting, may be erroneous due to the distortion of individual anatomy caused by other lung pathologies, such as atelectasis and pleural effusions, which often coexist in patients with PE (▶ Fig. 6.13).[13,51] This may help guide a reporting radiologist to the correct segmental artery should a CTPA be required to confirm the findings on a V/Q SPECT study.

6.7.3 Combining V/Q SPECT with CTPA

While most imaging facilities would typically use hybrid SPECT/CT scanners to combine the functional information provided by SPECT with the structural information provided by CT (usually done using low-dose protocols), another option is

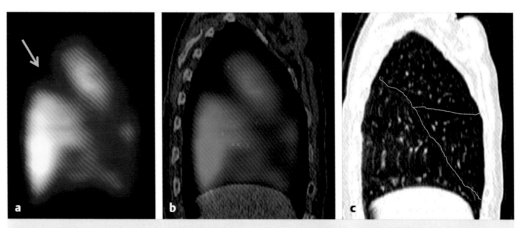

Fig. 6.12 (a) Sagittal perfusion SPECT slices show a linear perfusion reduction posteriorly (*arrow*). (b) SPECT/CT demonstrates that this corresponds with the oblique fissure. (c) The exact location of the oblique (and horizontal) fissures as demonstrated on the patient's CT is schematically drawn in yellow. SPECT/CT allows accurate characterization of anatomical structures (e.g., fissure and vessels), which may cause perfusion defects in SPECT imaging, thereby improving accuracy.

Perfusion SPECT   CTPA   Fused Perfusion SPECT/CTPA

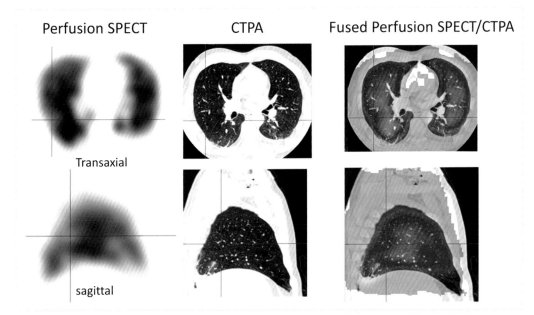

Transaxial

sagittal

Fig. 6.13 Representative perfusion SPECT, CTPA, and fused slices in a patient with PE and lower-lobe volume loss due to atelectasis. Prior to image fusion, the perfusion defect (red crosshairs) was localized to the superior segment of the right lower lobe; however, fusion accurately localized it to the posterior segment of the right upper lobe.

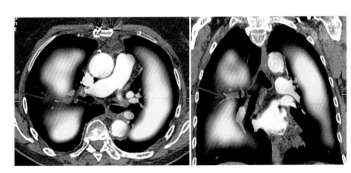

Fig. 6.14 Transaxial (left) and coronal (right) slice of a CTPA fused with a perfusion SPECT scan. A wedge-shaped perfusion defect is evident distal to the clot (*arrow*).

to fuse perfusion SPECT with diagnostic CTPA, performed either on the same hybrid scanner or another CT scanner using software fusion (▶ Fig. 6.14).[52] While this requires appropriate software programs and operator expertise, it can be of value in selected patients and may better guide the reporting radiologist to the site of a likely clot on CTPA.[53]

6.7.4 Using Perfusion SPECT/CT to Replace V/Q SPECT

As SPECT/CT can demonstrate various structural abnormalities, the need for a ventilation study has been questioned.[54] Several studies have demonstrated that specificity falls significantly if ventilation is omitted. Gradinscak et al showed that parenchymal abnormalities (usually subsegmental atelectasis) were noted on CT in 13% of V/Q SPECT mismatches.[55] Gutte et al demonstrated that perfusion-only SPECT/CT has a higher nondiagnostic rate (17%) and lower specificity than V/Q SPECT/CT (51% compared with 100%).[12] While perfusion-only SPECT/CT should be considered in sites without access to a suitable ventilation agent, limited literature suggests that performing a ventilation study does maximize specificity and reduce false-positive results.

6.8 Pitfalls

6.8.1 Technical Factors

Compared with planar imaging, technical factors are more likely to compromise the quality of SPECT imaging. These include the following:

- Misregistration between the ventilation and perfusion studies will complicate image interpretation and accurate defect localization. Software correction may be possible in some cases. Reporting specialists should identify and correct for misregistration prior to reporting the scan. Technologists should take great care during image acquisition to ensure that the image sets have been acquired with identical patient positioning.
- Suboptimal image processing will affect image quality and may affect the diagnostic accuracy of the study. Low count studies are particularly vulnerable, and studies may require reprocessing with different filters and reconstruction parameters prior to reporting (▶ Fig. 6.15).

6.8.2 Patient Factors

As with planar imaging, various patient-related variants may be seen on lung SPECT studies. These include the following:

- *Altered biodistribution due to patient positioning:* Patients should be supine when 99mTc-MAA is injected. Decreased radioactivity in the upper lobes on the lung perfusion scan is observed when patients are sitting, rather than lying supine, at the time of 99mTc-MAA injection.[56]

- *Stomach activity:* This is commonly due to swallowed radioaerosol/Technegas impacted in the mouth. The appearance is easily identified on the ventilation study (higher counts on perfusion SPECT may make it less visible).
- *Renal activity:* This is usually evident only when 99mTc-DTPA aerosol has been used as the ventilation agent in a patient with inflamed lungs and there has been subsequent absorption of the agent with excretion via the kidneys.
- *MAA clots:* These are seen when clots form in the needle or syringe in patients with difficult venous access. These produce focal areas of intense uptake on the perfusion images (▶ Fig. 6.16). A similar result may arise from failure to resuspend 99mTc-MAA particles prior to administration.[7]
- *Extrapulmonary uptake of MAA:* This is due to a right to left shunt.[57]
- *Mismatch due to mass compression of the pulmonary (or branch) artery:* This is a "false-positive" cause of mismatch and can be indistinguishable from a pulmonary embolus (▶ Fig. 6.17). SPECT/CT may be of value in detecting mass lesions causing vascular compression.[13]
- *Mismatch due to bullous lung disease:* Bullae can occasionally ventilate, allowing ingress of ventilation agents. When this occurs, a mismatch can be produced as the bullae are not perfused, leading to a false-positive scan (▶ Fig. 6.9).[11] SPECT/CT is particularly helpful in demonstrating bullae, thus showing the cause of the perfusion reduction. This reduces false-positive results and improves specificity.

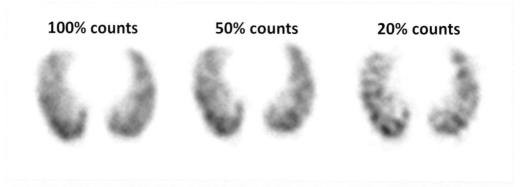

100% counts   **50% counts**   **20% counts**

Fig. 6.15 Transaxial perfusion images from a gated SPECT study where counts have been removed to simulate a low-count SPECT. Note that as count statistics are reduced (e.g., to 50% of original in the middle image, or to 20% of original in the right image), as would occur if a patient were injected with a reduced dose (e.g., due to extravasation or technical error), images become increasingly noisy, and image quality is compromised.

transaxial   coronal

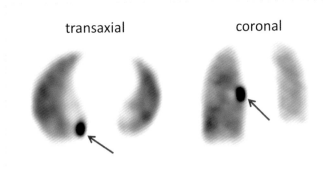

Fig. 6.16 Focal areas of intense uptake (*arrow*) on representative perfusion SPECT images, following formation of clots in the needle following an injection in a patient with difficult intravenous access.

Transaxial   Sagittal   Coronal

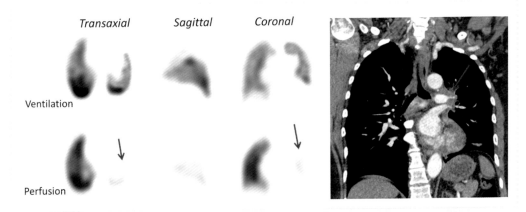

Ventilation

Perfusion

Fig. 6.17 Representative V and Q SPECT images (left) demonstrate mismatch in the left upper lobe (*arrow*). CT scan (right) shows a left hilar mass lesion (*arrow*). CT scanning done in conjunction with V/Q SPECT can account for false-positive causes of mismatch, such as in this case, in which the bronchus is patent but the pulmonary artery is occluded by the lung tumor.

- *Other false-positive causes of mismatch:* In addition to the aforementioned etiologies, nonembolic mismatch can also be seen with
  - septic, fat, and/or amniotic fluid embolism.
  - vasculitis.
  - asthma (rare).

In addition to the preceding pitfalls, there are certain artifacts and variants that are more commonly seen on SPECT imaging compared with conventional planar imaging or may impact image quality more significantly.

- Chronic obstructive pulmonary disease *(COPD) and central clumping:* Chronic airways disease leads to altered flow in the bronchi, often resulting in central impaction of tracer, regions of reduced ventilation peripherally, and areas of nonventilation/air trapping (▶ Fig. 6.2). This impacts larger ventilation particles (e.g., [99mTc]-DTPA) more than gases and Technegas. This can

reduce peripheral distribution within the lungs, resulting in SPECT studies of low counts and poor quality. Where possible, Technegas or [81mKr] should be used in such patients.

- *The "rind" artifact:* In some patients, ventilation scintigraphy results in the appearance of a band of increased radioactivity along the posterior (dependent) portion of the lungs (▶ Fig. 6.18). While this can be seen on planar ventilation images, it is more evident on SPECT images. We hypothesize that this is secondary to the development of transient dependent microatelectasis during the ventilation scanning phase.[58] Following administration of the ventilation agent (when there will be distribution of radioactivity to the lung periphery), dependent microatelectasis develops once the patient is placed supine on the scanning bed for the SPECT acquisition. This results in increased count density in dependent areas due to that section of lung being

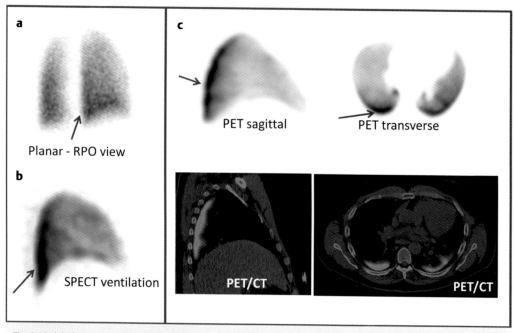

Fig. 6.18 (a) Planar right posterior oblique (RPO) ventilation scan demonstrates a mild linear increase in activity in the posterior/dependent lung (*arrow*). **(b)** Representative sagittal ventilation SPECT slice shows this more clearly (*arrow*). **(c)** A similar appearance is noted on representative sagittal and transverse slices from a positron emission tomography (PET) ventilation scan performed using ^{68}Ga-galligas as the ventilation agent. The posterior "rind" artifact is thought to be related to the development of transient dependent microatelectasis during the ventilation scanning acquisition causing count density to increase in dependent portions of the lungs due to compression of the dependent lung. This nonsegmental increase in ventilation, which predominantly affects the ventilation scan, is accentuated by tomographic imaging, such as V/Q SPECT and V/Q PET.

compressed.[59] This leads to a nonsegmental area of increased radioactivity in dependent zones. Avoiding deep inspiration during administration of the ventilation agent artifact may reduce the severity of the "rind."

- *Better visualization of fissures:* On SPECT imaging, it is common to see a linear reduction in radioactivity along the line of the oblique fissure (▶ Fig. 6.12). This can occasionally be noted on planar imaging but is more obvious on SPECT imaging due to improved resolution. This is more pronounced on the perfusion SPECT than on ventilation SPECT. This is likely due to the ability of the better ventilation agents, particularly Technegas, to distribute to the alveolar level (reaching the absolute peripheral margin of the lung, i.e., the pleural surface), whereas the

perfusion agent (Tc-99 m MAA) cannot reach beyond the terminal pulmonary arterioles.[60] SPECT/CT is helpful as the fissures are often seen; thus the cause of the nonsegmental linear perfusion reduction along the fissures can be confidently characterized.

- *Better visualization of anatomy:* Compared with planar imaging, SPECT has improved contrast and can remove overlying lung tissue. This results in improved visualization of anatomical structures, such as the larger vessels. Typically, these are better resolved on perfusion SPECT, due to a higher total number of counts and less noise, than on the ventilation study (▶ Fig. 6.19), which can lead to perfusion defects that are typically, but not always, mismatched. SPECT/CT can identify vessels and other anatomical structures,

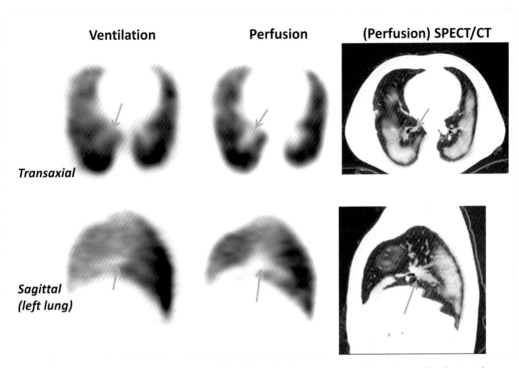

Ventilation **Perfusion** **(Perfusion) SPECT/CT**

Transaxial

Sagittal (left lung)

Fig. 6.19 Pulmonary vessels demonstrated on representative V and Q SPECT images (*arrow*). Note that these are better resolved on perfusion SPECT than ventilation SPECT imaging. SPECT/CT is helpful in showing physiological structures such as vessels and fissures.

thus explaining the etiology of the perfusion reduction.

- *Detection of smaller clots:* With its improved contrast resolution, SPECT (and SPECT/CT) can detect smaller clots than planar imaging. In particular, SPECT detects many more clots at the subsegmental level.[11] Whether small, subsegmental clots are significant enough to warrant anticoagulation has been the subject of controversy.[15,31,40,47] While large prospective outcome studies would be needed to answer this question, it should be emphasized that additional PEs detected by SPECT are not only at the subsegmental level (▶ Fig. 6.20).[11] Diagnosis of any PE, including small ones, may be of particular importance in patients with impaired

cardiopulmonary reserve, coexisting deep vein thrombosis (DVT), or recurrent small PE (with its risk of pulmonary hypertension).[40] The EANM criteria do report studies as positive for PE if there are two or more subsegmental clots, and there are increasing data validating these reporting criteria.[61]

6.9 Clinical Indications in Areas other than PE

V/Q SPECT and SPECT/CT have utility in areas other than PE.

- In patients undergoing lung volume reduction surgery, SPECT/CT can provide a more accurate assessment of relative perfusion (and

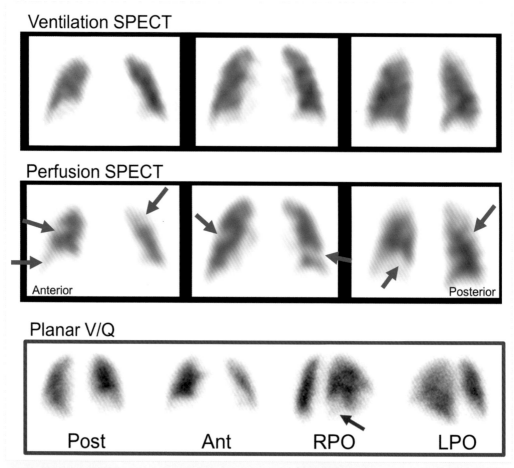

Fig. 6.20 Representative coronal ventilation (top row) and perfusion (middle row) SPECT slices show multiple mismatched defects (*blue arrows*) consistent with multiple PEs in a patient with extensive DVT. The planar V/Q scan (bottom row, representative images) obtained on the same day showed a clearly mismatched defect (right base, *red arrow*). However, other perfusion defects seen on SPECT are either less clearly or not seen on planar images, thereby potentially classifying the study as intermediate probability of PE. SPECT is more accurate than planar imaging and detects more PE at both the segmental and subsegmental levels.

ventilation) of individual segments than planar imaging (▶ Fig. 6.21).

- V/Q SPECT has also been shown to have use in the following areas[62]:
  - Predicting postoperative lung function following lung resection in patients with lung cancer.
  - Modifying radiotherapy fields to minimize radiation exposure to functioning lung.
  - Demonstrating regional changes of V/Q in asthma.
  - Estimating regional lung function in patients with interstitial pulmonary disease.

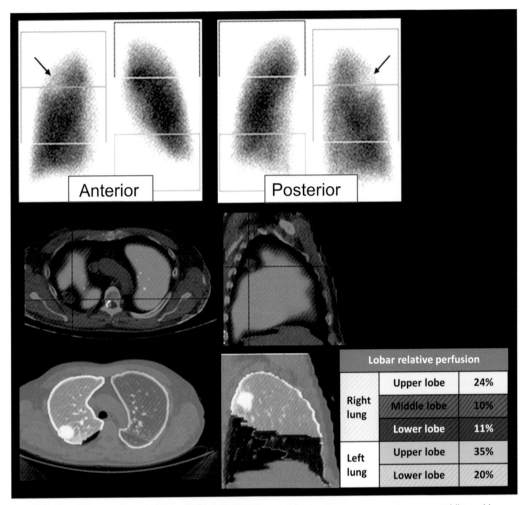

Fig. 6.21 Planar images (top row) in a patient with right lung carcinoma (*arrow*). Boxes over upper, middle, and lower thirds of each lung approximate relative contribution of each region; however, because of overlap of segments and differences in individual anatomy, accuracy is lacking. Fused perfusion SPECT/CT images (middle row) in transverse (left) and sagittal (right) planes show the perfusion defect caused by the tumor (red crosshairs) in the right upper lobe. The patient's individual CT scan can be used to generate patient-specific lobar slices (bottom row) in corresponding orthogonal planes. SPECT/CT allowed accurate determination of each lobe's relative contribution to overall ventilation (tabulated for each lobe).

References

[1] Wagner HN, Jr, Sabiston DC, Jr, McAfee JG, Tow D, Stern HS. Diagnosis of massive pulmonary embolism in man by radio-isotope scanning. N Engl J Med. 1964;271:377–384

[2] Morrell NW, Nijran KS, Jones BE, Biggs T, Seed WA. The underestimation of segmental defect size in radionuclide lung scanning. J Nucl Med. 1993;34(3):370–374

[3] Meignan MA. Lung ventilation/perfusion SPECT: the right technique for hard times. J Nucl Med. 2002;43(5):648–651

[4] Roach PJ, Schembri GP, Bailey DL. V/Q scanning using SPECT and SPECT/CT. J Nucl Med. 2013;54(9):1588–1596

[5] Roach PJ, Bailey DL, Harris BE. Enhancing lung scintigraphy with single-photon emission computed tomography. Semin Nucl Med. 2008;38(6):441–449

[6] Jögi J, Jonson B, Ekberg M, Bajc M. Ventilation-perfusion SPECT with 99mTc-DTPA versus Technegas: a head-to-head study in obstructive and nonobstructive disease. J Nucl Med. 2010;51(5):735–741

[7] Bajc M, Neilly JB, Miniati M, Schuemichen C, Meignan M, Jonson B, EANM Committee. EANM guidelines for ventilation/perfusion scintigraphy: part 1. Pulmonary imaging with ventilation/perfusion single photon emission tomography. Eur J Nucl Med Mol Imaging. 2009;36(8):1356–1370

[8] Bailey EA, Bailey DL, Roach PJ. V/Q imaging in 2010: a quick start guide. Semin Nucl Med. 2010;40(6):408–414

[9] Schembri GP, Miller AE, Smart R. Radiation dosimetry and safety issues in the investigation of pulmonary embolism. Semin Nucl Med. 2010;40(6):442–454

[10] Leblanc M, Leveillée F, Turcotte E. Prospective evaluation of the negative predictive value of V/Q SPECT using 99mTc-Technegas. Nucl Med Commun. 2007;28(8):667–672

[11] Reinartz P, Wildberger JE, Schaefer W, Nowak B, Mahnken AH, Buell U. Tomographic imaging in the diagnosis of pulmonary embolism: a comparison between V/Q lung scintigraphy in SPECT technique and multislice spiral CT. J Nucl Med. 2004;45(9):1501–1508

[12] Gutte H, Mortensen J, Jensen CV, et al. Detection of pulmonary embolism with combined ventilation-perfusion SPECT and low-dose CT: head-to-head comparison with multidetector CT angiography. J Nucl Med. 2009;50(12):1987–1992

[13] Roach PJ, Gradinscak DJ, Schembri GP, Bailey EA, Willowson KP, Bailey DL. SPECT/CT in V/Q scanning. Semin Nucl Med. 2010;40(6):455–466

[14] Ling IT, Naqvi HA, Siew TK, Loh NK, Ryan GF. SPECT ventilation perfusion scanning with the addition of low-dose CT for the investigation of suspected pulmonary embolism. Intern Med J. 2012;42(11):1257–1261

[15] Freeman LM. Don't bury the V/Q scan: it's as good as multidetector CT angiograms with a lot less radiation exposure. J Nucl Med. 2008;49(1):5–8

[16] Hurwitz LM, Yoshizumi TT, Goodman PC, et al. Radiation dose savings for adult pulmonary embolus 64-MDCT using bismuth breast shields, lower peak kilovoltage, and automatic tube current modulation. AJR Am J Roentgenol. 2009;192(1):244–253

[17] Delbeke D, Coleman RE, Guiberteau MJ, et al. Society of Nuclear Medicine (SNM). Procedure guideline for SPECT/CT imaging 1.0. J Nucl Med. 2006;47(7):1227–1234

[18] Roach PJ, Bailey DL, Schembri GP. Reinventing ventilation/perfusion lung scanning with SPECT. Nucl Med Commun. 2008;29(12):1023–1025

[19] Palmer J, Bitzén U, Jonson B, Bajc M. Comprehensive ventilation/perfusion SPECT. J Nucl Med. 2001;42(8):1288–1294

[20] Bailey DL, Schembri GP, Harris BE, Bailey EA, Cooper RA, Roach PJ. Generation of planar images from lung ventilation/perfusion SPECT. Ann Nucl Med. 200822(5):437–445

[21] Harris B, Bailey DL, Roach PJ, et al. A clinical comparison between traditional planar V/Q images and planar images generated from SPECT V/Q scintigraphy. Nucl Med Commun. 200829(4):323–330

[22] Bajc M, Olsson CG, Olsson B, Palmer J, Jonson B. Diagnostic evaluation of planar and tomographic ventilation/perfusion lung images in patients with suspected pulmonary emboli. Clin Physiol Funct Imaging. 2004;24(5):249–256

[23] Lemb M, Oei TH, Eifert H, Günther B. Technegas: a study of particle structure, size and distribution. Eur J Nucl Med. 1993;20(7):576–579

[24] Osborne DR, Jaszczak RJ, Greer K, Roggli V, Lischko M, Coleman RE. Detection of pulmonary emboli in dogs: comparison of single photon emission computed tomography, gamma camera imaging, and angiography. Radiology. 1983;146(2):493–497

[25] Bajc M, Bitzén U, Olsson B, Perez de Sá V, Palmer J, Jonson B. Lung ventilation/perfusion SPECT in the artificially embolized pig. J Nucl Med. 2002;43(5):640–647

[26] Magnussen JS, Chicco P, Palmer AW, et al. Single-photon emission tomography of a computerised model of pulmonary embolism. Eur J Nucl Med. 1999;26(11):1430–1438

[27] Collart JP, Roelants V, Vanpee D, et al. Is a lung perfusion scan obtained by using single photon emission computed tomography able to improve the radionuclide diagnosis of pulmonary embolism? Nucl Med Commun. 2002;23(11):1107–1113

[28] Le Roux PY, Palard X, Robin P, et al. Safety of ventilation/perfusion single photon emission computed tomography for pulmonary embolism diagnosis. Eur J Nucl Med Mol Imaging. 2014;41(10):1957–1964

[29] PIOPED Investigators. Value of the ventilation/perfusion scan in acute pulmonary embolism. Results of the prospective investigation of pulmonary embolism diagnosis (PIOPED). JAMA. 1990;263(20):2753–2759

[30] Strashun AM. A reduced role of V/Q scintigraphy in the diagnosis of acute pulmonary embolism. J Nucl Med. 2007;48(9):1405–1407

[31] Anderson DR, Kahn SR, Rodger MA, et al. Computed tomographic pulmonary angiography vs ventilation-perfusion lung scanning in patients with suspected pulmonary embolism: a randomized controlled trial. JAMA. 2007;298(23):2743–2753

[32] Stein PD, Fowler SE, Goodman LR, et al. PIOPED II Investigators. Multidetector computed tomography for acute pulmonary embolism. N Engl J Med. 2006;354(22):2317–2327

[33] Jones SE, Wittram C. The indeterminate CT pulmonary angiogram: imaging characteristics and patient clinical outcome. Radiology. 2005;237(1):329–337

[34] U-King-Im JM, Freeman SJ, Boylan T, Cheow HK, JM UK-I. Quality of CT pulmonary angiography for suspected pulmonary embolus in pregnancy. Eur Radiol. 2008;18(12):2709–2715

[35] Toney LK, Lewis DH, Richardson ML. Ventilation/perfusion scanning for acute pulmonary embolism: effect of direct communication on patient treatment outcomes. Clin Nucl Med. 2013;38(3):183–187

[36] Barrett BJ, Parfrey PS. Clinical practice. Preventing nephropathy induced by contrast medium. N Engl J Med. 2006;354(4):379–386

[37] Parker MS, Hui FK, Camacho MA, Chung JK, Broga DW, Sethi NN. Female breast radiation exposure during CT pulmonary angiography. AJR Am J Roentgenol. 2005;185(5):1228–1233

[38] ICRP. Radiation dose to patients from radiopharmaceuticals (addendum 2 to ICRP publication 53). Ann ICRP. 1998;28(3):1–126

[39] Jordan EJ, Godelman A, Levsky JM, Zalta B, Haramati LB. CT pulmonary angiography in pregnant and postpartum women: low yield, high dose. Clin Imaging. 201539(2):251–253

[40] Freeman LM, Glaser JE, Haramati LB. Planar ventilation-perfusion imaging for pulmonary embolism: the case for "outcomes" medicine. Semin Nucl Med. 2012;42(1):3–10

[41] Hall WB, Truitt SG, Scheunemann LP, et al. The prevalence of clinically relevant incidental findings on chest computed tomographic angiograms ordered to diagnose pulmonary embolism. Arch Intern Med. 2009;169(21):1961–1965

[42] Schattner A. Computed tomographic pulmonary angiography to diagnose acute pulmonary embolism: the good, the bad, and the ugly: comment on "The prevalence of clinically relevant incidental findings on chest computed tomographic angiograms ordered to diagnose pulmonary embolism". Arch Intern Med. 2009;169(21):1966–1968

[43] Chandra S, Sarkar PK, Chandra D, Ginsberg NE, Cohen RI. Finding an alternative diagnosis does not justify increased use of CT-pulmonary angiography. BMC Pulm Med. 2013;13:9

[44] Ridge CA, McDermott S, Freyne BJ, Brennan DJ, Collins CD, Skehan SJ. Pulmonary embolism in pregnancy: comparison

of pulmonary CT angiography and lung scintigraphy. AJR Am J Roentgenol. 2009;193(5):1223–1227

[45] Leblanc M, Paul N. V/Q SPECT and computed tomographic pulmonary angiography. Semin Nucl Med. 2010;40(6):426–441

[46] Miles S, Rogers KM, Thomas P, et al. A comparison of single-photon emission CT lung scintigraphy and CT pulmonary angiography for the diagnosis of pulmonary embolism. Chest. 2009;136(6):1546–1553

[47] Freeman LM, Haramati LB. V/Q scintigraphy: alive, well and equal to the challenge of CT angiography. Eur J Nucl Med Mol Imaging. 2009;36(3):499–504

[48] Miniati M, Pistolesi M, Marini C, et al. Value of perfusion lung scan in the diagnosis of pulmonary embolism: results of the Prospective Investigative Study of Acute Pulmonary Embolism Diagnosis (PISA-PED). Am J Respir Crit Care Med. 1996; 154(5):1387–1393

[49] Jögi J, Palmer J, Jonson B, Bajc M. Heart failure diagnostics based on ventilation/perfusion single photon emission computed tomography pattern and quantitative perfusion gradients. Nucl Med Commun. 2008;29(8):666–673

[50] Herald P, Roach P, Schembri GP. Does the addition of low dose CT improve diagnostic accuracy of V/Q SPECT scintigraphy? J Nucl Med. 2008;49 Suppl 1:91P

[51] Gradinscak DJ, Roach P, Schembri GP, Can CT. Coregistration improve the accuracy of segmental localisation on V/Q SPECT? Eur J Nucl Med Mol Imaging. 2009;36 Suppl 2:S463

[52] Harris B, Bailey D, Roach P, Bailey E, King G. Fusion imaging of computed tomographic pulmonary angiography and SPECT ventilation/perfusion scintigraphy: initial experience and potential benefit. Eur J Nucl Med Mol Imaging. 2007;34 (1):135–142

[53] Gradinscak DJ, Roach P, Schembri GP. Can Perfusion SPECT improve the accuracy of CTPA? Eur J Nucl Med Mol Imaging. 2009;36 Suppl 2:S463

[54] Lu Y, Lorenzoni A, Fox JJ, et al. Noncontrast perfusion single-photon emission CT/CT scanning: a new test for the expedited, high-accuracy diagnosis of acute pulmonary embolism. Chest. 2014;145(5):1079–1088

[55] Gradinscak DJ, Roach P, Schembri GP. Lung SPECT perfusion scintigraphy: can CT substitute for ventilation imaging? Eur J Nucl Med Mol Imaging. 2009;36 Suppl 2:S300

[56] Lau EM, Bailey DL, Bailey EA, et al. Pulmonary hypertension leads to a loss of gravity dependent redistribution of regional lung perfusion: a SPECT/CT study. Heart. 2014;100(1):47–53

[57] Kume N, Suga K, Uchisako H, Matsui M, Shimizu K, Matsunaga N. Abnormal extrapulmonary accumulation of 99mTc-MAA during lung perfusion scanning. Ann Nucl Med. 1995;9 (4):179–184

[58] Schembri G, Harris B, Roach P, et al. V/Q SPECT: What causes the posterior ventilation "rind" effect? Society of Nuclear Medicine Annual Meeting Abstracts. 2008;49(Suppl 1):91P

[59] Petersson J, Rohdin M, Sánchez-Crespo A, et al. Posture primarily affects lung tissue distribution with minor effect on blood flow and ventilation. Respir Physiol Neurobiol. 2007; 156(3):293–303

[60] Singhal S, Henderson R, Horsfield K, Harding K, Cumming G. Morphometry of the human pulmonary arterial tree. Circ Res. 1973;33(2):190–197

[61] Le Roux PY, Robin P, Delluc A, et al. V/Q SPECT interpretation for pulmonary embolism diagnosis: which criteria to use? J Nucl Med. 2013;54(7):1077–1081

[62] King GG, Harris B, Mahadev S. V/Q SPECT: utility for investigation of pulmonary physiology. Semin Nucl Med. 2010;40 (6):467–473

7 SPECT and SPECT/CT in Neoplastic Disease

Katherine A. Zukotynski, Victor H. Gerbaudo, and Chun K. Kim

7.1 Introduction

Planar imaging has been used for decades to detect sites of malignant disease, to plan therapy, and to assess response to treatment. More recently, multiplanar, multimodality imaging including single-photon emission computed tomography (SPECT), computed tomography (CT), magnetic resonance imaging (MRI), and hybrid imaging, such as SPECT/CT, have entered the realm of routine clinical care. SPECT improves the sensitivity and specificity of oncological planar scintigraphy studies and provides anatomical localization by generating multiplanar images. SPECT/CT can be even more helpful than SPECT alone since it combines the advantages of functional with anatomical imaging, improving anatomical localization of radiotracer uptake, and the characterization of physiological versus pathological sites of radiotracer uptake. The addition of SPECT and/or SPECT/CT to planar imaging tends to decrease the incidence of false-negative studies, increase reader confidence, and improve the concordance of intra- and interobserver interpretation of the findings. More recently, SPECT and SPECT/CT are being performed for preoperative imaging to guide biopsy and treatment, and are considered tools for quantitative measurements of tumor burden at baseline and following therapy. ▶ Fig. 7.1 and ▶ Fig. 7.2 illustrate the advantages of SPECT and its correlation with CT in the evaluation of a man with prostate cancer and lower back pain.

The application of SPECT and SPECT/CT to neoplastic disease has been discussed throughout several chapters in this book. In this chapter, we focus on SPECT and SPECT/CT in the context of lymphoscintigraphy, neuroendocrine tumors, scintimammography, and oncological therapy.

7.2 Lymphoscintigraphy in Oncology Patients

Lymphoscintigraphy is commonly performed in cancer patients to localize sentinel lymph nodes (SLNs) at the time of staging. The concept of the SLN was first proposed by Cabanas in 1977, who suggested the existence of a specific lymph node that appeared to be the primary site of metastasis in 100 men with penile carcinoma.[1] Specifically, *SLN* is the term used to describe the first lymph node to drain a site of malignancy. Through the years, several methods have been used to identify the SLN, including, among others, contrast lymphangiography, injection of isosulfan blue dye, and lymphoscintigraphy.

Lymphoscintigraphy may also be helpful in the evaluation of postoperative complications in oncology patients, such as lymphedema, lymphoceles (▶ Fig. 11.10 in Chapter 11 illustrates the value of SPECT/CT for the evaluation of a lymphocele), and the presence of a chyle leak, as well as for the characterization of primary lymphedema. Today,

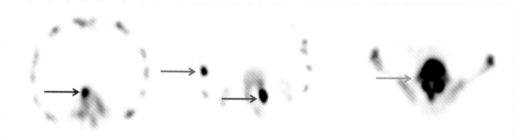

Fig. 7.1 Axial SPECT images from a bone scan of the spine of a man with prostate cancer and back pain show the following: degenerative change (*red arrow*; note that the anterolateral location on SPECT alone is suggestive of an osteophyte, while this finding was indeterminate on planar imaging; the specificity further improves with SPECT/CT), facet arthropathy (*blue arrow*; on SPECT alone, this may represent uptake in either the pedicle or the facet joint; SPECT/CT improves specificity), right rib metastasis (*green arrow*), and diffuse metastasis in a vertebral body (*orange arrow*; the anatomical location and appearance of radiotracer activity improves the specificity of the study).

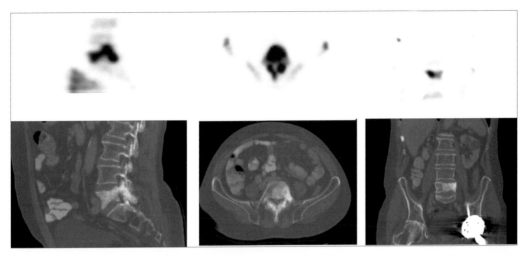

Fig. 7.2 Multiplanar SPECT images from a bone scan and corresponding CT images of a man with prostate cancer and back pain show diffuse sclerotic metastasis in a vertebral body.

lymphoscintigraphy is performed to inform therapy and reduce morbidity in patients with cancer.[2,3]

7.2.1 Technique

- Lymphoscintigraphy is used to identify lymphatic drainage pathways by planar and/or tomographic imaging following radiotracer administration.
- Lymphoscintigraphy is easy to perform and is safe and inexpensive, and it may be helpful in staging several cancer types, most often breast cancer and melanoma, and less commonly cervical, vulvar, and endometrial cancers.
- The radiotracers used include technetium-99m (^{99m}Tc)-sulfur colloid, ^{99m}Tc-antimony trisulphide, and ^{99m}Tc-rhenium sulphide, among others.[4] In North America, ^{99m}Tc-sulfur colloid is the most common.
- The particle size of ^{99m}Tc-sulfur colloid has a range of 0.1 to 1 μm.[4] Since 0.1–μm particles show rapid clearance from the interstitial space into the lymphatic channels with low capillary penetration, the radiotracer is commonly passed through a 0.22-μm filter prior to administration.
- No special patient preparation is necessary, and pregnancy is not a contraindication. It is generally recommended that breast-feeding should be suspended for 24 hours after radiopharmaceutical administration.

Sentinel Node Studies

The time needed to complete the procedure is generally less than 45 minutes and may be performed 30 minutes to several hours prior to surgery, although often it is done on the morning of or the afternoon prior to surgery. There is considerable variability in technique between centers and cancer types. In general, if the study is performed on the same day as surgery, a total amount of 15 to 30 MBq filtered ^{99m}Tc-sulfur colloid is divided into 0.5-mL volume injections. If the study is performed the day before surgery, up to 50 to 150 MBq may be used. Typically, one to four injections are administered symmetrically, intradermally about the areola in patients with breast cancer and adjacent to the tumor/excision site in patients with melanoma, penile, or vulvar cancer. Early dynamic images and delayed static images are obtained with imaging tailored to the indication/tumor type. A study by Uren et al of 209 patients with cutaneous melanoma of the trunk showed that more than 10% of patients had drainage to several lymph node groups, frequently on both sides of the midline.[5] Thus, in patients with trunk melanoma, imaging of both the right and left axillae and the groin is recommended. In patients with breast cancer, the breast that is injected and the ipsilateral axilla are imaged. During surgery, an intraoperative probe is used to identify the sentinel node as well as additional lymph nodes with radiotracer accumulation.

Other Indications (such as Lymphedema)

Two intradermal injections each of 0.05 mL of 18.5-MBq filtered ^{99m}Tc-sulfur colloid are given in the dorsum of the hands or feet. Static images of the extremities are obtained within 15 minutes of radiotracer administration, and delayed images are taken at multiple time intervals up to 4 hours following radiotracer injection. The imaging field of view should extend to include the liver.

7.2.2 Advantages of Including SPECT/CT in Sentinel Lymph Node Studies

- SPECT/CT improves the sensitivity and anatomical localization of planar lymphoscintigraphy for SLN detection. ▶ Fig. 7.3 shows a patient who underwent preoperative lymphoscintigraphy for a scalp melanoma. Planar images show radiotracer draining to the neck. SPECT/CT images show the anatomical location of several radioactive lymph nodes. A review of the literature by Hoogendam et al suggested that SPECT/CT improved SLN detection in patients with cervical cancer,[6] and a review by Vercellino et al indicated that SPECT/CT improved SLN detection in patients with breast cancer.[7] Mücke et al reported that SPECT/CT identified more lymph nodes than planar lymphoscintigraphy in patients with endometrial carcinoma.[8]
- The detection of multiple lymph nodes on SPECT/CT has been correlated with an increased likelihood of metastases.[9]
- The addition of preoperative SPECT/CT compared with SLN excision alone has been shown to be associated with a higher rate of disease-free survival.[10]
- Exact anatomical and three-dimensional localization on SPECT/CT may increase preoperative surgical confidence and may alter surgical approach and patient management (▶ Fig. 7.4).[11,12]
- Preoperative SPECT/CT in patients may be cost-effective compared with planar lymphoscintigraphy as a result of reduced operative time and hospital stay, among other things.[13,14] In addition, the use of SPECT/CT in patients with head and neck cutaneous malignancies resulted in better postoperative aesthetic results and lower morbidity.[14]

Other Indications

- Although SPECT/CT is most commonly performed for the localization of SLN in patients with malignant disease prior to therapy, sometimes it may be helpful for the evaluation of postoperative complications or for the characterization of suspected primary lymphedema.
- SPECT/CT allows more accurate identification of a chyle leakage site following surgery[15,16] and provides additional information about the presence of dermal backflow, the anatomical extent of the lymphatic disorder, and the detection of lymphatic vessels.[17]

7.2.3 Pearls

SPECT/CT is incorporated into lymphoscintigraphy studies for several reasons: (1) it improves the sensitivity and anatomical localization of SLNs; (2) it provides additional information about lymphatic vessels, lymphatic leakage sites, dermal backflow, and the extent of the lymphatic disorder; and (3) it is associated with higher preoperative surgical confidence, better postoperative aesthetic results, lower morbidity, and a higher rate of disease-free survival.

7.3 Neuroendocrine Neoplastic Disease

Pheochromocytoma, paraganglioma, and neuroblastoma are among the most common neuroendocrine tumors, and scintigraphy is frequently requested for their evaluation. However, the family of neuroendocrine tumors is large and includes entities such as pituitary adenoma, small cell lung cancer, carcinoid, pancreatic islet cell neoplasm, and medullary thyroid carcinoma, among others. Although symptoms of endocrine hyperfunction may be clinically apparent, often the disease is incidentally detected at the time of cross-sectional imaging for another indication. Functional imaging can be helpful to assess disease burden and plan therapy. It is commonly done using an ^{111}In-labeled somatostatin analogue, such as ^{111}In-pentetreotide and/or radioactive iodine (^{123}I or ^{131}I) labeled metaiodobenzylguanidine (MIBG).

SPECT or SPECT/CT is usually performed in addition to planar imaging to improve the sensitivity and specificity of the technique and to provide anatomical correlation for the functional imaging findings. SPECT/CT is particularly helpful in

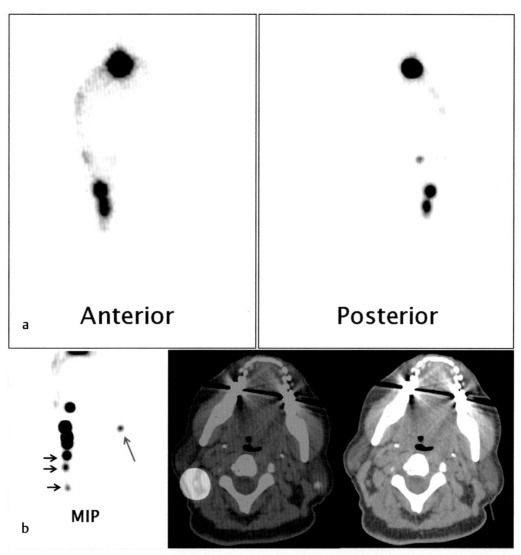

Fig. 7.3 **(a)** Filtered ^{99m}Tc-sulfur colloid was injected intradermally adjacent to a scalp melanoma. Static planar anterior and posterior images show radiotracer drainage to several lymph nodes in the neck. **(b)** The maximum intensity projection (MIP) (left), fused SPECT/CT (middle), and CT (right) images of the head and neck show the corresponding anatomical location of several radioactive lymph nodes (*black and red arrows*). Radiotracer drainage to a lymph node in the left neck (*red arrow*) is seen on SPECT/CT but was not seen on the planar images, suggesting improved sensitivity. Furthermore, given its location (medial to the parotid gland), the surgical approach was altered, which would not have been possible with planar imaging alone.

detecting and localizing small lesions that may not be seen on planar imaging and in differentiating tumor uptake from physiological radiotracer activity.[18] In a study of 72 patients evaluated with ^{111}In-pentetreotide for suspected neuroendocrine disease, the addition of SPECT/CT improved disease detection and localization, resulting in a change in image interpretation in 32% of cases and a change in management in 14% of patients.[19] In a study of 54 patients with neuroendocrine tumors, the addition of SPECT/CT improved the specificity of image interpretation and resulted in a change in management in 28% of patients.[20] ▶ Fig. 7.5 illustrates the benefit of SPECT/CT in the localization of a pancreatic neuroendocrine tumor.

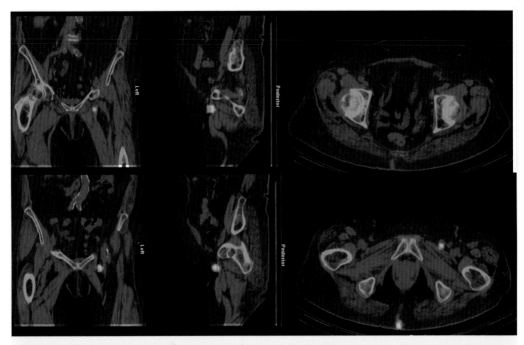

Fig. 7.4 Lymphoscintigraphy in a patient with vulvar cancer. Fused SPECT/CT clearly shows the anatomical location of radioactive lymph nodes, including a radioactive left inguinal lymph node and a left external iliac node, helping the surgeons with planning.

7.3.1 Somatostatin Receptor Imaging

- Somatostatin is a naturally occurring neuropolypeptide. Although endogenous somatostatin has a biological half-life of a few minutes, synthetic analogues have been designed with longer half-lives and improved imaging characteristics. Today, ^{111}In-labeled OctreoScan (pentetreotide) is the most common radioactive somatostatin analogue probe used in clinical practice. It has greater stability than previously synthesized somatostatin analogues and has high renal excretion and limited gastrointestinal activity.[21]
- There are several somatostatin receptor subtypes, and ^{111}In-pentetreotide preferentially binds to subtypes II and V.
- Most neuroendocrine tumors express somatostatin receptors, and the administration of radiolabeled somatostatin analogues followed by planar imaging, SPECT, and/or SPECT/CT can be helpful in detecting the site of primary disease and determining overall disease burden.
- ^{111}In-pentetreotide-positive disease suggests improved symptom control with cold octreotide.

Radionuclide therapy using [131]I- or ^{90}Y-labeled octreotide has been used with limited success.
- ^{111}In-pentetreotide uptake is not specific to neuroendocrine tumors, and the intensity of radiotracer uptake does not characterize tumor histology. Nonneuroendocrine neoplastic diseases can express somatostatin receptors as well. For example, meningiomas (▶ Fig. 7.6), gliomas, lymphoma, breast cancer, and renal cell carcinoma show variable radiolabeled somatostatin analogue uptake, depending on the concentration of somatostatin receptors present. Nonneoplastic processes may also express somatostatin receptors, such as infection (e.g., tuberculosis) or inflammation (e.g., sarcoidosis and inflammatory bowel disease).

Technique

- Prior to imaging, patients should be hydrated and may be given a laxative to decrease bowel activity. Furthermore, patients are often on a cold somatostatin analogue since somatostatin receptor binding has an inhibitory effect on hormone secretion, which can result in improved symptom control. Cold somatostatin analogue

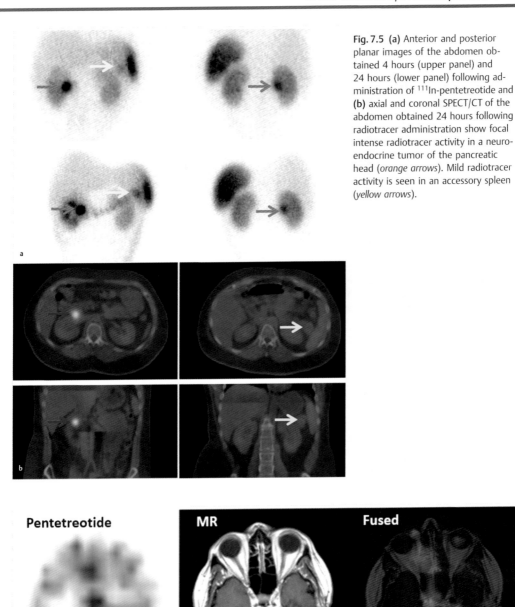

Fig. 7.5 **(a)** Anterior and posterior planar images of the abdomen obtained 4 hours (upper panel) and 24 hours (lower panel) following administration of ^{111}In-pentetreotide and **(b)** axial and coronal SPECT/CT of the abdomen obtained 24 hours following radiotracer administration show focal intense radiotracer activity in a neuroendocrine tumor of the pancreatic head (*orange arrows*). Mild radiotracer activity is seen in an accessory spleen (*yellow arrows*).

Pentetreotide MR Fused

Fig. 7.6 A 60-year-old woman with vague left facial pain and occasional dizziness. Axial SPECT image obtained following ^{111}In-pentetreotide administration, contrast-enhanced MR image, and fused SPECT/MR image show focal radiotracer uptake correlating with an enhancing mass with dural tail extending along the left tentorium at the cerebellopontine angle. Pathology following surgical resection confirmed a meningioma. (Courtesy of Samuel E. Almodóvar, MD.)

should be discontinued prior to imaging, for which consultation with the referring clinician is suggested.

- Intravenously, 111 to 222 MBq ^{111}In-pentetreotide is administered. When SPECT or SPECT/CT is performed, generally a higher administered activity is preferred (~ 222 MBq) to improve image quality.
- Planar whole-body images and SPECT (or SPECT/CT) are acquired at 24 hours. Imaging at 4 hours is optional, and imaging at 48 hours may be obtained for clarification of sites of equivocal activity.[22]
- The normal biodistribution of radiotracer includes activity in the blood pool, thyroid tissue, kidneys, spleen, liver, gallbladder, and gastrointestinal and genitourinary tracts. Activity in the gastrointestinal and genitourinary tracts tends to change over time. Radiotracer uptake at sites of disease is variable and depends on the tumor somatostatin receptors subtype expressed.

Pearls

- ^{111}In-pentetreotide is particularly helpful in detecting carcinoid tumors (sensitivity: 85–95%) and gastrinomas (sensitivity: 75–93%) and in the evaluation of pheochromocytoma, neuroblastoma, and paraganglioma, where the sensitivity is estimated to exceed 85%. It is less effective for insulinomas (sensitivity: 50–60%), and its limited utility in medullary thyroid cancer is well known (sensitivity: 65–70%).[21]
- SPECT/CT can improve sensitivity and disease localization and reduce false-positive results.

7.3.2 Metaiodobenzylguanidine Imaging

- Although most neuroendocrine tumors express somatostatin receptors, some of these tumors are more easily imaged with MIBG.
- MIBG is a guanethidine analogue that is taken up by the sympathomedullary system, with 75 to 90% being excreted by the kidneys.[23]
- MIBG can be labeled with either ^{123}I or [131]I. [123]I labeling is preferred because of the shorter half-life, lack of beta emission, and lower radiation compared with [131]I. Furthermore, there is an improved count rate with ^{123}I, resulting from a higher injected dose compared to ^{131}I, thus making it preferable for SPECT. In general, medium-

energy collimators are used for ^{123}I-MIBG imaging.

Technique

- Prior to imaging, the patient is given supersaturated potassium iodide (SSKI) to block uptake of free radioiodine by the thyroid gland. Although a single dose of SSKI at the time of radiotracer administration may be sufficient to block thyroid uptake, often SSKI is given for 2 to 3 days, starting the day before radiotracer administration. Furthermore, since several drugs, such as phenylephrine, tricyclic antidepressants, and labetalol, among others, interfere with MIBG uptake, the referring clinician should be contacted prior to patient imaging.
- ^{131}I-MIBG is most commonly performed in pediatric patients, and the amount of radiotracer activity administered is calculated using a weight-based approach, namely, 0.14 mCi/kg (5.2 MBq/kg), with a minimum dose of 1 mCi (37 MBq) and a maximum dose of 10 mCi (370 MBq).
- Planar whole-body images and SPECT (or SPECT/CT) are acquired 24 hours following radiotracer administration. Lateral images of the skull may be helpful, and delayed images at 48 hours after radiotracer administration may be obtained, as needed, for clarification of sites of equivocal activity on the earlier images.[24] SPECT or SPECT/CT can increase the sensitivity and diagnostic accuracy of the study while improving anatomical localization.
- The normal biodistribution of radiotracer includes activity in the blood pool, salivary glands, olfactory mucosa, thyroid tissue, myocardium, adrenal glands, kidneys, liver, and gastrointestinal and genitourinary tracts. Rarely, lung activity or uptake associated with metabolically active brown adipose tissue may be seen.

Pearls

- MIBG is particularly helpful in evaluating neuroblastoma and pheochromocytoma. Somatostatin receptor imaging may be superior to MIBG imaging for evaluating paraganglioma and is preferred for carcinoid tumors.
- SPECT or SPECT/CT is helpful to differentiate sites of radiotracer uptake associated with disease from physiological activity, particularly in the retroperitoneum and the upper abdomen. Activity in the liver is often heterogeneous, and SPECT

or SPECT/CT can be very helpful to characterize the presence of hepatic metastases.

The subsequent section of this chapter focuses on the most common neuroendocrine tumors imaged in the adult nuclear medicine clinical practice, namely, pheochromocytoma and paraganglioma. These shall serve as illustrative examples of the benefits of including SPECT and SPECT/CT in imaging neuroendocrine disease.

7.3.3 Pheochromocytoma and Paraganglioma

- Pheochromocytomas are rare tumors, predominantly of adults, that originate from neural crest cells and are associated with the adrenal medulla. Paragangliomas (also known as extra-adrenal pheochromocytoma) originate from neural crest cells, consisting of secretory

and nonsecretory phenotypes, in an extra-adrenal location. Typically, sympathetic paragangliomas secrete norepinephrine, while parasympathetic paragangliomas are nonsecretory.[25,26] Extra-adrenal sympathetic paragangliomas are commonly found in the mediastinum (▶ Fig. 7.7), the infradiaphragmatic para-aortic region, or the organ of Zuckerkandl, and tend to be associated with metastases.[27]

Extra-adrenal parasympathetic, nonsecretory paragangliomas are often found in the head and neck (▶ Fig. 7.8), where they tend to be locally aggressive, with extension into adjacent bone and intracranial structures.[28] The incidence of metastatic disease and prognosis varies depending on tumor type, location of tumor origin, and extent of disease, among other factors.[26,29] It is thought that approximately 2 to 10% of pheochromocytomas

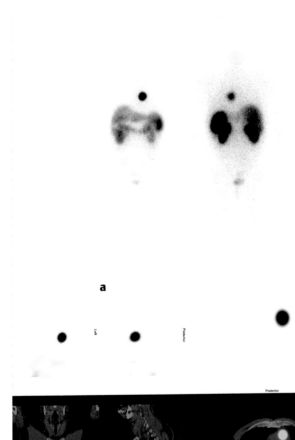

Fig. 7.7 **(a)** Anterior and posterior planar whole-body images and **(b)** multiplanar SPECT and fused SPECT/CT images obtained following intravenous administration of ^{111}In-pentetreotide in a patient with headache, palpitations, and sweating revealed no abnormal radiotracer activity in the region of the adrenal glands but showed intense focal uptake in the anterior mediastinum, which was found to be a sympathetic paraganglioma.

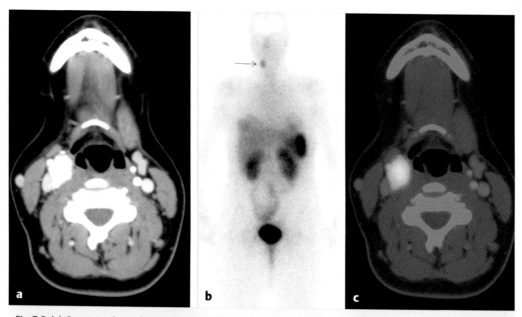

Fig. 7.8 (a) Contrast-enhanced axial CT neck performed on a 24-year-old woman demonstrates an avidly enhancing mass deep to the medial side of the right carotid artery bifurcation, and a clinical suspicion of carotid body tumor was raised. (b) The anterior whole-body ^{111}In-pentetreotide image shows focal increased uptake in the right neck. (c) An axial SPECT image electronically fused to the diagnostic CT shows the increased uptake corresponding to the enhancing mass. The final diagnosis was a parasympathetic paraganglioma. (Courtesy of Samuel E. Almodóvar, MD.)

metastasize, while 20 to 70% of extra-adrenal paragangliomas metastasize.[30]

- *Genetic considerations:* Pheochromocytomas and paragangliomas can occur sporadically or may be secondary to genetic mutations. For example, mutations in succinate dehydrogenase have been linked to the paraganglioma syndromes I–IV.[26] Different genetic mutations may predispose patients to specific malignancies, and there are several such mutations associated with pheochromocytomas and paragangliomas. For example, von Hippel–Lindau disease is associated with gene mutations linked with central nervous system hemangioblastomas, renal cysts, renal cell carcinoma, pancreatic cysts, retinal angiomas, and pheochromocytomas. Carney–Stratakis syndrome describes the association of familial paraganglioma and gastrointestinal tumors. Other syndromes that include either pheochromocytomas or paragangliomas among their constellations of findings include multiple endocrine neoplasia, neurofibromatosis type I, and Sturge–Weber syndrome, among others.[26]
- *Clinical considerations:* The clinical suspicion of a neuroendocrine tumor begins with the patient history and is confirmed with biochemical testing. Pheochromocytomas and paragangliomas

can have similar clinical features. Symptoms, when present, often include hypertension, tachycardia, palpitations, perspiration, pallor, headache, and nonspecific abdominal or flank pain. Ideally, the biochemical diagnosis has been made prior to imaging being requested. Clinical management relies on a combination of surgical resection, radiation therapy, and chemotherapy in malignant tumors.

- *Imaging considerations:* Concurrent functional imaging with ^{111}In-octreotide or ^{123}I-MIBG planar imaging with SPECT or SPECT/CT and anatomical imaging with diagnostic CT (often using nonionic iodinated contrast) can be useful to confirm the diagnosis, evaluate for metastases, and assess disease burden. MRI is reserved for problem solving. Positron emission tomography (PET) with somatostatin analogues is being used clinically in Europe but is not yet approved for clinical use in the United States. Final diagnosis depends on the combination of history, urinary or circulating catecholamines/metabolites, imaging, and histopathology. Prognosis varies depending on tumor type, location, and extent.
- ^{111}In-octreotide is often the first radiotracer used for patients with a suspected paraganglioma (► Fig. 7.7 and ► Fig. 7.8). ^{111}In-octreotide

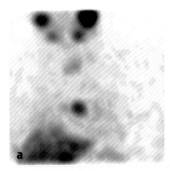
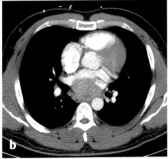
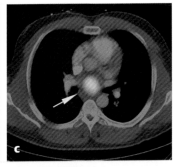

Fig. 7.9 A 34-year-old man with recent onset of uncontrolled hypertension suspected of having pheochromocytoma. **(a)** Anterior planar ^{123}I-MIBG image, **(b)** axial contrast-enhanced CT, and **(c)** axial SPECT fused to the separately acquired CT show focally increased ^{123}I-MIBG uptake corresponding to a large, mildly enhancing posterior mediastinal mass on the contrast-enhanced CT (*arrow*), consistent with a paraganglioma. (Courtesy of Samuel E. Almodóvar, MD.)

has high sensitivity for detecting metastatic disease, and can be positive in tumors that are not MIBG-avid.[25,31] If the ^{111}In-octreotide scan is negative, then an ^{123}I-MIBG scan may be helpful (▶ Fig. 7.9).

○ Anatomical imaging modalities can be used to evaluate disease burden. On CT, pheochromocytomas and paragangliomas present as avidly contrast-enhancing masses with delayed washout and density greater than 10 Hounsfield units (HU) prior to contrast administration. Internal hemorrhage may be seen, and cystic change, necrosis, and internal calcifications are common.[25,32] While there is a theoretical risk of precipitating a hypertensive crisis following the use of intravenous iodinated contrast, no adverse events were reported in a retrospective study of 25 patients with paragangliomas and pheochromocytomas who received nonionic iodinated contrast.[33] CT with contrast is often performed in these patients. On MRI, pheochromocytomas tend to show T2 prolongation and variable but typically intense contrast enhancement. The appearance can be heterogeneous due to the presence of cystic change and hemorrhage, with no dropout of signal on opposed phase imaging due to the absence of microscopic fat.[34,35]

○ PET has been investigated for the evaluation of patients with pheochromocytomas or paragangliomas. There are several radiotracers that can be used with PET, including fluorine-18 fluorodeoxyglucose (^{18}F-FDG), (^{18}F-L-dihydroxyphenylalanine [^{18}F-DOPA]), and ^{18}F-dopamine. Although ^{18}F-FDG PET has a high sensitivity for metastatic disease, the

specificity is less than that of ^{111}In-octreotide or ^{123}I-MIBG with SPECT or SPECT/CT.[31] To date, PET remains investigational, playing a complementary role for the evaluation of this patient population.

Pearls

• There is no consensus on the order in which imaging tests should be done for patients with suspected neural crest tumors. Although a biochemical diagnosis is key, ^{111}In-octreotide and/or ^{123}I-MIBG and SPECT (or SPECT/CT), as well as CT and/or MRI, can be helpful in the evaluation and staging of these malignancies.

7.4 SPECT and SPECT/CT in Pre- and Posttherapy Evaluation

SPECT and SPECT/CT can be helpful in the pretherapy evaluation of patients with neoplastic disease to detect disease spread and aid in the selection of effective therapy with potentially reduced radiation toxicity. SPECT and SPECT/CT can also be helpful in the posttherapy evaluation of patients.[35]

7.4.1 Scintimammography and SPECT

• The addition of SPECT to planar scintimammography with ^{99m}Tc-sestamibi improves the accuracy of the study for the detection of disease extent and therapy response. DeCesare et al prospectively studied 172 women with a solid breast lesion under 3 cm in size at the time of

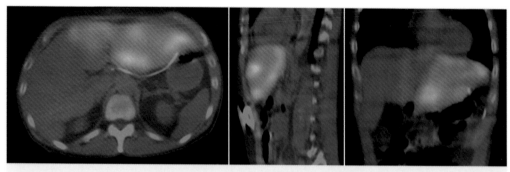

Fig. 7.10 Multiplanar SPECT/CT images obtained following the injection of ^{99m}Tc-MAA into a hepatic artery infusion pump show radiopharmaceutical delivery to hepatic segments 2, 3, and 4 only.

staging and found that scintimammography with SPECT was not only sensitive (100%) and specific (93.5%) for differentiating between benign and malignant lesions, but also helpful in the detection of axillary lymph node spread with a sensitivity and specificity of 86% and 98%, respectively.[36]

- Spanu et al found the addition of SPECT to planar scintimammography in patients with locally advanced primary breast cancer following neo-adjuvant chemotherapy or hormonotherapy improved the sensitivity of the study for detecting residual disease.[37]

Pitfall

The detection of microscopic disease, especially in axillary lymph nodes, is limited, regardless of the use of SPECT. Therefore, a SPECT/CT scintimammography negative for axillary metastasis does not obviate the need for SLN mapping.

7.4.2 SPECT and SPECT/CT for Targeted Radioembolization and Chemotherapy

The utilization of targeted radioembolization and chemotherapy for the treatment of hepatic disease is becoming increasingly prevalent in clinical nuclear medicine practice. Prior to therapy, ^{99m}Tc-labeled macroaggregated albumin (MAA) is injected into the hepatic artery, either directly or via a hepatic artery infusion pump, and imaging is performed. This is done in order to assess the extent of radiopharmaceutical uptake by liver disease, hepatic vascularization, and the presence of arteriovenous shunts between hepatic arteries and extrahepatic organs, such as the lungs, stomach, or duodenum, as well as to establish pump placement and exclude a leak. SPECT/CT can provide additional helpful anatomical information in this setting, as illustrated in ▶ Fig. 7.10 and ▶ Fig. 7.11.

7.4.3 SPECT and SPECT/CT for Dosimetry Planning

Recently, several studies have suggested the use of sequential SPECT/CT studies to determine the tumor-absorbed dose of a radiopharmaceutical and tailor targeted radionuclide therapy to achieve maximum effect with limited toxicity. In 2013, Jackson et al proposed an automated voxelized dosimetry technique using serial quantitative SPECT/CT images that would allow physicians to determine the radioactivity required for a therapeutic effect while limiting radiation toxicity to normal tissue.[38] In a recent study of 24 patients with metastatic pancreatic neuroendocrine cancer treated with radionuclide therapy, SPECT/CT was used to determine the tumor-absorbed dose of radiopharmaceutical, and a significant correlation was found between the absorbed dose and tumor reduction.[39] A study conducted by Garin et al of 41 patients with hepatocellular carcinoma and portal vein thrombosis showed that ^{99m}Tc-MAA SPECT/CT personalized dosimetry with intensification using yttrium-90 (^{90}Y)-loaded glass microspheres was associated with improved overall survival.[40] Kao et al showed that tumor dose estimated by ^{99m}Tc-MAA SPECT/CT correlated well with that of ^{90}Y-resin microspheres calculated by post-^{90}Y PET.[41]

Pearls

- Personalized dosimetry using SPECT/CT can minimize toxicity associated with targeted therapy and may be associated with improved survival.

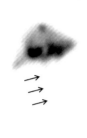
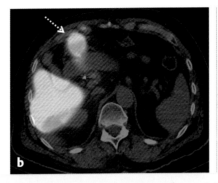

a **b** **c**

Fig. 7.11 ^{99m}Tc-MAA was injected into the hepatic artery of a patient with metastatic colon cancer to the liver. **(a)** The anterior planar image shows several sites of focal increased radiotracer accumulation in the liver corresponding to known metastatic disease as well as mild diffuse activity in the normal parenchyma. Although no significant pulmonary activity was present, there was linear extrahepatic activity (*black arrows*) extending inferiorly to the lower abdomen. **(b)** This linear activity was anteriorly located on SPECT/CT (a single axial slice is shown) in the distribution of the hepatic falciform artery (*white arrow*). While coil embolization of extrahepatic vessels is often performed prior to ^{90}Y administration, it was felt this would be challenging in this particular case. Instead, given the superficial location of the vessel, cold-induced vasoconstriction was attempted by applying ice immediately prior to ^{90}Y radioembolization. **(c)** A post-^{90}Y bremsstrahlung image showed no obvious activity in the distribution of the falciform artery.

7.5 Conclusion

Scintigraphic imaging for patients with neoplastic disease is a helpful tool to detect disease and determine disease extent, plan therapy, and assess treatment response. Over the years, it has become increasingly clear that SPECT and SPECT/CT can improve the sensitivity and specificity of a planar scintigraphy study and provide anatomical localization that can change patient management. As our interest in targeted radionuclide therapy grows, it is likely that SPECT/CT will play an even more important role in the pretherapy evaluation of patients with cancer as a tool enabling us to choose the most effective therapy with the least morbidity.

References

[1] Cabanas RM. An approach for the treatment of penile carcinoma. Cancer. 1977;39(2):456–466

[2] Moncayo VM, Aarsvold JN, Alazraki NP. Lymphoscintigraphy and sentinel nodes. J Nucl Med. 2015;56(6):901–907

[3] Uren RF, Howman-Giles R, Chung D, Thompson JF. Imaging sentinel lymph nodes. Cancer J. 2015;21(1):25–32

[4] Giammarile F, Alazraki N, Aarsvold JN, et al. The EANM and SNMMI practice guideline for lymphoscintigraphy and sentinel node localization in breast cancer. Eur J Nucl Med Mol Imaging. 2013;40(12):1932–1947

[5] Uren RF, Howman-Giles RB, Shaw HM, Thompson JF, McCarthy WH. Lymphoscintigraphy in high-risk melanoma of the trunk: predicting draining node groups, defining lymphatic channels and locating the sentinel node. J Nucl Med. 1993; 34(9):1435–1440

[6] Hoogendam JP, Veldhuis WB, Hobbelink MG, Verheijen RH, van den Bosch MA, Zweemer RP. 99mTc SPECT-CT versus planar lymphoscintigraphy for preoperative sentinel lymph node detection in cervical cancer: a systematic review and metaanalysis. J Nucl Med. 2015;56(5):675–680

[7] Vercellino L, Ohnona J, Groheux D, et al. Role of SPECT/CT in sentinel lymph node detection in patients with breast cancer. Clin Nucl Med. 2014;39(5):431–436

[8] Mücke J, Klapdor R, Schneider M, et al. Isthmocervical labelling and SPECT/CT for optimized sentinel detection in endometrial cancer: technique, experience and results. Gynecol Oncol. 2014;134(2):287–292

[9] Tomiguchi M, Yamamoto-Ibusuki M, Yamamoto Y, et al. Prediction of sentinel lymph node status using single-photon emission computed tomography (SPECT)/computed tomography (CT) imaging of breast cancer. Surg Today. 2016;46 (2):214–223

[10] Stoffels I, Boy C, Pöppel T, et al. Association between sentinel lymph node excision with or without preoperative SPECT/CT and metastatic node detection and disease-free survival in melanoma. JAMA. 2012;308(10):1007–1014

[11] Bluemel C, Rubello D, Colletti PM, de Bree R, Herrmann K. Sentinel lymph node biopsy in oral and oropharyngeal squamous cell carcinoma: current status and unresolved challenges. Eur J Nucl Med Mol Imaging. 2015;42(9):1469–1480

[12] Balasubramanian Harisankar CN, Mittal BR, Bhattacharya A, Dhaliwal LK. Utility of SPECT/CT in sentinel lymph node detection in a case of vulvar carcinoma. Mol Imaging Radionucl Ther. 2013;22(3):106–108

[13] Stoffels I, Müller M, Geisel MH, et al. Cost-effectiveness of preoperative SPECT/CT combined with lymphoscintigraphy vs. lymphoscintigraphy for sentinel lymph node excision in patients with cutaneous malignant melanoma. Eur J Nucl Med Mol Imaging. 2014;41(9):1723–1731

[14] Klode J, Poeppel T, Boy C, et al. Advantages of preoperative hybrid SPECT/CT in detection of sentinel lymph nodes in cutaneous head and neck malignancies. J Eur Acad Dermatol Venereol. 2011;25(10):1213–1221

[15] Thang SP, Tong AK, Ng DC. Postmastectomy/axillary node dissection chyloma: the additional value of SPECT/CT lymphoscintigraphy. J Breast Cancer. 2014;17(3):291–294

[16] Das J, Thambudorai R, Ray S. Lymphoscintigraphy combined with single-photon emission computed tomography-computed tomography (SPECT-CT): a very effective imaging approach for identification of the site of leak in postoperative chylothorax. Indian J Nucl Med. 2015;30(2):177–179

[17] Weiss M, Baumeister RG, Frick A, Wallmichrath J, Bartenstein P, Rominger A. Primary lymphedema of the lower limb: the clinical utility of single photon emission computed tomography/CT. Korean J Radiol. 2015;16(1):188–195

[18] Bar-Shalom R, Keidar Z, Krausz Y. Prospective image fusion: the role of SPECT/CT and PET/CT. In: Henkin RE, ed. Nuclear Medicine. 2nd ed. Vol. 2. Philadelphia, PA: Mosby Elsevier; 2006:1527–1544

[19] Krausz Y, Keidar Z, Kogan I, et al. SPECT/CT hybrid imaging with 111 In-pentetreotide in assessment of neuroendocrine tumours. Clin Endocrinol (Oxf). 2003;59(5):565–573

[20] Pfannenberg AC, Eschmann SM, Horger M, et al. Benefit of anatomical-functional image fusion in the diagnostic work-up of neuroendocrine neoplasms. Eur J Nucl Med Mol Imaging. 2003;30(6):835–843

[21] Mettler FA, Guiberteau MJ, eds. Non-PET neoplasm imaging and radioimmunotherapy. In: Essentials of Nuclear Medicine Imaging. 6th ed. Philadelphia, PA: Elsevier Saunders; 2012:351–353

[22] Balon HR, Brown TLY, Goldsmith SJ, et al. Society of Nuclear Medicine. The SNM practice guideline for somatostatin receptor scintigraphy 2.0. J Nucl Med Technol. 2011;39(4):317–324

[23] Mettler FA, Guiberteau MJ, eds. Genitourinary system and adrenal glands. In: Essentials of Nuclear Medicine Imaging. 6th ed. Philadelphia, PA: Elsevier Saunders; 2012:341–343

[24] Sharp S, Gelfand MJ, Shulkin BL. Neuroblastoma: functional imaging. In: Treves ST, ed. Pediatric Nuclear Medicine and Molecular Imaging. 4th ed. New York, NY: Springer; 2014:429–447

[25] Blake MA, Kalra MK, Maher MM, et al. Pheochromocytoma: an imaging chameleon. Radiographics. 2004;24 Suppl 1:S87–S99

[26] Opocher G, Schiavi F. Genetics of pheochromocytomas and paragangliomas. Best Pract Res Clin Endocrinol Metab. 2010; 24(6):943–956

[27] Ayala-Ramirez M, Feng L, Johnson MM, et al. Clinical risk factors for malignancy and overall survival in patients with pheochromocytomas and sympathetic paragangliomas: primary tumor size and primary tumor location as prognostic indicators. J Clin Endocrinol Metab. 2011;96(3):717–725

[28] Rao AB, Koeller KK, Adair CF. From the archives of the AFIP. Paragangliomas of the head and neck: radiologic-pathologic correlation. Armed Forces Institute of Pathology. Radiographics. 1999;19(6):1605–1632

[29] Chrisoulidou A, Kaltsas G, Ilias I, Grossman AB. The diagnosis and management of malignant phaeochromocytoma and paraganglioma. Endocr Relat Cancer. 2007;14(3):569–585

[30] Wen J, Li HZ, Ji ZG, Mao QZ, Shi BB, Yan WG. A decade of clinical experience with extra-adrenal paragangliomas of retroperitoneum: report of 67 cases and a literature review. Urol Ann. 2010;2(1):12–16

[31] Intenzo CM, Jabbour S, Lin HC, et al. Scintigraphic imaging of body neuroendocrine tumors. Radiographics. 2007;27 (5):1355–1369

[32] Motta-Ramirez GA, Remer EM, Herts BR, Gill IS, Hamrahian AH. Comparison of CT findings in symptomatic and incidentally discovered pheochromocytomas. AJR Am J Roentgenol. 2005;185(3):684–688

[33] Bessell-Browne R, O'Malley ME. CT of pheochromocytoma and paraganglioma: risk of adverse events with i.v. administration of nonionic contrast material. AJR Am J Roentgenol. 2007;188(4):970–974

[34] Varghese JC, Hahn PF, Papanicolaou N, Mayo-Smith WW, Gaa JA, Lee MJ. MR differentiation of phaeochromocytoma from other adrenal lesions based on qualitative analysis of T2 relaxation times. Clin Radiol. 1997;52(8):603–606

[35] Bural GG, Muthukrishnan A, Oborski MJ, Mountz JM. Improved benefit of SPECT/CT compared to SPECT alone for the accurate localization of endocrine and neuroendocrine tumors. Mol Imaging Radionucl Ther. 2012;21(3):91–96

[36] DeCesare A, De Vincentis G, Gervasi S, et al. Single-photon-emission computed tomography (SPECT) with technetium-99 m sestamibi in the diagnosis of small breast cancer and axillary lymph node involvement. World J Surg. 2011;35 (12):2668–2672

[37] Spanu A, Farris A, Chessa F, et al. Planar scintimammography and SPECT in neoadjuvant chemo or hormonotherapy response evaluation in locally advanced primary breast cancer. Int J Oncol. 2008;32(6):1275–1283

[38] Jackson PA, Beauregard JM, Hofman MS, Kron T, Hogg A, Hicks RJ. An automated voxelized dosimetry tool for radionuclide therapy based on serial quantitative SPECT/CT imaging. Med Phys. 2013;40(11):112503

[39] Ilan E, Sandström M, Wassberg C, et al. Dose response of pancreatic neuroendocrine tumors treated with peptide receptor radionuclide therapy using 177Lu-DOTATATE. J Nucl Med. 2015;56(2):177–182

[40] Garin E, Rolland Y, Edeline J, et al. Personalized dosimetry with intensification using 90Y-loaded glass microsphere radioembolization induces prolonged overall survival in hepatocellular carcinoma patients with portal vein thrombosis. J Nucl Med. 2015;56(3):339–346

[41] Kao YH, Steinberg JD, Tay YS, et al. Post-radioembolization yttrium-90 PET/CT – part 2: dose-response and tumor predictive dosimetry for resin microspheres. EJNMMI Res. 2013;3(1):57

8 SPECT and SPECT/CT for the Skeletal System

Hyewon Hyun, Chun K. Kim, and Katherine A. Zukotynski

8.1 Introduction

Skeletal scintigraphy is one of the most commonly requested general nuclear medicine studies due to its wide availability, ease of performance, low cost, and ability to assess the entire skeletal system. Often, abnormalities can be identified on skeletal scintigraphy earlier than on anatomical imaging. Since radiotracer uptake in the skeleton occurs as a result of osteoblastic activity, it can be seen in traumatic, infectious, and neoplastic conditions. Thus, although the sensitivity of skeletal scintigraphy is high, correlation with clinical history and additional imaging is crucial for accurate image interpretation (▶ Fig. 8.1). Single-photon emission computed tomography (SPECT; ▶ Fig. 8.2) and SPECT/computed tomography (SPECT/CT; ▶ Fig. 8.3) can improve image contrast

as well as cross-sectional anatomical detail, resulting in higher sensitivity, specificity, diagnostic accuracy, and reader confidence compared with planar skeletal scintigraphy alone.

Although adding CT to SPECT increases the radiation dose to the patient, the benefits often far outweigh the risks associated with the additional radiation exposure. The CT data can be used for attenuation and scatter correction, thus improving the quality of SPECT. The addition of CT has allowed us to clarify SPECT findings and has also increased our ability to determine the anatomical location and extent of disease and enabled concurrent evaluation of anatomical and metabolic changes, thereby assisting with surgical planning and determination of appropriate management. Today, some of the most common indications for skeletal scintigraphy with SPECT or SPECT/CT

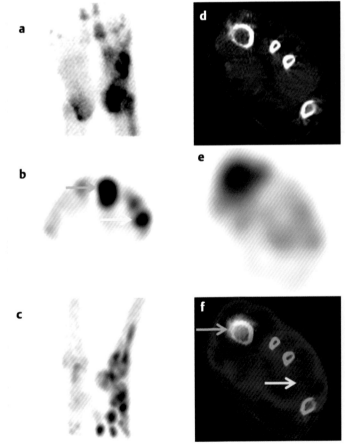

Fig. 8.1 A 74-year-old man with left foot pain due to simultaneous metastatic lung cancer and osteomyelitis shown with SPECT/CT. **(a)** Skeletal phase planar, **(b)** axial SPECT, and **(c)** Maximum intensity projection (MIP) images from a skeletal scintigraphy study of the feet show multifocal radiotracer uptake at sites of active osteoblastic turnover. Although skeletal scintigraphy with SPECT helps to detect and localize several sites of osseous disease, it cannot reliably distinguish osteomyelitis from metastatic disease. **(d)** Axial CT, **(e)** SPECT, and **(f)** fused SPECT/CT images from a 99mTc-labeled WBC study focusing on the left midfoot show that the osteoblastic turnover in the region of the left first metatarsal head (*orange arrow* in **b**) correlates with intense white blood cell accumulation at a site of active osteomyelitis (*orange arrow* in **f**), while the osteoblastic turnover in the region of the left fourth metatarsal head (*yellow arrow* in **b**) correlates with a destructive mass at a site of lung cancer metastasis (*yellow arrow* in **f**).

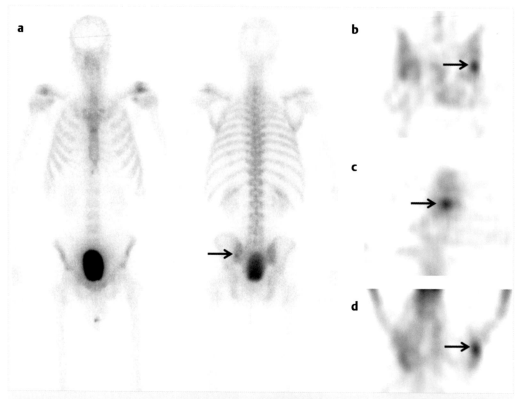

Fig. 8.2 A 65-year-old man with prostate cancer and rising prostate-specific antigen. SPECT helped to detect a left iliac bone metastasis adjacent to the sacroiliac joint (SIJ), which was equivocal on planar bone scintigraphy. **(a)** Anterior and posterior projection skeletal phase whole-body images from a skeletal scintigraphy study show subtle active osteoblastic turnover in the left iliac bone adjacent to the SIJ (arrow) that is indeterminate for osseous metastasis. **(b)** Coronal, **(c)** sagittal, and **(d)** axial SPECT images from the skeletal scintigraphy study improve the contrast of the metabolically active osseous metastasis (*arrows*) and localize it to the left iliac bone.

include evaluation of suspected radiographically occult fractures and stress changes; postsurgical complications, such as pain and hardware instability; and suspected neoplastic disease. Skeletal scintigraphy with SPECT or SPECT/CT is also often used when magnetic resonance imaging (MRI) cannot be performed because of contraindications or a high likelihood of artifact.

8.1.1 Technique

Bone is made up of a crystalline lattice consisting of calcium, phosphate, and hydroxyl ions that form hydroxyapatite. Bone-targeting radiopharmaceuticals are analogues of calcium, hydroxyl groups, or phosphates and are taken up in osteoblasts at the time of bone remodeling or healing.[1] Among them, technetium-99 m (^{99m}Tc)-labeled methylene diphosphonate (MDP) is the most widely used radiopharmaceutical for skeletal scintigraphy.

Images are typically acquired as either a single- or a three-phase study. No patient preparation is required prior to the study.

- In a three-phase bone scan, angiographic phase (blood flow) images are acquired by dynamic imaging, usually for 60 seconds, immediately after the injection of 740 to 925 MBq (20–25 mCi) of ^{99m}Tc-MDP to assess perfusion to the area of interest. Tissue phase (blood pool) static images are acquired once the dynamic imaging has been completed and are used to assess hyperemia or the amount of activity that extravasates into the soft tissue in the area of interest. Skeletal phase imaging is performed 2 to 4 hours afterward to assess skeletal uptake. Three-phase bone scans are often done to evaluate traumatic injury where knowledge regarding perfusion is needed, such as in cases of suspected complex regional pain syndrome or osteomyelitis. They are also useful for the evaluation of neoplastic

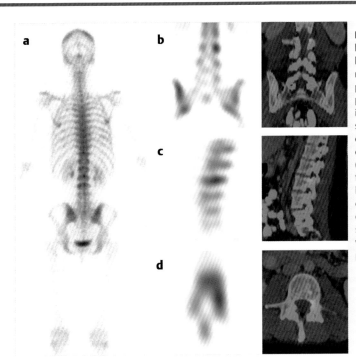

Fig. 8.3 A 50-year-old woman with breast cancer for staging. SPECT/CT helped identify an L3 vertebral body metastasis, which was equivocal on planar bone scintigraphy. **(a)** Posterior projection skeletal phase whole-body image from a skeletal scintigraphy study shows subtle osteoblastic turnover in L3 that is indeterminate for osseous metastasis. **(b)** Coronal, **(c)** sagittal, and **(d)** axial SPECT and fused SPECT/CT images from the skeletal scintigraphy study improve the contrast of the metabolically active osseous metastasis and localize the site of disease to the junction of the L3 vertebral body posteriorly and the left pedicle.

osseous disease, such as for a suspected osteoid osteoma, among other pathologies.

- In a single-phase bone scan, only skeletal phase imaging is performed. Single-phase bone scans are commonly done for follow-up of patients with known osseous metastases.
- SPECT or SPECT/CT is obtained at the time of skeletal phase imaging as needed and is usually targeted to a site of abnormality on planar images or to improve the sensitivity and specificity in a region of clinical concern. SPECT is typically acquired using a 128 × 128 matrix with 25 seconds per step, iterative reconstruction, and resolution recovery. Images are displayed in coronal, sagittal, and axial projections alongside a rotating maximum intensity projection (MIP) image. For the CT portion of the study, the typical kVp range is 80 to 110 kVp and slice thickness is 2 to 2.5 mm with overlapping cuts; however, the CT may be tailored to the clinical question, varying from very low dose for attenuation correction, to low dose for anatomical correlation, to normal dose for more precise anatomical imaging when needed. Intravenous contrast administration is not performed, and dose modulation is applied to minimize radiation exposure. Also, radiation exposure can be minimized by avoiding the use of CT when unlikely to provide additional value to SPECT. Bone and soft tissue windows as well

as reformats in coronal and sagittal projections are available for studies with three-dimensional rendering as required. Fused and nonfused SPECT and CT images are reviewed. Since CT images are rapidly acquired (in a matter of seconds), motion is rarely an issue. SPECT typically requires 12 to 15 minutes to complete and can lead to potential misregistration artifact between the CT and SPECT images. Thus it is important to ensure that patients are comfortably positioned whenever possible.

8.1.2 Pearls

- Intense activity in the bladder can cause artifact on reconstructed SPECT images, including streak artifact and "cold" areas close to the bladder due to pixel overload (▶ Fig. 8.4). Therefore, if the patient cannot void and there is clinical concern for sacral, pelvic bone, or proximal femoral abnormality, bladder catheterization may be helpful.

8.2 Trauma/Arthropathy/ Unexplained Pain

Skeletal scintigraphy has long been used for the evaluation of traumatic injury, and there are a

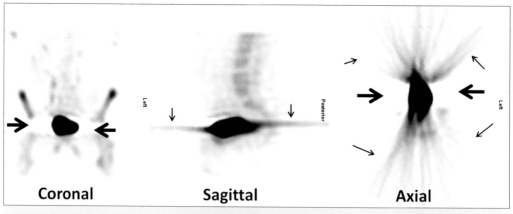

Coronal   **Sagittal**   **Axial**

Fig. 8.4 Streak artifact (small arrows on the sagittal and axial images) and "cold" areas close to the bladder (large arrows on the coronal and axial images) are caused by intense bladder activity.

number of indications as to when SPECT or SPECT/CT should be considered. In particular, SPECT or SPECT/CT can be particularly useful (1) to diagnose a clinically suspected fracture in the setting of negative anatomical imaging, (2) to diagnose a cause of mechanical back pain or pars stress, and (3) for the evaluation of pain after surgical intervention when MRI is subject to significant artifact. Whole-body skeletal scintigraphy with additional SPECT or SPECT/CT where needed is also good to provide a rapid whole-body assessment with limited radiation exposure for the detection of multifocal traumatic injury that may be difficult to obtain using anatomical imaging modalities, such as radiographs, CT, or MRI.

8.2.1 Fractures

Skeletal scintigraphy with SPECT or SPECT/CT is helpful in patients with pain, a clinical history of trauma or osseous stress, and negative diagnostic imaging. Stress injury occurs following repetitive activity causing marrow edema and microtrabecular fractures that ultimately coalesce to form a cortical break. Skeletal scintigraphy is exquisitely sensitive for stress injury and fractures. Indeed, active osteoblastic turnover can be seen prior to anatomical changes and often correlates with the site of pain.[2,3] SPECT/CT has improved diagnostic accuracy compared with planar imaging alone or with SPECT and can be particularly helpful to localize abnormalities in patients with radiographically occult stress fractures (▶ Fig. 8.5) or osteochondral defects (▶ Fig. 8.6). Linke et al studied 71 patients with extremity pain and found that

planar imaging and SPECT/CT led to a different diagnosis compared with planar imaging and SPECT in 23 patients ($p < 0.01$).[4] Scheyerer et al found improved diagnosis of occult pelvic fractures on SPECT/CT compared with radiographs and CT,[5] while Allainmat et al found improved diagnosis of occult wrist fractures on SPECT/CT compared with CT.[6] MRI is sensitive for bone marrow edema; however, the extent of edema is protocol dependent, and image interpretation can be difficult and/or misleading. Skeletal scintigraphy with SPECT or SPECT/CT can also identify ongoing active osteoblastic turnover, which can be useful to suggest when healing is complete as well as the presence of nonunion. Active osteoblastic turnover 12 to 18 months after a fracture is suggestive of nonunion.[2]

8.2.2 Back Pain

SPECT or SPECT/CT is recommended for the evaluation of back pain. SPECT has been shown to have improved specificity compared with planar skeletal scintigraphy, particularly for the evaluation of lesions in the lumbar spine.[7,8] CT increases the specificity still further.[9] Moderately to markedly active facet arthropathy is generally evident on planar images, demonstrating a characteristic appearance.[10] However, mild facet arthropathy may not be apparent on planar images, while it is clearly evident on SPECT or SPECT/CT (▶ Fig. 8.7). Skeletal scintigraphy with SPECT or SPECT/CT may also be helpful to identify active osteoblastic turnover at sites of pain associated with transitional vertebra or stress to the region of the pars interarticularis.[2]

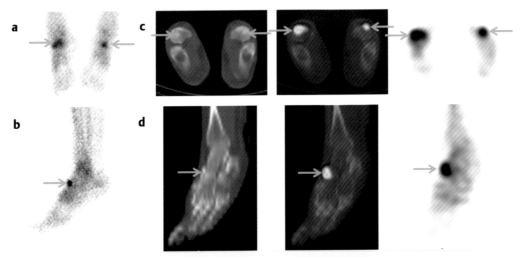

Fig. 8.5 A 29-year-old athletic woman with bilateral foot pain and negative radiographs. SPECT/CT confirmed stress fractures of bilateral navicular bones suggested on planar skeletal scintigraphy. **(a)** Skeletal phase images of both feet in the anterior projection and **(b)** lateral projection of the left foot show active osteoblastic turnover in the region of both the right and left navicular bone (*arrows*). **(c)** Axial CT, fused SPECT/CT, and SPECT images of both feet as well as **(d)** sagittal CT, fused SPECT/CT, and SPECT images of the left foot show metabolically active osteoblastic turnover in both the right and left navicular bone correlating with subtle sclerosis on CT at sites of bilateral navicular stress fractures (*arrows*). Stress is often associated with athletes who engage in forceful push-offs for sprinting or jumping. Symptoms can be nonspecific. Although radiographs are often the first imaging study performed, the sensitivity of skeletal scintigraphy is significantly higher. Navicular bone stress fractures are at high risk of delayed union and nonunion, in part, related to the relatively avascular central area, making early diagnosis and management important for good long-term results and early resumption of physical activity.[29]

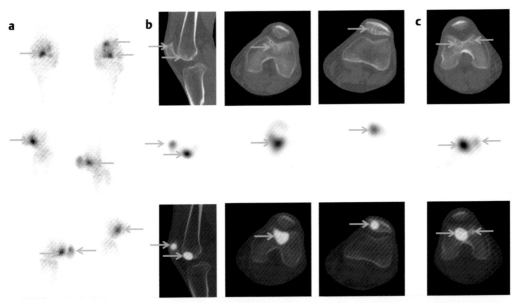

Fig. 8.6 A 20-year-old athletic woman with bilateral knee pain and negative radiographs. SPECT/CT clarified the location and extent of several osteochondral defects involving the left patella and both femora. **(a)** Skeletal phase images in anterior and lateral projections of both knees show several sites of active osteoblastic turnover in the knees (*arrows*). **(b)** Sagittal and axial CT, SPECT, and fused SPECT/CT images of the left knee localize osteochondral defects in the left patella and femur (*arrows*). **(c)** Axial CT, SPECT, and fused SPECT/CT images of the right knee localize additional osteochondral defects (*arrows*). Articular cartilage abnormalities of the knees are common in active patients, and early, accurate characterization of size and location is helpful to ensure appropriate management.[30]

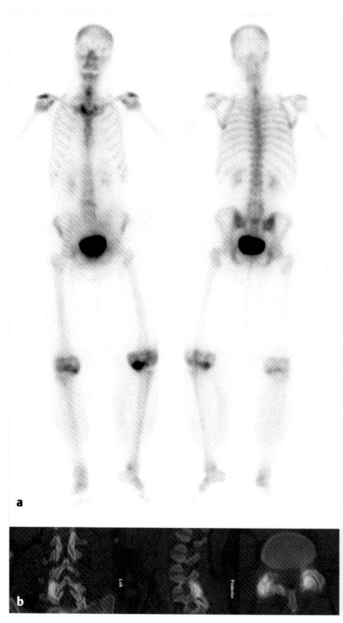

Fig. 8.7 A 57-year-old woman with low back pain. **(a)** Planar images show mild irregular tracer activity in the lower lumbar spine but no obvious focal abnormalities. **(b)** SPECT/CT shows intense tracer uptake in the bilateral facet joints, right greater than left, at the L4/L5 level.

8.2.3 Accessory Ossicles

Skeletal scintigraphy with SPECT/CT may be helpful to precisely localize the site of active osteoblastic turnover to an accessory ossicle. Active osteoblastic turnover associated with an accessory ossicle may suggest a cause of pain (stress, fracture, inflammation, etc.) versus absent activity, which is more commonly associated with a normal anatomical variant, an important distinction if surgical resection is considered.[2]

8.2.4 Soft Tissue Injury

Soft tissues are typically more reliably evaluated using MRI than skeletal scintigraphy with SPECT or SPECT/CT. Furthermore, although SPECT/CT may be helpful to determine the extent of an osteochondral defect, MRI is preferred for the evaluation of soft tissue injury in most large joints and in the spine.[2] In a retrospective study of the Israel Defense Forces database between 2005 and 2009, 330 subjects who had undergone both SPECT and MRI of the knee prior to arthroscopy were identified.[11] SPECT was 61% sensitive, 54% specific, and 58% accurate for the detection of knee pathology and had poor correlation with arthroscopic findings. MRI was 95% sensitive, 67% specific, and 85% accurate for the detection of knee pathology and correlated with arthroscopic findings far better than SPECT.

8.2.5 Pearls

- Skeletal scintigraphy with SPECT or SPECT/CT is very helpful in detecting and localizing osseous

stress and/or fractures, while MRI is the imaging modality of choice to detect and characterize soft tissue abnormalities.
- Skeletal scintigraphy with SPECT or SPECT/CT can be a helpful addition to white blood cell (WBC) imaging if traumatic injury is suspected in addition to osteomyelitis (▸ Fig. 8.8).
- SPECT and SPECT/CT may localize tumoral calcinosis, a benign condition resulting in soft tissue calcification that can occur following trauma and that can enlarge with time.[12]

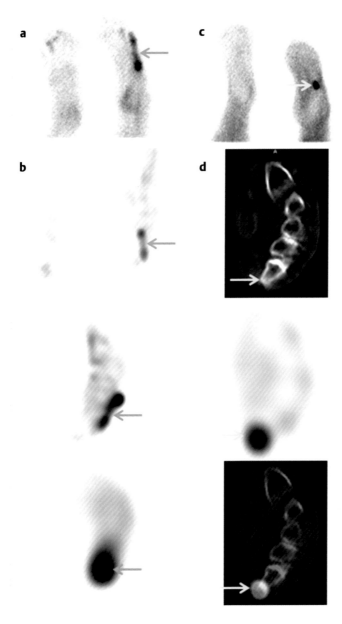

Fig. 8.8 A 70-year-old diabetic man with left foot trauma and ulceration at the base of the left fifth metatarsal bone. Skeletal scintigraphy with SPECT helped clarify the location and extent of traumatic injury, while a ^{99m}Tc-labeled WBC study with SPECT/CT confirmed the location and extent of simultaneous osteomyelitis. **(a)** Skeletal phase image of both feet from a skeletal scintigraphy study shows several sites of active osteoblastic turnover, most pronounced throughout the right fifth metatarsal bone (*orange arrow*). **(b)** MIP, sagittal, and axial SPECT images from this study, focusing on the left foot, show intense active osteoblastic turnover throughout the fifth metatarsal bone (*orange arrows*). **(c)** Planar and **(d)** axial CT, SPECT, and fused SPECT/CT images from the WBC study show active infection in the base of the fifth metatarsal bone at a site of soft tissue ulceration (*yellow arrows*). Active osteoblastic turnover elsewhere in both feet was likely related to a combination of traumatic injury and degenerative change.

- Radiotracer uptake in soft tissue with or without radiographic calcification may occur after traumatic injury. SPECT/CT can clarify focal soft tissue uptake immediately adjacent to bone, which may be misinterpreted as a bone lesion based on planar images alone (▶ Fig. 8.9).

8.3 Presurgical Planning and Postintervention Complications

The addition of hybrid imaging has increased our ability to plan surgical intervention and detect complications following therapy.

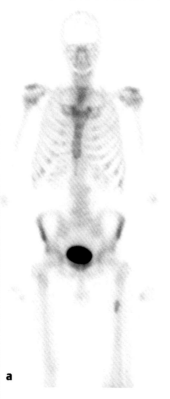

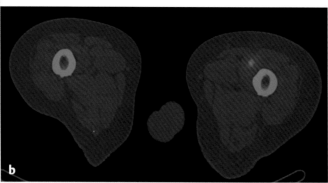

Fig. 8.9 A 67-year-old man with prostate cancer. **(a)** Planar image shows focally increased tracer uptake overlying the left femur. **(b)** On SPECT/CT, this was found to be in the soft tissue.

8.3.1 Surgical Planning

Skeletal scintigraphy with SPECT/CT is helpful in determining the anatomical location of active degenerative/arthritic change and can be used to plan the extent of fusion needed, allowing surgery to be limited to the involved joints. Also, SPECT/CT can help guide surgical intervention for osteochondral defects by showing the extent of associated active osteoblastic turnover.[2]

8.3.2 Infection

Skeletal scintigraphy with SPECT/CT can be a helpful addition to WBC imaging to determine the location of infection following surgery (▸ Fig. 8.10).

8.3.3 Postsurgical Assessment

Skeletal scintigraphy with SPECT or SPECT/CT can define the extent of osteoblastic turnover and pinpoint the cause of pain in postsurgical patients (▸ Fig. 8.11). Furthermore, SPECT is less often affected by artifact compared with CT and MRI. Active osteoblastic turnover within the first 6 to 12 months following surgery suggests bone healing, while absent uptake may be a harbinger of subsequent instability and pain. Indeed, active osteoblastic turnover has been seen at sites of bone remodeling up to 18 months postsurgery, long after the radiographic appearance suggests healing. Active osteoblastic turnover associated with facet arthropathy at the level just above or below spinal fusion may suggest ongoing spinal

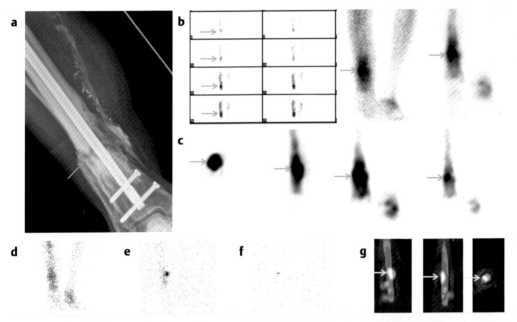

Fig. 8.10 A 73-year-old man with a history of a traumatic right distal tibial fracture. Skeletal scintigraphy with SPECT is helpful to identify the extent of active osteoblastic turnover, while WBC imaging with SPECT/CT pinpoints the site of active osteomyelitis. **(a)** Radiograph of the right distal tibia shows an intramedullary rod transfixing the distal tibial fracture with no significant bridging across the fracture, consistent with nonunion (*orange arrow*) and heterotopic ossification. **(b)** Angiographic, tissue phase, and skeletal phase skeletal scintigraphy images of the lower extremities show hyperemia and active osteoblastic turnover in the right distal tibia (*orange arrow*). **(c)** Axial, sagittal, coronal, and MIP images from the skeletal scintigraphy SPECT show active osteoblastic turnover in the right tibia distally, most intense in the region of the nonunited fracture (*orange arrow*). **(d)** ^{99m}Tc-sulfur colloid bone marrow scan, **(e)** matched In-111 WBC scan, and **(f)** subtracted images show focal active infection in the region of the right distal tibia (*yellow arrows*). **(g)** Coronal, sagittal, and axial fused SPECT/CT images from the WBC study confirm the site of active infection in the distal tibia, correlating with the site of most intense osteoblastic turnover.

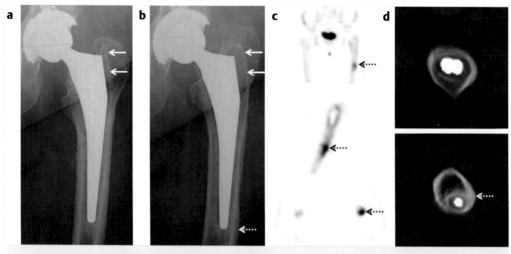

Fig. 8.11 A 58-year-old woman with left hip pain, approximately 3 years following a total left hip arthroplasty. SPECT helps to localize the extent of active osteoblastic turnover and pinpoints the site of maximal active stress at the distal tip of the femoral prosthesis. Radiographs at **(a)** 12 months and **(b)** 48 months following the right total hip arthroplasty show loosening of the femoral component of the left hip prosthesis evidenced by increasing periprosthetic lucency (*solid arrows*) and increased sclerosis adjacent to the femoral prosthesis tip (*dotted arrow*). **(c)** Coronal, sagittal, and axial SPECT images from a skeletal scintigraphy study of both hips show active osteoblastic turnover adjacent to the left femoral prosthesis shaft with focal intense active osteoblastic turnover in the region of the left femoral prosthesis tip (*dotted arrow*). **(d)** Axial CT images in the region of the mid femoral prosthesis show circumferential lucency consistent with loosening, while in the region of the femoral prosthesis tip asymmetric osseous sclerosis suggests a stress fracture (*dotted arrow*). SPECT or SPECT/CT can be helpful to identify loosening of total hip replacements.[31]

instability, while absent activity shortly following placement of a graft is suggestive of graft failure.[2]

8.4 Neoplastic Disease

Most bone tumors show some degree of radio-tracer uptake on skeletal scintigraphy. SPECT or SPECT/CT is increasingly performed for the evaluation of neoplastic disease, either benign (▶ Fig. 8.12) or malignant (▶ Fig. 8.13), due to the improved sensitivity, specificity, and reader confidence compared with planar skeletal scintigraphy. SPECT and/or SPECT/CT may significantly improve

detection of subtle radiographic or CT lesions (▶ Fig. 8.14). Furthermore, hybrid imaging can anatomically localize sites of osseous disease (▶ Fig. 8.15) and may identify unanticipated sites of osseous or nonosseous neoplastic disease (▶ Fig. 8.16).

• SPECT, and even more so SPECT/CT or SPECT fused with diagnostic CT, significantly improve the detection, localization, and characterization of neoplastic osseous disease. Furthermore, SPECT/CT may be helpful to assess cortical integrity in cases of unsuspected osseous metastatic disease to weight-bearing bones (▶ Fig. 8.17).

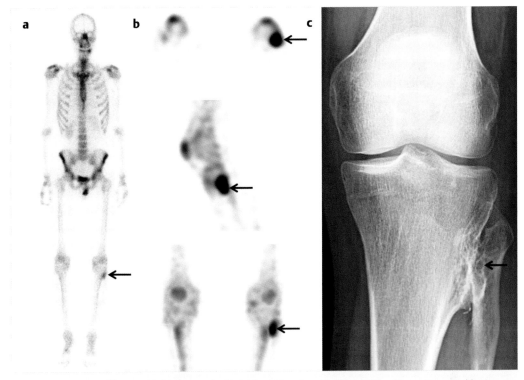

Fig. 8.12 A 25-year-old man with left knee pain. Skeletal scintigraphy with SPECT/CT localizes active osteoblastic turnover in an osteochondroma of the left lateral tibial metadiaphysis. (**a**) Whole-body skeletal phase image shows focal radiotracer uptake in the region of the left lateral tibial metadiaphysis (*arrow*). (**b**) Axial, sagittal, and coronal SPECT images localize the focal radiotracer uptake to the left posterolateral tibial metadiaphysis (*arrow*), adjacent to the fibula. (**c**) Correlating radiograph shows the active osteoblastic turnover is in an osteochondroma (*arrow*). An osteochondroma (exostosis) is a common benign bone tumor that typically arises from the femur or tibia in patients under 30 years of age.[32] Active osteoblastic turnover suggests growth at the cartilaginous cap. In this case, pain and active growth of the osteochondroma prompted surgical removal.

Even-Sapir et al found higher sensitivity and specificity for osseous disease on SPECT compared with planar scintigraphy in 44 men with high-risk prostate cancer.[13] Abikhzer et al found improved sensitivity and reader confidence on SPECT compared with planar imaging in 92 women with breast cancer.[14] Zhang et al evaluated 48 patients with bone tumors (32 malignant and 16 benign) using SPECT/CT and three-phase bone scintigraphy prior to surgical resection. The addition of SPECT/CT to planar scintigraphy improved the sensitivity (100% vs. 97%) and specificity (81% vs. 31%).[15] Palmedo et al studied 353 patients and found similar sensitivity for SPECT and SPECT/CT but higher specificity for SPECT/CT compared with SPECT (94% vs. 71%, respectively).[16] Horger et al found that SPECT/CT was able to correctly classify 88 of 104 lesions (85%) compared with 37 of 104 (36%) on SPECT in 47 patients with osseous disease.[17]

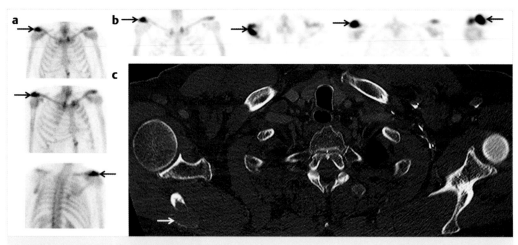

Fig. 8.13 A 59-year-old man with locally advanced esophageal cancer and right scapular pain for evaluation of osseous disease. Skeletal scintigraphy with SPECT localizes active osteoblastic turnover to a destructive right scapular metastasis. **(a)** Skeletal phase images in anterior, RAO, and RPO projections of the thorax show active osteoblastic turnover in the region of the right scapula (*arrows*). **(b)** MIP, axial, coronal, and sagittal SPECT images localize the active osteoblastic turnover to the right scapular spine (arrows). **(c)** Diagnostic CT image shows a destructive osseous metastasis in the right scapular spine correlating with the active osteoblastic turnover (*arrow*). This was the only site of osseous metastatic disease.

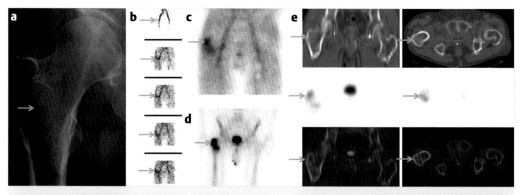

Fig. 8.14 A 76-year-old man with prostate cancer and subtle sclerosis on radiographs and CT at a site of osseous metastasis identified and localized on skeletal scintigraphy with SPECT/CT. **(a)** Radiograph of the right proximal femur shows subtle sclerosis in the intertrochanteric region (*arrow*). **(b)** Angiographic, **(c)** tissue phase, and **(d)** skeletal phase images from a skeletal scintigraphy study show hyperemia and active osteoblastic turnover in the intertrochanteric region of the right femur (arrows). **(e)** Coronal and axial CT, SPECT, and fused SPECT/CT images of the hips show focal osteoblastic turnover correlating with subtle intertrochanteric sclerosis of the right femur at a site of metastatic disease (*arrows*).

SPECT fused with diagnostic CT also provides superior osseous lesion characterization compared to SPECT and/or planar scintigraphy.[18]

- SPECT and SPECT/CT improve the detection and characterization of nonosseous disease. Wuest et al found that 7% of patients who had SPECT/CT of the thoracic spine at the time of staging had unsuspected sites of nonosseous disease.[19]

- ^{18}F-NaF (sodium fluoride) positron emission tomography (PET)/CT and MRI are slightly more sensitive and specific than skeletal scintigraphy, even when combined with SPECT, particularly with lytic disease. In a study of 10 patients with metastatic renal cell carcinoma to bone, ^{18}F-NaF PET/CT was more sensitive for the detection of osseous lesions than diagnostic CT or bone

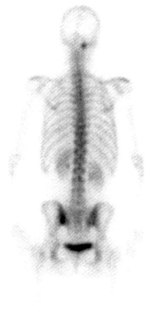

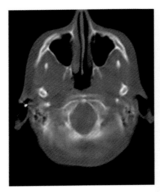

Fig. 8.15 A 50-year-old woman with breast cancer for evaluation of osseous metastasis. SPECT/CT localizes a site of osseous metastatic disease to the right occipital bone. **(a)** Posterior projection whole-body skeletal phase image shows focal radiotracer uptake in the right skull base, left sacral wing, and left lesser trochanter. **(b)** CT, SPECT, and fused SPECT/CT images of the skull base show that the site of active osteoblastic turnover localizes to the right occipital bone at a site of osseous metastasis.

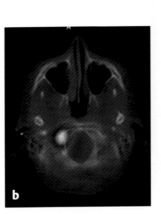

a   b

scintigraphy with SPECT of the pelvis.[20] In a meta-analysis, Shen et al concluded that MRI was superior to planar skeletal scintigraphy with SPECT for diagnosing bone metastases in men with prostate cancer: the pooled sensitivities were 97% versus 79% and pooled specificities were 95% versus 82%.[21]

8.4.1 Pearls

- The addition of SPECT or SPECT/CT to planar skeletal scintigraphy can be particularly helpful to improve diagnostic accuracy and confidence in identifying and characterizing developmental bone defects (▶ Fig. 8.18), benign versus malignant features of osseous disease, and spine pathology.
- A bone scan is done at the time of breast and prostate cancer staging only if the patient is symptomatic or considered to be at increased risk for metastases. SPECT or SPECT/CT can be helpful to detect occult fractures in these patients, particularly when planar imaging is normal and there is a high pretest likelihood of metastases.

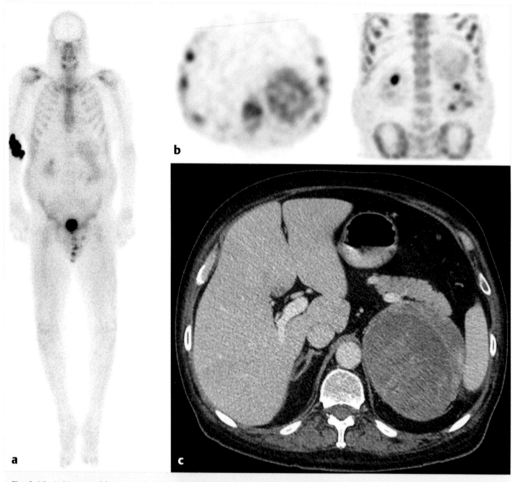

Fig. 8.16 A 61-year-old man with left rib pain for evaluation of osseous disease. Skeletal scintigraphy with SPECT localizes the abnormality to the left upper abdomen in the region of the adrenal gland. **(a)** Skeletal phase whole-body image in the anterior projection shows radiotracer uptake in the left upper abdomen. **(b)** Axial SPECT and MIP images localize the radiotracer uptake to the left adrenal fossa. **(c)** Diagnostic CT shows a complex soft tissue mass associated with the left adrenal gland that was subsequently proven to be an adrenal cortical carcinoma on pathology.

- Bone scan with SPECT has limited sensitivity for lytic metastases, such as those from lung cancer, renal cell carcinoma, thyroid cancer, or multiple myeloma. SPECT/CT may increase the sensitivity as lytic lesions can be detected by CT. In general, fluorine-18 fluorodeoxyglucose PET/CT is preferred for lung cancer staging. ^{18}F-NaF PET/CT and MRI are also helpful for the detection and characterization of neoplastic osseous disease, although their most appropriate use remains a topic of research.

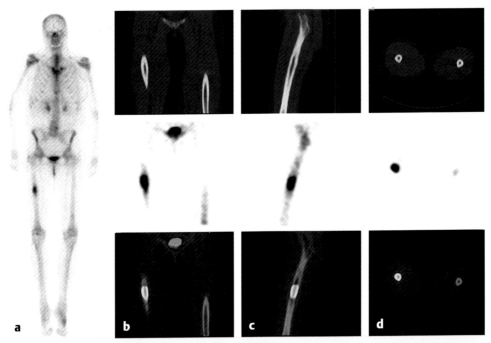

Fig. 8.17 A 51-year-old woman with previously resected melanoma of the right upper extremity and right leg pain for further evaluation following negative radiographs. Planar skeletal scintigraphy detected the new solitary osseous metastasis in the right femoral diaphysis at the site of pain. SPECT/CT localized the metastasis to the intramedullary canal and showed intact cortical integrity. **(a)** Anterior projection whole-body skeletal phase image and **(b)** coronal, **(c)** sagittal, and **(d)** axial CT, SPECT, and fused SPECT/CT images show the solitary osseous metastasis in the right femoral diaphysis with preserved cortical integrity. Malignancy associated with melanoma, renal cancer, and lung cancer has a predilection to metastasize to the extremities. Older age, aggressive histology, and more comorbidities are associated with higher postoperative risk following pathological fracture fixation.[33]

- A "flare" phenomenon may be seen on SPECT or SPECT/CT. This occurs within 3 months and lasts up to 6 months after chemotherapy or hormonal therapy. It manifests as apparent interval worsening of disease with more intense uptake of known lesions that correspond to healing osteoblastic activity. This phenomenon may or may not be accompanied by apparent "new" lesions. After 6 months, such findings reflect progression of disease.

8.5 Special Considerations

8.5.1 Solitary Focal Lesions: Advantages of SPECT and SPECT/CT

- Focal calvarial activity is seen in less than 1% of bone scans and is most commonly due to small cartilaginous rests, sutural foramina, or enlarged pacchionian granulations.[22] Even if there is a known history of malignancy, solitary focal calvarial or solitary focal rib lesions

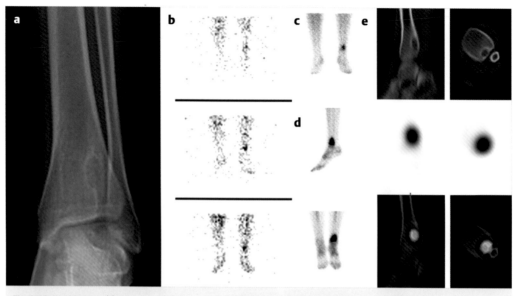

Fig. 8.18 An 18-year-old woman with left ankle pain. Skeletal scintigraphy with SPECT/CT pinpoints the active osteoblastic turnover to a nonossifying fibroma. **(a)** Radiograph of the left ankle shows a lytic lesion in the left distal tibia with a well-defined, thin, sclerotic rim (characteristic of nonaggressive osseous lesions). **(b)** Angiographic, **(c)** tissue phase, and **(d)** skeletal phase images from a skeletal scintigraphy study of the lower extremities show hyperemia and active osteoblastic turnover in the distal left tibia. **(e)** Sagittal and axial CT, SPECT, and fused SPECT/CT images from the skeletal scintigraphy study localize the active osteoblastic turnover to the lytic lesion with thin sclerotic rim consistent with a nonossifying fibroma. A nonossifying fibroma is a common benign fibrous bone lesion thought to be a developmental defect, typically found in the long bones, such as the femur or tibia of children and young adults. At the time of ossification, a nonossifying fibroma can show intense osteoblastic turnover on skeletal scintigraphy. These lesions are typically followed-up conservatively.[34]

are suspicious for benign variants or traumatic injury, respectively. Rarely, SPECT/CT will show a correlating abnormality suggestive of metastasis. If the site of focal activity is equivocal following skeletal scintigraphy and will change patient management should this be malignant, correlative diagnostic imaging for further characterization or short interval follow-up bone scan to establish stability is suggested.

- If there is a known history of malignancy, a solitary focal site of radiotracer uptake in the spine

or sternum (▶ Fig. 8.19) is suspicious for metastasis.

8.5.2 Pediatric Imaging

- Skeletal scintigraphy with SPECT or SPECT/CT is becoming the standard of care in the evaluation of pediatric back pain, sports-related injury, and neoplastic disease, such as osseous metastases from neuroblastoma. The addition of CT may decrease the need for additional imaging studies

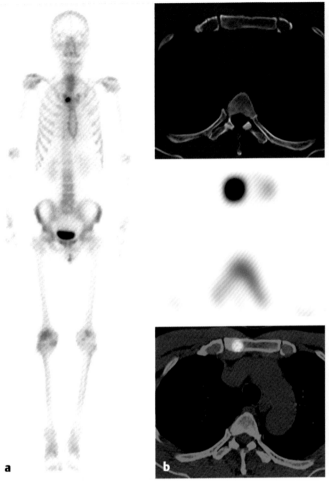

Fig. 8.19 A 50-year-old woman with breast cancer for evaluation of osseous disease. Skeletal scintigraphy with SPECT localizes a solitary osseous metastasis to the right lateral manubrium. **(a)** Skeletal phase whole-body image in the anterior projection shows focal radiotracer uptake in the manubrium. **(b)** Axial CT, SPECT, and fused SPECT/CT images of the manubrium show intense focal radiotracer uptake reflecting active osteoblastic turnover correlating with a mixed lytic and sclerotic osseous metastasis in the right lateral manubrium on CT.

and sedation; however, each study should be tailored to the patient to optimize value while minimizing radiation exposure. Children younger than 6 years who require diagnostic quality CT for coregistration with SPECT may need sedation, although sedation is rarely required for SPECT/CT of musculoskeletal disorders.[23] Typically, a noncontrast, nonattenuation-corrected limited CT is performed over the area of interest to clarify an area of abnormality while minimizing radiation exposure.

- SPECT or SPECT/CT can be particularly helpful for the evaluation of back pain related to transitional vertebrae or stress in the region of the pars interarticularis (▶ Fig. 8.20).[24,25] Connolly et al studied 48 children (6–19 years of age) and identified increased activity associated with a transitional vertebra in 81% on planar skeletal scintigraphy with SPECT compared with conventional radiographs, CT, and MRI that showed an abnormality in 21%, 55%, and 63%, respectively.[26] In a study of 213 children with low back pain by Gregory et al, 68% had an abnormality on SPECT/CT.[27]

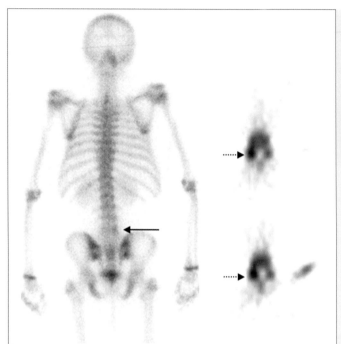

Fig. 8.20 A 16-year-old boy with low back pain. Posterior planar image (left) shows mildly increased radiotracer uptake in the lower lumbar spine (*solid arrow*). Selected axial SPECT images show clearly increased uptake in the right pars region (*dotted arrows*), consistent with active osteoblastic turnover and stress at a site of spondylolysis.

- Mandibular asymmetry may be due to generalized mandibular hypertrophy or condylar hyperplasia (i.e., overgrowth) or hemifacial microsomia (i.e., undergrowth). Treatment may vary depending on the cause of the mandibular asymmetry. Skeletal scintigraphy with SPECT or SPECT/CT can be particularly helpful for surgical planning for mandibular growth asymmetry (► Fig. 8.21).[28]

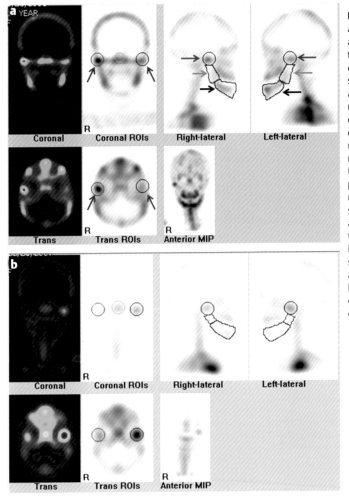

Fig. 8.21 (a) Red, blue, and black arrows indicate the condyle, ramus, and body of the mandible, respectively, in a 16-year-old girl with mandibular asymmetry. Compared to standard values obtained from an age- and sex-matched control group, the radiotracer uptake value normalized to external standard counts was significantly low in the left condyle and normal in the right condyle, bilateral rami, and body of the mandible. The final diagnosis was left condylar hypoplasia. (b) A 12-year-old girl with mandibular asymmetry. Compared to standard values obtained from the age- and sex-matched control group, the radiotracer uptake value normalized to external standard counts was significantly high in the left condyle and normal in the right condyle, bilateral rami, and body of the mandible. The final diagnosis was left condylar hyperplasia.

References

[1] Zhong ZA, Peck A, Li S, et al. (99m)TC-Methylene diphosphonate uptake at injury site correlates with osteoblast differentiation and mineralization during bone healing in mice. Bone Res. 2015;3:15013

[2] Scharf SC. Bone SPECT/CT in skeletal trauma. Semin Nucl Med. 2015;45(1):47–57

[3] Al-faham Z, Rydberg JN, Oliver Wong CY. Use of SPECT/CT with 99mTc-MDP bone scintigraphy to diagnose sacral insufficiency fracture. J Nucl Med Technol. 2014;42(3):240–241

[4] Linke R, Kuwert T, Uder M, Forst R, Wuest W. Skeletal SPECT/CT of the peripheral extremities. AJR Am J Roentgenol. 2010;194(4):W329–W335

[5] Scheyerer MJ, Hüllner M, Pietsch C, Werner CM, Veit-Haibach P. Evaluation of pelvic ring injuries using SPECT/CT. Skeletal Radiol. 2015;44(2):217–222

[6] Allainmat L, Aubault M, Noël V, Baulieu F, Laulan J, Eder V. Use of hybrid SPECT/CT for diagnosis of radiographic occult fractures of the wrist. Clin Nucl Med. 2013;38(6):e246–e251

[7] Nadel HR. Bone scan update. Semin Nucl Med. 2007;37(5):332–339

[8] Even-Sapir E, Flusser G, Lerman H, Lievshitz G, Metser U. SPECT/multislice low-dose CT: a clinically relevant constituent in the imaging algorithm of nononcologic patients referred for bone scintigraphy. J Nucl Med. 2007;48(2):319–324

[9] Treglia G, Focacci C, Caldarella C, et al. The role of nuclear medicine in the diagnosis of spondylodiscitis. Eur Rev Med Pharmacol Sci. 2012;16 Suppl 2:20–25

[10] Kim CK, Park KW. Characteristic appearance of facet osteoarthritis of the lower lumbar spine on planar bone scintigraphy with a high negative predictive value for metastasis. Clin Nucl Med. 2008;33(4):251–254

[11] Wertman M, Milgrom C, Agar G, Milgrom Y, Yalom N, Finestone AS. Comparison of knee SPECT and MRI in evaluating meniscus injuries in soldiers. Isr Med Assoc J. 2014;16(11):703–706

[12] Kamaleshwaran KK, Asokumar P, Malaikkal A, Mohanan V, Shinto AS. Hybrid single-photon emission computed tomography/computed tomography imaging features of tumoral calcinosis in technetium-99 m methylene diphosphonate bone scintigraphy. World J Nucl Med. 2015;14(2):137–139

[13] Even-Sapir E, Metser U, Mishani E, Lievshitz G, Lerman H, Leibovitch I. The detection of bone metastases in patients with high-risk prostate cancer: 99mTc-MDP planar bone scintigraphy, single- and multi-field-of-view SPECT, 18F-fluoride PET, and 18F-fluoride PET/CT. J Nucl Med. 2006;47(2):287–297

[14] Abikhzer G, Gourevich K, Kagna O, et al. Whole-body bone SPECT in breast cancer patients: the future bone scan protocol? Nucl Med Commun. 2016;37(3):247–253

[15] Zhang Y, Shi H, Li B, et al. Diagnostic value of 99mTc-MDP SPECT/spiral CT combined with three-phase bone scintigraphy in assessing suspected bone tumors in patients with no malignant history. Nucl Med Commun. 2015;36(7):686–694

[16] Palmedo H, Marx C, Ebert A, et al. Whole-body SPECT/CT for bone scintigraphy: diagnostic value and effect on patient management in oncological patients. Eur J Nucl Med Mol Imaging. 2014;41(1):59–67

[17] Horger M, Eschmann SM, Pfannenberg C, et al. Evaluation of combined transmission and emission tomography for classification of skeletal lesions. AJR Am J Roentgenol. 2004;183 (3):655–661

[18] Strobel K, Burger C, Seifert B, Husarik DB, Soyka JD, Hany TF. Characterization of focal bone lesions in the axial skeleton: performance of planar bone scintigraphy compared with SPECT and SPECT fused with CT. AJR Am J Roentgenol. 2007; 188(5):W467–W474

[19] Wuest W, Lell M, May MS, et al. Thoracic non-osseous lesions in cancer patients detected in low-dose CT images acquired as part of skeletal SPECT/CT examinations. Nucl Med (Stuttg). 2015;54(4):173–177

[20] Gerety EL, Lawrence EM, Wason J, et al. Prospective study evaluating the relative sensitivity of 18F-NaF PET/CT for detecting skeletal metastases from renal cell carcinoma in comparison to multidetector CT and 99mTc-MDP bone scintigraphy, using an adaptive trial design. Ann Oncol. 2015;26 (10):2113–2118

[21] Shen G, Deng H, Hu S, Jia Z. Comparison of choline-PET/CT, MRI, SPECT, and bone scintigraphy in the diagnosis of bone metastases in patients with prostate cancer: a meta-analysis. Skeletal Radiol. 2014;43(11):1503–1513

[22] Harbert J, Desai R. Small calvarial bone scan foci—normal variations. J Nucl Med. 1985;26(10):1144–1148

[23] Nadel HR. SPECT/CT in pediatric patient management. Eur J Nucl Med Mol Imaging. 2014;41 Suppl 1:S104–S114

[24] Miller R, Beck NA, Sampson NR, Zhu X, Flynn JM, Drummond D. Imaging modalities for low back pain in children: a review of spondyloysis and undiagnosed mechanical back pain. J Pediatr Orthop. 2013;33(3):282–288

[25] Campbell RS, Grainger AJ, Hide IG, Papastefanou S, Greenough CG. Juvenile spondylolysis: a comparative analysis of CT, SPECT and MRI. Skeletal Radiol. 2005;34(2):63–73

[26] Connolly LP, d'Hemecourt PA, Connolly SA, Drubach LA, Micheli LJ, Treves ST. Skeletal scintigraphy of young patients with low-back pain and a lumbosacral transitional vertebra. J Nucl Med. 2003;44(6):909–914

[27] Gregory PL, Batt ME, Kerslake RW, Webb JK. Single photon emission computerized tomography and reverse gantry computerized tomography findings in patients with back pain investigated for spondylolysis. Clin J Sport Med. 2005;15 (2):79–86

[28] Fahey FH, Abramson ZR, Padwa BL, et al. Use of (99m)Tc-MDP SPECT for assessment of mandibular growth: development of normal values. Eur J Nucl Med Mol Imaging. 2010; 37(5):1002–1010

[29] Hossain M, Clutton J, Ridgewell M, Lyons K, Perera A. Stress fractures of the foot. Clin Sports Med. 2015;34(4):769–790

[30] Prince MR, King AH, Stuart MJ, Dahm DL, Krych AJ. Treatment of patellofemoral cartilage lesions in the young, active patient. J Knee Surg. 2015;28(4):285–295

[31] Tam HH, Bhaludin B, Rahman F, Weller A, Ejindu V, Parthipun A. SPECT-CT in total hip arthroplasty. Clin Radiol. 2014;69 (1):82–95

[32] Hakim DN, Pelly T, Kulendran M, Caris JA. Benign tumours of the bone: a review. J Bone Oncol. 2015;4(2):37–41

[33] Tsuda Y, Yasunaga H, Horiguchi H, Fushimi K, Kawano H, Tanaka S. Complications and postoperative mortality rate after surgery for pathologic femur fracture related to bone metastasis: analysis of a nationwide database. Ann Surg Oncol. 2016;23(3):801–810

[34] Hod N, Levi Y, Fire G, et al. Scintigraphic characteristics of non-ossifying fibroma in military recruits undergoing bone scintigraphy for suspected stress fractures and lower limb pains. Nucl Med Commun. 2007;28(1):25–33

9 SPECT/CT for Infection and Inflammation

Christopher J. Palestro

9.1 Introduction

The detection and localization of inflammation and infection with nuclear medicine techniques have been studied for nearly half a century. A major advantage of radionuclide, or functional, imaging tests compared to anatomical imaging tests is the ability to provide information early in the course of a disease process, that is, prior to the development of anatomical or structural changes. Functional imaging unfortunately does not always provide the anatomical detail necessary to differentiate physiological from pathological processes. This limitation has been largely overcome with the introduction of hybrid imaging, which is redefining the diagnostic workup of patients with suspected or known infection and inflammation. In addition to improving diagnostic accuracy, hybrid imaging also affects patient management. This chapter reviews the role of single-photon emission computed tomography/computed tomography (SPECT/CT) in inflammation and infection.

9.2 Procedures

9.2.1 Bone Scintigraphy

Bone scintigraphy is performed with technetium-99 m (^{99m}Tc)-labeled diphosphonates. Radiopharmaceutical uptake depends on blood flow and the rate of new bone formation. The procedure is usually performed as a three-phase bone scan for suspected osteomyelitis: the flow, or perfusion, phase acquired immediately after radiopharmaceutical injection, followed immediately by the blood pool, or soft tissue, phase. The third, or bone, phase is performed 2 to 4 hours later. On three-phase bone scintigraphy, osteomyelitis typically presents as focal hyperperfusion, focal hyperemia, and focal bone uptake (▶ Fig. 9.1). It is important to remember that abnormalities on bone scintigraphy reflect the rate of new bone formation in general, not infection specifically.[1]

Advantages

- Widely available.
- Relatively inexpensive.
- Rapidly completed (2–4 hours).
- Extremely sensitive: becomes positive within 2 days after onset of symptoms.
- Accuracy exceeds 90% in the setting of unviolated bone.

Disadvantage

- Decreased specificity in the presence of underlying bony conditions (fracture, orthopaedic hardware, neuropathic joint, tumor, and so on).

9.2.2 Gallium-67 Imaging

Gallium-67 (^{67}Ga) has a half-life of 78 hours and emits gamma radiation with four energy peaks suitable for imaging: 93 keV (40%), 184 keV (24%), 296 keV (22%), and 388 keV (7%). By 24 hours after injection, 10 to 25% of the administered dose is excreted via the kidneys. Beyond 24 hours, the

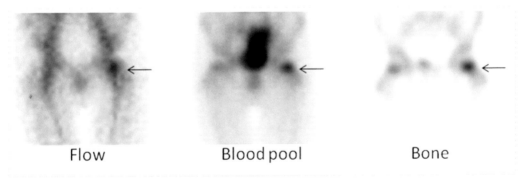

Fig. 9.1 Left femoral osteomyelitis. There is focal hyperperfusion, focal hyperemia, and focally increased bone uptake (*arrows*) of radiopharmaceutical in the left femoral head/neck of a 3-year-old child. This is a classic presentation of osteomyelitis on three-phase bone scintigraphy.

colon is the principal excretory pathway. At 48 to 72 hours after injection, when imaging is usually performed, about 75% of the injected dose remains in the body, distributed among soft tissues, liver, and bone/bone marrow (▶ Fig. 9.2). This "normal" distribution, however, is subject to considerable variation. Nasopharyngeal and lacrimal gland activity can be prominent. Breast uptake can be intense in pregnant and lactating women as well as in other hyperprolactinemic states. Normally, healing surgical incisions concentrate ^{67}Ga for variable time periods. The biodistribution can be altered by blood transfusions and the magnetic resonance imaging (MRI) contrast agent gadolinium, with increased skeletal and urinary tract and decreased hepatic and colonic activity.[2]

[67]Ga uptake in inflammation and infection likely depends on several factors. Approximately 99% of circulating gallium is in the plasma, nearly all transferrin bound. The increased blood flow and vascular membrane permeability associated with inflammation result in increased ^{67}Ga delivery and accumulation at inflammatory sites. Lactoferrin, another plasma protein, is present in high concentrations in inflammatory exudates. [67]Ga is presumably transported via transferrin to inflammatory foci, where it dissociates from transferrin and complexes with lactoferrin. Bacteria are also involved in ^{67}Ga uptake in infection, probably through nonspecific binding and facilitated diffusion. Small-molecule metal chelates known as siderophores, which are produced by bacteria, are ^{67}Ga-avid. The siderophore–[67]Ga complex is transported into the bacterium, from which it cannot be released without destruction of the entire molecule. Some ^{67}Ga may be bound to leukocytes and transported by leukocytes to inflammatory foci,

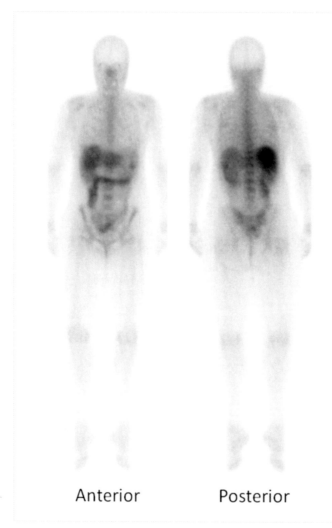

Anterior   Posterior

Fig. 9.2 Normal ^{67}Ga scan. Anterior and posterior whole-body images obtained about 48 hours postinjection. Activity is distributed among soft tissues, including the bowel, liver, and bone/bone marrow.

but this is probably a relatively unimportant mechanism. There are ample data confirming ^{67}Ga accumulation in infection, even in the absence of circulating white cells.[2]

Advantages

- Detects inflammation and infection.
- Sensitive in immunocompromised individuals.

Disadvantages

- Nonspecific accumulation in tumor, at sites of recent surgery, and at sites of new bone formation.
- A delay of 24 to 72 hours between injection and imaging.
- Variable biodistribution.
- Low-resolution images.

9.2.3 In Vitro Labeled Leukocyte Imaging

In vitro leukocyte (white blood cell [WBC]) labeling is most often performed with either ^{111}In-oxyquinolone or ^{99m}Tc-exametazime (HMPAO). Labeled leukocyte uptake depends on intact chemotaxis, which is not an issue with routine in vitro labeling procedures, the number and types of cells labeled, and the cellular component of a particular inflammatory response. A total circulating WBC count of at least 2,000/u is needed to obtain satisfactory images. Usually, the majority of leukocytes labeled are neutrophils, and the procedure is most sensitive for identifying neutrophil-mediated inflammatory processes, such as bacterial infections. WBC imaging is less useful for those illnesses in which the predominant cellular response is not neutrophilic, that is, sarcoidosis.[3]

Regardless of whether the white cells are labeled with ^{111}In or ^{99m}Tc, images obtained shortly after injection are characterized by intense pulmonary activity. This activity, which clears rapidly and reaches background levels within 4 hours after injection, is probably due to leukocyte activation during labeling, which impedes cellular movement through the pulmonary vascular bed, slowing passage through the lungs.[3]

^{111}In-WBC

The usual adult administered activity is 10 to 20 MBq (0.3–0.5 mCi). Imaging is typically performed 18 to 30 hours after injection. The advantages of using ^{111}In as the radiolabel include label stability and, at 24 hours postinjection, a normal distribution of activity limited to the liver, spleen, and bone marrow (▶ Fig. 9.3). The 67-hour half-life of ^{111}In allows for delayed imaging. Patients with musculoskeletal infection may need to undergo bone marrow scintigraphy, which can be performed while the patient's cells are being labeled, as part of a simultaneous dual-isotope acquisition with ^{111}In-WBC imaging, or after completion of the ^{111}In-WBC study. Disadvantages include suboptimal photon energies, low-resolution images, and the 18- to 30-hour interval between injection and imaging.[3]

^{99m}Tc-WBC

The usual administered activity is 185 to 370 MBq (5–10 mCi). The normal biodistribution of ^{99m}Tc-WBC is more variable than that of ^{111}In-WBC. In addition to the reticuloendothelial system, activity is normally present in the urinary tract, large bowel (within 4 hours after injection), blood pool, and occasionally the gallbladder (▶ Fig. 9.4). The time interval between injection and imaging varies with the indication; imaging is usually performed within a few hours after injection.[3]

Advantages of using ^{99m}Tc as the radiolabel include a photon energy that is optimal for imaging using current instrumentation, a high photon flux, and the ability to detect abnormalities within a few hours after injection. This is especially important when performing SPECT/CT. Disadvantages include urinary tract activity, which appears shortly after injection, and bowel activity, which appears by 4 hours after injection. The instability of the label and short half-life of ^{99m}Tc are disadvantages when delayed 24-hour imaging is needed. Simultaneous dual-isotope imaging, of course, is not possible, and when bone or bone marrow imaging is necessary, an interval of 48 to 72 hours is required between the two tests.[3]

White Blood Cell/Marrow Imaging

WBC imaging, which is the radionuclide test of choice for diagnosing most cases of complicating osteomyelitis, must often be performed in conjunction with bone marrow imaging to maximize accuracy. This is because leukocytes accumulate in both infection and in the bone marrow. The normal distribution of hematopoietically active bone marrow in adults is very variable. Systemic diseases cause generalized alterations in marrow distribution,

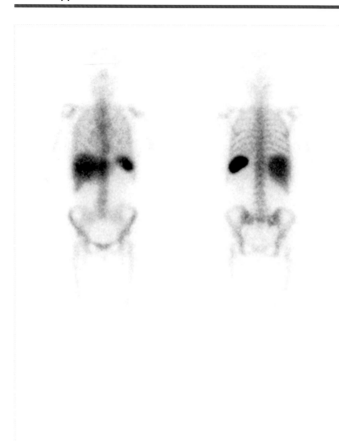

Anterior   Posterior

while fractures, orthopaedic hardware, neuropathic joints, trauma, and heterotopic bone cause localized alterations. In children, the normal distribution of hematopoietically active marrow varies with age. It is not always possible to determine if activity on a WBC image indicates infection or bone marrow. This difficulty can be overcome by performing [99mTc]-sulfur colloid bone marrow (marrow) imaging. Leukocytes and sulfur colloid both accumulate in bone marrow; leukocytes also accumulate in infection, while sulfur colloid does not. WBC/marrow imaging is positive for infection when activity is present on the WBC image without corresponding activity on the marrow image (▶ Fig. 9.5, ▶ Fig. 9.6). The overall accuracy of WBC/marrow imaging is approximately 90%.[4]

Advantages of White Blood Cell Imaging

- Specific for neutrophil-mediated processes, such as bacterial infections.
- Accurately diagnoses complicating osteomyelitis.

Disadvantages of White Blood Cell Imaging

- Labor-intensive labeling process.
- Not always available.
- Usually needs to be combined with bone marrow imaging for musculoskeletal infection.
- Difficult to perform in leukopenic patients and children.

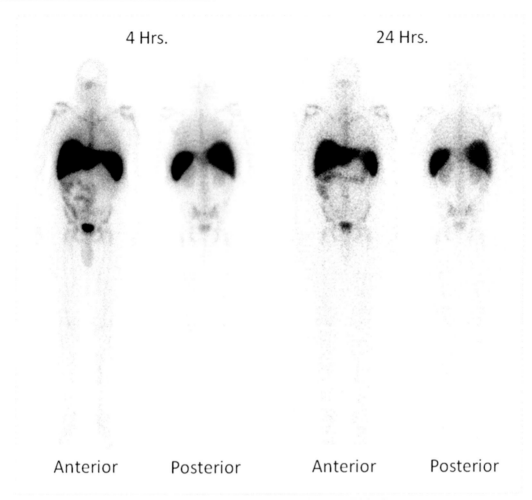

4 Hrs.

24 Hrs.

Anterior   Posterior   Anterior   Posterior

Fig. 9.4 Normal ^{99m}Tc-labeled autologous leukocyte scan at 4 and 24 hours postinjection. In addition to reticuloendothelial system uptake of labeled leukocytes, small bowel and urinary tract activities are present on the 4-hour images. At 24 hours, urinary tract activity persists, and bowel activity has moved into the colon. Image quality has deteriorated by 24 hours due to the short half-life of ^{99m}Tc. It is important to recognize that bowel and urinary tract activities are secondary to elution of ^{99m}Tc from the leukocytes, not labeled leukocyte accumulation in these structures.

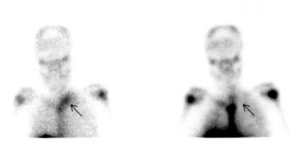

^{111}In-WBC ^{99m}Tc sulfur colloid

Fig. 9.5 On the ^{111}In-labeled autologous leukocyte image (left), the left clavicle (*arrow*) is slightly larger and more intense than the right clavicle. On the bone marrow image (right), there is a well-defined photopenic defect (*arrow*) in the medial half of the left clavicle. The combined study is positive for osteomyelitis.

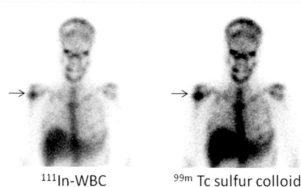

Fig. 9.6 Focal hypercellular marrow. Interpreted in isolation, the increased activity in the right humeral head (*arrow*) on the ^{111}In-labeled leukocyte image performed on a patient with sickle cell disease (left) could easily be mistaken for osteomyelitis. On the bone marrow image (right), the distribution of activity in the right humeral head (*arrow*) is virtually identical to that on the labeled leukocyte image. The combined study is negative for osteomyelitis. The intensity of uptake on labeled leukocyte images is not useful for determining the presence or absence of osteomyelitis.

^{111}In-WBC   [99m]Tc sulfur colloid

9.2.4 In Vivo Labeled Leukocytes

In vivo techniques for WBC labeling using antigranulocyte antibodies and antibody fragments have been explored as alternatives to the in vitro labeling procedure. Besilesomab is a murine monoclonal G1 immunoglobulin that binds to the normal cross-reactive antigen (NCA)-95 antigen on leukocytes. About 10% of the injected activity is neutrophil bound at 45 minutes after injection; 20% of the activity circulates freely in the blood. Studies usually become positive by 6 hours after injection, although delayed imaging may increase lesion detection. Up to 40% of the injected dose accumulates in the bone marrow, which can obscure small foci of infection.[1] Besilesomab incites a human antimurine antibody (HAMA) response in up to 30% of individuals receiving this agent. Patients should be prescreened for HAMA. A positive result is a contraindication to the procedure. Because of immunogenicity concerns, patients should not undergo repeat studies with this agent.[5]

Antibody fragments do not induce a HAMA response and are a potential alternative to whole antibodies. Sulesomab is a 50-kD fragment antigen binding (Fab´) portion of a murine monoclonal IgG1 class antibody that binds to NCA-90 present on leukocytes. NCA-90 is also present on the macrophage–monocyte cell lineage, in normal colonic mucosa, and in colonic adenocarcinoma. The exact uptake mechanisms of sulesomab are somewhat controversial. Some data suggest that sulesomab not only binds to circulating neutrophils, which then migrate to foci of infection, but also crosses permeable capillary membranes and binds to leukocytes already present at sites of infection. Other data, however, suggest that sulesomab does not bind to circulating leukocytes; rather, it accumulates nonspecifically through increased capillary membrane permeability.[5]

9.2.5 Other Radiopharmaceuticals

Radiolabeled synthetic fragments of ubiquicidin, a human antimicrobial peptide that targets bacteria, possess the ability to differentiate infection from sterile inflammation and may be useful for monitoring the efficacy of antibacterial agents in certain infections.[5]

Biotin is used as a growth factor by certain bacteria. ^{111}In-labeled biotin has been used in the evaluation of patients with suspected spinal infections.[5]

9.3 Specific Indications

Adding SPECT/CT to conventional scintigraphic imaging of infection and inflammation increases reader confidence and improves accuracy by increasing the specificity of the test and better defining the location and extent of the infection (▶ Fig. 9.7). SPECT/CT has proven to be especially useful in the evaluation of cardiovascular and musculoskeletal infections.

9.3.1 Cardiovascular Infections

Infective Endocarditis

Imaging plays a key role in the diagnosis of infective endocarditis (IE). Echocardiography is useful for diagnosis, risk stratification, prognosis, guiding treatment (medical vs. surgical), and monitoring response to treatment. The major echocardiographic

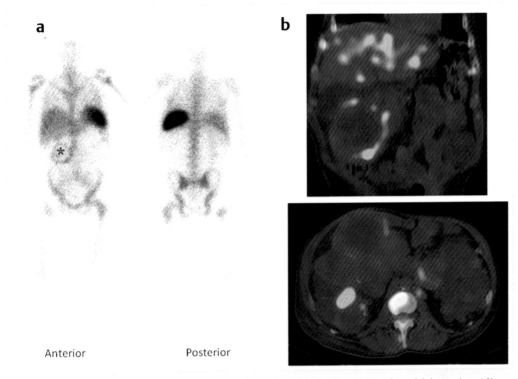

a Anterior   Posterior

b

Fig. 9.7 Infected renal cyst. **(a)** There is a circumferential area of increased activity in the right midabdomen (*asterisk*) on the ^{111}In-labeled autologous leukocyte whole-body scan. More precise localization of this focus is not possible. **(b)** On the coronal and axial SPECT/CT images, the abnormal activity is localized to a renal cyst (*asterisk*) in a patient with polycystic kidney disease.

criteria for IE are vegetation and abscess. The sensitivity for diagnosis of vegetations is 75% for transthoracic echocardiography (TTE) and 85 to 90% for transesophageal echocardiography (TEE). Abscess is the second most typical finding associated with IE. The sensitivities of TTE and TEE for detecting abscesses are about 50 and 90%, respectively. Although echocardiography is the primary imaging modality used to diagnose IE, there are limitations to the test. Atypical findings are frequent, and the test may be false-negative in up to 15% of patients in whom there are preexisting conditions, such as mitral valve prolapse, and in the presence of prosthetic valves.[6]

Until recently, the use of radionuclide imaging in suspected IE was limited. The development of hybrid imaging has stimulated renewed interest in radionuclide imaging for diagnosing IE and its complications. Although most investigations have focused on fluorine-18 fluorodeoxyglucose (^{18}F-FDG) positron emission tomography/CT (PET/CT), labeled leukocyte SPECT/CT shows considerable promise. Erba et al[7] assessed the value of ^{99m}Tc-WBC scintigraphy including SPECT/CT in 131 consecutive patients with suspected IE. Results were correlated with TTE or TEE, blood cultures, and the Duke criteria. These investigators reported that ^{99m}Tc-WBC SPECT/CT was 96% (46/51) sensitive and 100% specific (80/80) for IE. Extracardiac uptake of ^{99m}Tc-WBC was present in nearly half of the patients with IE. ^{99m}Tc-WBC SPECT/CT was useful in patients with possible IE by the Duke criteria. The scan was especially valuable in patients with negative or difficult-to-interpret echocardiograms. Three patients with marantic vegetations who had false-positive echocardiograms were true negative on ^{99m}Tc-WBC SPECT/CT. These investigators concluded that ^{99m}Tc-WBC SPECT/CT reduces the rate of misdiagnosis of IE when combined with standard diagnostic tests when clinical suspicion is high but echocardiography is inconclusive; when there is a need to differentiate between septic and sterile vegetations detected on echocardiography; when echocardiographic, laboratory, and clinical data are contradictory, and when valve involvement (especially prosthetic valves) needs to be excluded during febrile episodes, sepsis, or postoperative infections.

IE is a serious complication of valve replacement that occurs in up to 6% of patients with prosthetic valves. The diagnosis of IE by echocardiography is more difficult when a prosthetic valve is involved than when a native valve is involved. The Duke criteria are less helpful in prosthetic valve endocarditis (PVE) because of lower sensitivity. TEE is mandatory in the evaluation of suspected PVE because of its higher sensitivity and specificity for the detection of vegetations, abscesses, and perivalvular lesions in patients with prosthetic valves.[6] Hyafil et al[8] studied 42 patients with suspected PVE and reported that patient management was affected by the results of ^{99m}Tc-WBC SPECT/CT in 12 (29%) patients (▶ Fig. 9.8).

The development of severe prosthetic dehiscence requiring cardiac surgery was closely related to the extent of perivalvular infection, and in this investigation, ^{99m}Tc-WBC SPECT/CT was more accurate than echocardiography for delineating the extent of infection in perivalvular regions. These investigators also found that intensity of ^{99m}Tc-WBC uptake might be useful to distinguish between those patients needing surgery and those for whom medical therapy is sufficient. They concluded that ^{99m}Tc-WBC SPECT/CT is useful in patients with suspected PVE and inconclusive TEE.

Cardiovascular Implantable Electronic Device Infection

The use of cardiovascular implantable electronic devices (CIEDs), such as pacemakers, cardioverter-defibrillators, and ventricular assist devices, has increased significantly over the past several years. As with any foreign object implanted in the human body, there is the potential for infection. The rate of CIED-related infection ranges from 1 to 7% and is associated with significant morbidity and mortality. The diagnosis of CIED infection is based on results of blood cultures of and cultures of pocket exudates and TEE, which is used to define the likelihood of disease according to the Duke criteria. These criteria, which were developed for the diagnosis of IE, may not be adequate for CIED-related infection.[9]

Most CIED infections originate in the surgical pocket and, if untreated, may extend through the catheter leads, resulting in endocarditis and systemic infection. The extent of infection may be underestimated in patients who present with manifestations of local infection at the site of the device implantation, and sophisticated imaging tests are playing an increasingly important role in diagnosing and determining the extent of the infection. While several nuclear medicine techniques have been used to evaluate CIED infection, the introduction of hybrid imaging has demonstrated the true value of these studies.[9] ^{99m}Tc-WBC SPECT/CT is useful for defining the presence and extent of CIED and left-ventricular-assist device infection, resulting in improved patient care. Erba et al[9] investigated ^{99m}Tc-WBC SPECT/CT in 63 consecutive patients with possible CIED infection, all of whom underwent clinical examination, blood chemistry, microbiology, and echocardiography of the cardiac region/venous pathways of the device. Thirty-two (51%) patients were diagnosed with infection. The sensitivity of ^{99m}Tc-WBC SPECT/CT was 94% for both detection and localization of CIED-associated infection (▶ Fig. 9.9), and specificity was 100%.

Pocket infection was often associated with lead involvement; the intracardiac portion of the lead(s) more frequently exhibited ^{99m}Tc-WBC uptake and

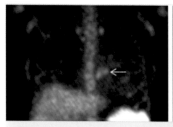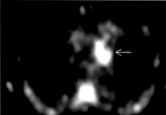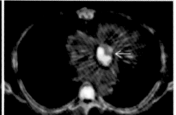

Fig. 9.8 Infected prosthetic aortic valve. There is focal accumulation of ^{99m}Tc-labeled autologous leukocytes in the left midchest (*arrow*) on the maximum intensity projection image (left). The axial SPECT image (center) localizes the activity to the vicinity of the heart (*arrow*). On the fused SPECT/CT image (right), the abnormal activity involves the prosthetic valve (*arrow*). (Case courtesy of Professor P. Erba.)

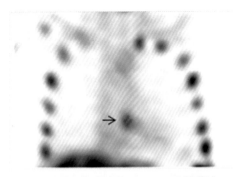 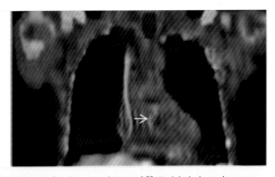

Fig. 9.9 CIED infection. On the coronal SPECT image (left), there is focal accumulation of ^{99m}Tc-labeled autologous leukocytes in the region of the heart *(arrow)*. On the fused SPECT/CT coronal image (right), the abnormal activity is localized to an intracardiac lead of the CIED *(arrow)*. (Case courtesy of Professor P. Erba.)

presented the highest rate of complications, infectious endocarditis, and septic embolism. Echocardiography was 90% specific but only 81% sensitive when intracardiac lead infection only was considered. The Duke criteria had 31% sensitivity for the definite category (100% specificity) and 81% sensitivity and 77% specificity when definite and possible categories were included. The authors concluded that ^{99m}Tc-WBC SPECT/CT is useful for confirming the presence of CIED-associated infection, defining the extent of device involvement, and detecting associated complications with a positive predictive value of 100%. The test also reliably excluded device-associated infection during a febrile episode and sepsis, with a 95% negative predictive value.

Litzler et al[10] performed 13 ^{99m}Tc-WBC SPECT/CT studies on eight consecutive patients with implanted left-ventricular-assist devices to assess suspected device-related infection and to evaluate the efficacy of antibiotic treatment. ^{99m}Tc-WBC SPECT/CT was positive for infection in all eight patients with infection, while planar imaging was positive in six of the eight patients. SPECT/CT provided relevant information on the exact location and the extent of infection in all eight patients. Distant foci of infection were identified in 3 of the 13 patients. The authors concluded that ^{99m}Tc-WBC SPECT/CT not only accurately diagnoses left-ventricular-assist-device-related infection but also provides information on both the location and the extent of the infection—information that could lead to improved therapeutic strategies.

Prosthetic Vascular Graft Infection

The rate of infection following placement of a prosthetic vascular graft is less than 5%; the rate

of morbidity and mortality range from about 20 to 75%. Imaging studies are often performed to confirm the diagnosis. Morphological studies, such as CT, MRI, and sonography, provide direct visualization of perigraft abnormalities and facilitate aspiration of fluid but cannot always differentiate normal postoperative changes from infection, especially in the early postoperative period. Several investigations support the use of labeled leukocyte imaging for diagnosing prosthetic vascular graft infection. The sensitivity of the test is not adversely affected by antibiotic therapy or duration of symptoms. False-positive results have been associated with lymphoceles, perigraft hematomas, thrombosed grafts, bleeding, and pseudoaneurysms. Labeled leukocyte accumulation in uninfected grafts less than 1 month old has also been reported.[3]

Recent data indicate that ^{99m}Tc-WBC SPECT/CT is a useful diagnostic test in suspected prosthetic vascular graft infection.[11,12,13] Erba et al[12] evaluated the diagnostic performance of ^{99m}Tc-WBC SPECT/CT in 55 consecutive patients suspected of having late or a low-grade late prosthetic vascular graft infection. Forty-seven (85%) of the 55 patients had infected vascular grafts. SPECT/CT was both more sensitive (100 vs. 81.5%) and more specific (100 vs. 62.5%) than SPECT alone. These investigators observed that ^{99m}Tc-WBC SPECT/CT is useful for detecting, localizing, and defining the extent of prosthetic vascular graft infection (▶ Fig. 9.10).

Advantages (^{99m}Tc-WBC SPECT/CT)

- Differentiates between sterile and septic vegetations.

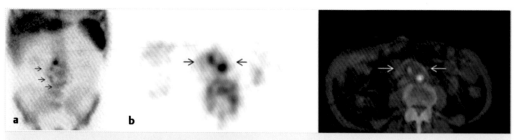

Fig. 9.10 Infected aortoiliac prosthetic vascular graft. **(a)** There is irregularly increased accumulation of ^{99m}Tc-labeled autologous leukocytes overlying the lumbar spine (*arrows*) on the anterior planar image. **(b)** On the axial SPECT (left) and fused SPECT/CT (right) images, the abnormal labeled leukocyte activity is localized to the vascular graft (*arrows*). (Case courtesy of Professor P. Erba.)

- Useful for diagnosing prosthetic heart valve infection.
- Accurately diagnoses CIED infection, defines extent of device involvement, and detects distant foci of infection.
- Useful for detecting, localizing, and defining the extent of prosthetic vascular graft infection.

Disadvantage

- There are limited data available.

9.3.2 Musculoskeletal Infection

SPECT/CT is extremely useful in patients with suspected musculoskeletal infection. This hybrid imaging technique, by precisely localizing radiopharmaceutical uptake, facilitates the differentiation between soft tissue and bone infection, thus guiding patient management (▶ Fig. 9.11). Furthermore, in patients without infection, SPECT/CT can help identify the cause of an individual's symptoms. Horger et al[14] compared three-phase bone scintigraphy with SPECT versus SPECT/CT in 31 patients, including 9 patients with osteomyelitis. Although the sensitivity of both tests was 78%, SPECT/CT was significantly more specific (86%) than SPECT (50%; $p < 0.05$). The superior specificity achieved with SPECT/CT was due to improved anatomical localization of radiopharmaceutical uptake and due to the identification of conditions besides infection that were responsible for abnormal radiopharmaceutical accumulation.

Bar-Shalom et al[13] reported that SPECT/CT was helpful in about half of the 32 patients who underwent ^{67}Ga or ^{111}In-WBC imaging for suspected musculoskeletal infection by providing precise anatomical localization of radiopharmaceutical uptake and delineating the extent of the infection.

Filippi and Schillaci[15] compared ^{99m}Tc-WBC SPECT and SPECT/CT in 28 patients with suspected musculoskeletal infection. The accuracy of the test improved from 64% for SPECT to 100% for SPECT/CT. SPECT/CT altered study interpretation in more than one-third of the patients by precisely localizing foci of labeled leukocyte accumulation: excluding osteomyelitis in seven patients and providing more precise delineation of the extent of infection in three patients.

Horger et al[16] compared ^{99m}Tc-besilesomab SPECT and SPECT/CT in 27 patients suspected of having osteomyelitis superimposed on previous trauma. The accuracy of the test improved from 59% with SPECT to 97% with SPECT/CT. SPECT/CT was especially useful in the appendicular skeleton for differentiating soft tissue infection from osteomyelitis. Interobserver agreement was stronger for SPECT/CT ($k = 1.0$) than for SPECT ($k = 0.68$).

Skull and Facial Bones

The anatomy of the skull and facial bones is complex, and accurate localization of radiopharmaceutical uptake, even with SPECT, can be an arduous task. Moschilla et al[17] reported on the value of ^{67}Ga SPECT/CT in skull and skull base infections and found that the CT component overcomes the inherent limitations of poor spatial resolution and variable distribution associated with [67]Ga. The improved radiopharmaceutical localization provided by SPECT/CT obviates the need to routinely perform bone scintigraphy in these cases. Furthermore, SPECT/CT improved diagnostic confidence and test accuracy.

Chakraborty et al[18] retrospectively reviewed three-phase bone scintigraphy and SPECT/CT for diagnosing skull base osteomyelitis in 20 patients with diabetes. Hyperperfusion and hyperemia were present in 9 and 10 patients, respectively; delayed

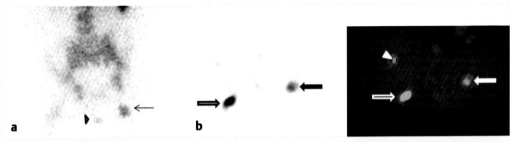

Fig. 9.11 Soft tissue infection upper thighs. (**a**) There is one focus of abnormal accumulation of ^{111}In-labeled autologous leukocyte in the right upper thigh (*arrow*) and a second, less intense focus in the left upper thigh (*arrowhead*) on this posterior planar image. It is not possible to determine whether or not the bones are involved. (**b**) On the axial SPECT (left) and fused SPECT/CT (right) images, the right thigh focus (*open arrow*) is confined to the soft tissues, well away from the bones. The left thigh focus in (**a**, *arrowhead*) is also confined to the soft tissues on SPECT/CT (slice not shown). A focus of activity on the left side (*closed arrow*) represents marrow activity in the left femur. The radioopaque density in the right femur (*arrowhead*) on the fused SPECT/CT image is an intramedullary rod.

bone images showed increased bone uptake in 19 of the 20 patients. Hybrid SPECT/CT of the skull localized areas of increased tracer uptake to the mastoid part of the temporal bone in 15 patients and the petrous part in 11, the sphenoid bone in 3 patients, and the zygomatic in 1, with the CT portion of the study detecting destructive changes in 5 patients. Three-phase bone scintigraphy with SPECT/CT was positive for skull base osteomyelitis in 10 of the 20 patients, changing management in 4 patients.

Sharma et al[19] compared planar bone imaging to SPECT, SPECT/CT, and CT in 13 patients with known or suspected skull base osteomyelitis. Accuracy was highest for SPECT/CT (92%) and lowest for planar bone imaging (46%). Bolouri et al[20] compared orthopantomography, CT, planar bone scintigraphy, and SPECT/CT for diagnosing osteomyelitis of the jaw in 42 patients. They found that SPECT/CT was superior to CT alone and orthopantomography and was slightly more specific than planar bone imaging.

We routinely perform ^{111}In-WBC/marrow imaging for skull and facial bone infections and have found SPECT/CT to be an invaluable adjunct in these cases. Many of the patients have a history of head and neck tumors and are referred to differentiate osteoradionecrosis from osteomyelitis. The success of WBC/marrow imaging depends on accurate localization of WBC activity to bone or soft tissue. Unfortunately, as a result of previous surgery or radiation, anatomical landmarks are lacking, making it difficult to determine whether WBC activity involves bone or is confined to the soft tissues. With SPECT/CT, however, foci of WBC accumulation can be precisely localized, allowing for a definitive conclusion about whether or not osteomyelitis is present (▶ Fig. 9.12).

Spinal Osteomyelitis/Discitis

Spinal osteomyelitis/discitis has a predilection for the elderly and accounts for less than 10% of all cases of osteomyelitis. Infection is usually confined to the vertebral body and intervertebral disc; the posterior elements are involved in up to 20% of cases. Soft tissue abscesses often accompany these infections. Radionuclide imaging is a useful adjunct to MRI, which is currently the best imaging test available for spinal infection. The best radionuclide test for spinal infection undoubtedly is ^{18}F-FDG PET/CT. When ^{18}F-FDG PET/CT is not available, ^{67}Ga imaging probably is the best alternative.[1]

Data on ^{67}Ga SPECT/CT for diagnosing spinal infection are scant. Liévano et al[21] reported that ^{67}Ga SPECT/CT precisely localized focal radiopharmaceutical uptake seen on planar images, thereby avoiding a false-positive diagnosis of spinal osteomyelitis. Domínguez et al[22] reported that hybrid imaging improves disease detection. Fuster et al[23] reported that ^{67}Ga SPECT/CT helped identify soft tissue involvement in more than half of the patients with spinal osteomyelitis. SPECT/CT improves localization of radiopharmaceutical accumulation, facilitates the differentiation of soft tissue from bony infection, and can identify abnormalities, besides infection, that may be responsible for the patient's symptoms.

There are few data about the reliability of ^{67}Ga imaging, with or without SPECT/CT, in patients who have recently undergone spinal surgery, have spinal hardware in place, or have a coexistent malignancy. In these circumstances, the test, especially when positive, should be interpreted cautiously.

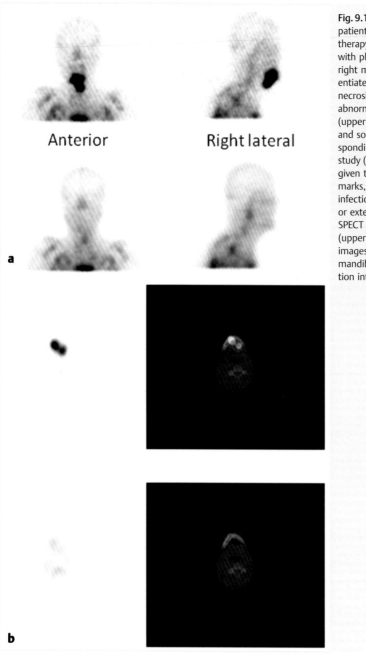

Fig. 9.12 Mandibular osteomyelitis. A patient who had undergone radiation therapy and surgery for oral cancer, with placement of hardware in the right mandible, was referred to differentiate osteomyelitis from osteoradionecrosis. (a) There is a large area of abnormal labeled leukocyte activity (upper images) overlying the lower jaw and soft tissues. There is no corresponding activity on the bone marrow study (lower images). It is not possible, given the paucity of anatomical landmarks, to determine whether the infection is confined to the soft tissues or extends into the bone. (b) Axial SPECT and SPECT/CT labeled leukocyte (upper) and bone marrow (lower) images confirm osteomyelitis of the mandible with extension of the infection into the floor of the mouth.

Prosthetic Joint Infection

Aseptic loosening, the most common cause of prosthetic failure, is usually caused by an inflammatory reaction to one or more of the prosthetic components and is accompanied by an intense leukocytic response consisting primarily of histiocytes and giant cells and, occasionally, lymphocytes and plasma cells. Aseptic loosening is usually managed by a single-stage exchange arthroplasty.[1]

Infection, an uncommon complication of prosthetic joint surgery, develops in up to 2% of primary implants and up to 5% of revision implants.

Risk factors for infection include native bone quality, complexity of the surgery, diabetes, rheumatoid arthritis, and immune status of the patient. Approximately one-third of prosthetic joint infections develop within 3 months (early), another one-third within 1 year (delayed), and the remainder more than 1 year (late) after surgery. Early and delayed infections are probably caused by organisms introduced at surgery; late infection is more likely secondary to hematogenous spread.[1]

The inflammatory reaction accompanying the infected prosthesis can be similar to that present in aseptic loosening, with one important difference. Neutrophils, which are rarely present in aseptic loosening, are invariably present, and usually in large numbers, in infection. The treatment of the infected joint replacement is more involved than that of the aseptically loosened device and consists of an excisional arthroplasty, with weeks to months of antimicrobial therapy, followed by a revision arthroplasty.[1]

Differentiating aseptic loosening from infection of a prosthetic joint, which is extremely important because their treatments are very different, can be challenging. Clinical signs of infection are often absent. Elevated circulating leukocytes, erythrocyte sedimentation rate, and C-reactive protein are suggestive, but not diagnostic, of infection. Joint aspiration and culture, the definitive preoperative diagnostic procedure, is specific, but sensitivity is variable. Plain radiographs are not specific, and hardware-induced artifacts limit, to some degree, CT and MRI.[1]

Radionuclide imaging is extremely useful in the evaluation of the painful joint replacement, especially when infection is suspected. The most widely and often the initial radionuclide test performed is bone scintigraphy. Though sensitive, bone scintigraphy is not specific, and with an accuracy ranging from 50 to 70%, it is most useful for screening purposes. Performing the test as a three-phase study does not improve accuracy.[1]

[67]Ga imaging has been used to improve the specificity of bone scintigraphy. [67]Ga, either alone or in combination with bone scintigraphy, has an accuracy between 60 and 80%, which is only a modest improvement over bone scintigraphy alone, and has fallen into disuse. At the present time, the best available imaging test for diagnosing prosthetic joint infection is WBC/marrow imaging, with an accuracy of about 90% (▶ Fig. 9.13). All of the studies published over the past 3 decades confirm that this test is highly specific for diagnosing joint replacement infection. In nearly all of the

investigations, the test has proved to be sensitive as well.[1]

Tam et al[24] reported that the CT component of bone SPECT/CT may reveal areas of lucency with associated periosteal reaction, which correspond to areas of increased activity on planar bone images. Soft tissue abnormalities, including joint distension, fluid-filled bursae, and intramuscular fluid collections in muscles, findings that can be up to 100% sensitive and up to 87% specific for infection, can be identified on the CT component. Al-Nabhani et al[25] performed bone SPECT/CT on 69 patients with a painful knee arthroplasty and found that the test provided useful information in more than 80% of the patients, helping to confirm mechanical loosening and excluding other causes of pain, such as infection. Filippi and Schillaci[15] compared ^{99m}Tc-WBC imaging with SPECT and SPECT/CT in 13 patients with prosthetic joints. Although planar imaging correctly identified all eight infected and all five uninfected prostheses (100% accuracy), SPECT/CT provided additional important information. In five patients with a hip replacement, SPECT/CT made it possible to differentiate between periprosthetic and soft tissue WBC accumulation. In another patient with an infected hip replacement, SPECT/CT detected WBC accumulation along the femoral stem of the prosthesis as well as in the adjacent soft tissues. In two patients with a knee prosthesis, SPECT/CT correctly localized WBC accumulation to the synovium, thus excluding prosthetic infection. The accuracy improved from 64% for scintigraphy with SPECT to 100% for SPECT/CT. The authors concluded that SPECT/CT is a useful clinical tool to image bone and joint infections because it precisely localizes foci of WBC accumulation and facilitates the differentiation of soft tissue from bone infection.

Kim et al[26] retrospectively reviewed ^{99m}Tc-WBC scans performed on 164 patients with lower extremity joint arthroplasties (71 hip, 93 knee), 89 of whom were infected. The sensitivity, specificity, and accuracy of planar imaging were 82.0, 88.0, and 84.8%, respectively. When planar images were combined with SPECT, sensitivity increased to 91%, specificity was unchanged at 88%, and accuracy increased to 89.6%. When planar images were combined with SPECT/CT, sensitivity, specificity, and accuracy all increased to 93.3%. The authors found that the main contribution of SPECT/CT was precise localization of the anatomical site of the infection and delineation of the extent of the infection (▶ Fig. 9.13).

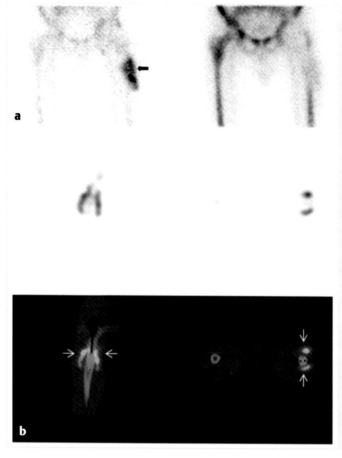

Fig. 9.13 Infected left hip arthroplasty. (a) There is intense activity along the lateral aspect of the femoral component of the prosthesis (*arrow*) on the anterior image from the ^{111}In-labeled autologous leukocyte study (left), with no corresponding activity on the bone marrow image (right). The study confirms the presence of infection but provides only limited information about its extent. (b) Sagittal (left) and axial (right) SPECT and fused SPECT/CT images demonstrate that the infection extends into the soft tissues around the prosthesis both anteriorly and posteriorly (*arrows*). This information is very useful for surgical planning. (Reproduced with permission from Palestro CJ. Continuing Education on Radionuclide Imaging of Musculoskeletal Infection: A Review. J Nucl Med.)

Kaisidis et al[27] evaluated hip prostheses with [99mTc]-sulesomab and reported that SPECT/CT corroborated planar imaging results in three patients. Graute et al[28] reported on 31 patients with suspected lower extremity prosthetic joint infection who underwent [99mTc]-besilesomab planar and SPECT/CT imaging. Nine of the 31 prostheses were infected. Sensitivity, specificity, and accuracy for planar imaging alone were 66, 60, and 61%, respectively. When planar images were interpreted together with SPECT, sensitivity increased to 89%, while specificity and accuracy decreased to 45% and 58%, respectively. When planar images were interpreted together with SPECT/CT, sensitivity remained at 89%, while specificity and accuracy increased to 73 and 77%, respectively.

The impact of SPECT/CT on the diagnosis of prosthetic joint infection is potentially significant. The examination could provide information, not only about the presence but also about the extent of infection. Joint aspiration and culture could be performed at the same time. The test could provide information about other causes of prosthetic failure in patients without infection.[29,30] Patients could potentially be spared the need to undergo multiple imaging tests at different times and possibly different locations, and a diagnosis could be made in a more expeditious, cost-effective manner.

Diabetic Foot Infection

Imaging tests are an essential part of the diagnostic evaluation of diabetic patients with foot infections. WBC imaging is the radionuclide "gold standard" for diagnosing pedal osteomyelitis in this population. The sensitivity of planar ^{111}In-WBC imaging ranges from 72 to 100% and the specificity from 67 to 100%. The sensitivity and specificity of planar [99mTc]-WBC range from 86 to 93% and from 80 to 98%, respectively.[1] The accuracy of WBC imaging is limited by poor image resolution and the small size of the structures being evaluated. Several investigators have used SPECT/CT in an effort to improve the accuracy of the test.[31,32,35]

Heiba et al[32] investigated dual-isotope SPECT/CT using ^{111}In-WBC, bone scintigraphy, and, when necessary, bone marrow imaging in 213 patients with diabetes, including 38 patients with osteomyelitis. Simultaneous dual-isotope (^{111}In-WBC + ^{99m}Tc-MDP) SPECT/CT was significantly more accurate than both planar imaging and single-isotope bone or ^{111}In-WBC SPECT/CT. Because of the inherently poor resolution with ^{111}In-WBC imaging and the small structures being evaluated, it was not always possible, even with the CT component of the examination, to distinguish between soft tissue and bone infection. The addition of bone SPECT/CT permitted precise localization of labeled leukocyte accumulation, improving both accuracy and confidence of diagnosis. In another investigation, dual-isotope SPECT/CT was more accurate than conventional imaging for diagnosing and localizing infection in patients with diabetes

helped guide patient management, and was associated with a shorter length of hospitalization compared to conventional imaging.[33]

An alternative to dual-isotope SPECT/CT is to use ^{99m}Tc-WBC rather than ^{111}In-WBC. ^{99m}Tc-WBC image resolution is superior, and both labeling and imaging can be performed on the same day. Filippi et al[34] performed ^{99m}Tc-WBC SPECT/CT on 17 patients with diabetes, with 19 clinically suspected sites of infection. Planar imaging was performed at 30 minutes, and 4 and 24 hours postinjection. SPECT/CT, which was performed at 6 hours postinjection, changed study interpretation in more than half of the patients by excluding osteomyelitis in six sites, confirming osteomyelitis in one site, and better defining the extent of the infection in three sites (▶ Fig. 9.14).

Erdman et al[35] developed a standardized scoring system, the Composite Severity Index (CSI), based on ^{99m}Tc-WBC SPECT/CT. These investigators found that the likelihood of a favorable outcome varied

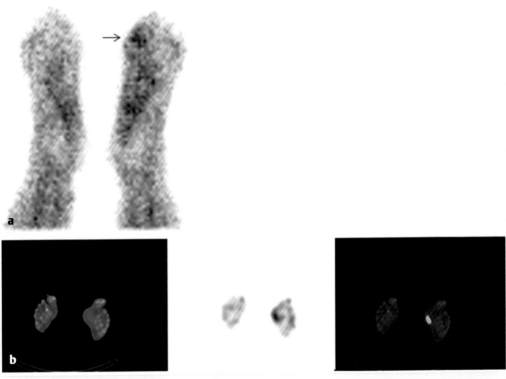

Fig. 9.14 Soft-tissue infection left foot. (**a**) There is a poorly defined focus of increased activity (*arrow*) underlying the first metatarsal of the left foot on this plantar image from a ^{99m}Tc-labeled leukocyte study performed on a patient with diabetes. There is no way to determine whether or not the bone is involved. (**b**) Coronal images from the SPECT/CT confirm that the infection is confined to the soft tissues and does not extend into the bone. (Reproduced with permission from, Palestro CJ. Continuing Education on Radionuclide Imaging of Musculoskeletal Infection: A Review. J Nucl Med.)

inversely with the CSI score. The CSI score was more accurate at predicting outcome than simply classifying studies as positive or negative for osteomyelitis.

Although ^{67}Ga imaging has been used infrequently in the evaluation of diabetic patients with foot infections, recent data suggest a possible role for ^{67}Ga SPECT/CT in this population. In an investigation of 55 patients with diabetes with uninfected pedal ulcers, Aslangul et al[36] reported that the test was 88% sensitive and 93.6% specific for diagnosing pedal osteomyelitis.

Most investigations have focused on diagnosing diabetic pedal osteomyelitis. Recent data suggest that ^{99m}Tc-WBC SPECT/CT may be useful for monitoring treatment response. Vouillarmet et al[37] used ^{99m}Tc-WBC SPECT/CT to monitor response to treatment in 29 patients with diabetes with pedal osteomyelitis, all of whom were in clinical remission at the time of imaging. ^{99m}Tc-WBC SPECT/CT was negative in 22 patients. The test was positive in 7 patients, including 5 who relapsed. Sensitivity, specificity, positive predictive value, and negative predictive value for osteomyelitis relapse were 80, 33, 20, and 89%, respectively, for radiographs; 100, 12.5, 15.5, and 100%, respectively, for three-phase bone scintigraphy; and 100, 91.5, 71.5, and 100%, respectively, for ^{99m}Tc-WBC SPECT/CT. The authors concluded that a negative ^{99m}Tc-WBC SPECT/CT is a good indicator of diabetic foot osteomyelitis remission and might be useful to guide antibiotic therapy. Lazaga et al[38] reported that ^{99m}Tc-WBC appears to be useful for monitoring response to therapy in patients with diabetes with pedal osteomyelitis.

Pearls

- Bone scintigraphy has a high negative predictive value and can be used as a screening test in suspected musculoskeletal infection.
- [67]Ga is the preferred single-photon emitting radiopharmaceutical for spinal osteomyelitis/discitis.
- In vitro labeled leukocyte imaging is the preferred radionuclide test for complicating osteomyelitis, except for spinal infections.
- Accuracy of ^{111}In-WBC and ^{99m}Tc-WBC is improved by performing complementary bone marrow imaging.
- SPECT/CT improves the accuracy of diagnosing musculoskeletal infection by precisely localizing areas of radiopharmaceutical uptake.

- SPECT/CT can help delineate the extent of the infection.
- SPECT/CT facilitates the differentiation between soft tissue and bone infection, thus guiding patient management.
- SPECT/CT can help identify the causes, besides infection, of an individual's symptoms.

Pitfalls

- A positive three-phase bone scan cannot automatically be equated with infection.
- In patients with underlying malignancy, orthopaedic hardware, or recent surgery, ^{67}Ga imaging is most useful when it is negative.
- ^{111}In-WBC and ^{99m}Tc-WBC imaging are not useful for diagnosing spinal osteomyelitis/diskitis.

References

[1] Palestro CJ. Radionuclide imaging of osteomyelitis. Semin Nucl Med. 2015;45(1):32–46

[2] Palestro CJ, Love C. Radionuclide imaging of musculoskeletal infection: conventional agents. Semin Musculoskelet Radiol. 2007;11(4):335–352

[3] Palestro CJ, Love C, Bhargava KK. Labeled leukocyte imaging: current status and future directions. Q J Nucl Med Mol Imaging. 2009;53(1):105–123

[4] Palestro CJ, Love C, Tronco GG, et al. Combined labeled leukocyte and technetium-99 m sulfur colloid bone marrow imaging for diagnosing musculoskeletal infection: principles, technique, interpretation, indications and limitations. Radiographics. 2006;26:859–870

[5] Palestro CJ, Glaudemans AWJM, Dierckx RAJO. Multiagent imaging of inflammation and infection with radionuclides. Clin Transl Imaging. 2013;1:385–396

[6] Bruun NE, Habib G, Thuny F, Sogaard P. Cardiac imaging in infectious endocarditis. Eur Heart J. 2014;35(10):624–632

[7] Erba PA, Conti U, Lazzeri E, et al. Added value of 99mTc-HMPAO-labeled leukocyte SPECT/CT in the characterization and management of patients with infectious endocarditis. J Nucl Med. 2012;53(8):1235–1243

[8] Hyafil F, Rouzet F, Lepage L, et al. Role of radiolabelled leucocyte scintigraphy in patients with a suspicion of prosthetic valve endocarditis and inconclusive echocardiography. Eur Heart J Cardiovasc Imaging. 2013;14(6):586–594

[9] Erba PA, Sollini M, Conti U, et al. Radiolabeled WBC scintigraphy in the diagnostic workup of patients with suspected device-related infections. JACC Cardiovasc Imaging. 2013;6 (10):1075–1086

[10] Litzler PY, Manrique A, Etienne M, et al. Leukocyte SPECT/CT for detecting infection of left-ventricular-assist devices: preliminary results. J Nucl Med. 2010;51(7):1044–1048

[11] Lou L, Alibhai KN, Winkelaar GB, et al. 99mTc-WBC scintigraphy with SPECT/CT in the evaluation of arterial graft infection. Nucl Med Commun. 2010;31(5):411–416

[12] Erba PA, Leo G, Sollini M, et al. Radiolabelled leucocyte scintigraphy versus conventional radiological imaging for the management of late, low-grade vascular prosthesis infections. Eur J Nucl Med Mol Imaging. 2014;41(2):357–368

[13] Bar-Shalom R, Yefremov N, Guralnik L, et al. SPECT/CT using 67Ga and 111In-labeled leukocyte scintigraphy for diagnosis of infection. J Nucl Med. 2006;47(4):587–594

[14] Horger M, Eschmann SM, Pfannenberg C, et al. Added value of SPECT/CT in patients suspected of having bone infection: preliminary results. Arch Orthop Trauma Surg. 2007;127 (3):211–221

[15] Filippi L, Schillaci O. Tc-99 m HMPAO-labeled leukocyte scintigraphy for bone and joint infections. J Nucl Med. 2006; 47:1908–1913

[16] Horger M, Eschmann SM, Pfannenberg C, et al. The value of SPET/CT in chronic osteomyelitis. Eur J Nucl Med Mol Imaging. 2003;30(12):1665–1673

[17] Moschilla G, Thompson J, Turner JH. Co-registered gallium-67 SPECT/CT imaging in the diagnosis of infection and monitoring treatment. World J Nucl Med. 2006;5:32–39

[18] Chakraborty D, Bhattacharya A, Gupta AK, Panda NK, Das A, Mittal BR. Skull base osteomyelitis in otitis externa: the utility of triphasic and single photon emission computed tomography/computed tomography bone scintigraphy. Indian J Nucl Med. 2013;28(2):65–69

[19] Sharma P, Agarwal KK, Kumar S, Singh H, Bal C, Malhotra A. Utility of (99m)Tc-MDP hybrid SPECT-CT for diagnosis of skull base osteomyelitis: comparison with planar bone scintigraphy, SPECT, and CT. Jpn J Radiol. 2013;31:81–88

[20] Bolouri C, Merwald M, Huellner MW, et al. Performance of orthopantomography, planar scintigraphy, CT alone and SPECT/CT in patients with suspected osteomyelitis of the jaw. Eur J Nucl Med Mol Imaging. 2013;40(3):411–417

[21] Liévano P, De la Cueva L, Navarro P, Arroyo E, Añaños M, Abós MD. 67Ga SPECT/low-dose CT. A case report of spondylodiscitis and Schmorl's node [in Spanish]. Rev Esp Med Nucl. 2009;28(6):288–290

[22] Domínguez ML, Lorente R, Rayo JI, et al. SPECT-CT with 67Ga-citrate in the management of spondylodiscitis. Rev Esp Med Nucl Imagen Mol. 2012;31(1):34–39

[23] Fuster D, Solà O, Soriano A, et al. A prospective study comparing whole-body FDG PET/CT to combined planar bone scan with 67Ga SPECT/CT in the diagnosis of spondylodiskitis. Clin Nucl Med. 2012;37(9):827–832

[24] Tam HH, Bhaludin B, Rahman F, Weller A, Ejindu V, Parthipun A. SPECT-CT in total hip arthroplasty. Clin Radiol. 2014;69 (1):82–95

[25] Al-Nabhani K, Michopoulou S, Allie R, et al. Painful knee prosthesis: can we help with bone SPECT/CT? Nucl Med Commun. 2014;35(2):182–188

[26] Kim HO, Na SJ, Oh SJ, et al. Usefulness of adding SPECT/CT to 99mTc-hexamethylpropylene amine oxime (HMPAO)-labeled leukocyte imaging for diagnosing prosthetic joint infections. J Comput Assist Tomogr. 2014;38(2):313–319

[27] Kaisidis A, Megas P, Apostolopoulos D, et al. Diagnosis of septic loosening of hip prosthesis with LeukoScan. SPECT scan with 99mTc-labeled monoclonal antibodies [in German]. Orthopade. 2005;34(5):462–469

[28] Graute V, Feist M, Lehner S, et al. Detection of low-grade prosthetic joint infections using 99mTc-antigranulocyte SPECT/CT: initial clinical results. Eur J Nucl Med Mol Imaging. 2010;37(9):1751–1759

[29] Hirschmann MT, Iranpour F, Konala P, et al. A novel standardized algorithm for evaluating patients with painful total knee arthroplasty using combined single photon emission tomography and conventional computerized tomography. Knee Surg Sports Traumatol Arthrosc. 2010;18(7):939–944

[30] Hirschmann MT, Konala P, Iranpour F, Kerner A, Rasch H, Friederich NF. Clinical value of SPECT/CT for evaluation of patients with painful knees after total knee arthroplasty—a new dimension of diagnostics? BMC Musculoskelet Disord. 2011;12:36

[31] Przybylski MM, Holloway S, Vyce SD, Obando A. Diagnosing osteomyelitis in the diabetic foot: a pilot study to examine the sensitivity and specificity of Tc99 m white blood cell-labelled single photon emission computed tomography/computed tomography. Int Wound J. 2016;13(3):382–389

[32] Heiba SI, Kolker D, Mocherla B, et al. The optimized evaluation of diabetic foot infection by dual isotope SPECT/CT imaging protocol. J Foot Ankle Surg. 2010;49(6):529–536

[33] Heiba S, Kolker D, Ong L, et al. Dual-isotope SPECT/CT impact on hospitalized patients with suspected diabetic foot infection: saving limbs, lives, and resources. Nucl Med Commun. 2013;34(9):877–884

[34] Filippi L, Uccioli L, Giurato L, Schillaci O. Diabetic foot infection: usefulness of SPECT/CT for 99mTc-HMPAO-labeled leukocyte imaging. J Nucl Med. 2009;50(7):1042–1046

[35] Erdman WA, Buethe J, Bhore R, et al. Indexing severity of diabetic foot infection with 99mTc-WBC SPECT/CT hybrid imaging. Diabetes Care. 2012;35(9):1826–1831

[36] Aslangul E, M'bemba J, Caillat-Vigneron N, et al. Diagnosing diabetic foot osteomyelitis in patients without signs of soft tissue infection by coupling hybrid 67Ga SPECT/CT with bedside percutaneous bone puncture. Diabetes Care. 2013;36 (8):2203–2210

[37] Vouillarmet J, Morelec I, Thivolet C. Assessing diabetic foot osteomyelitis remission with white blood cell SPECT/CT imaging. Diabet Med. 2014;31(9):1093–1099

[38] Lazaga F, Van Asten SA, Nichols A, et al. Hybrid imaging with 99mTc-WBC SPECT/CT to monitor the effect of therapy in diabetic foot osteomyelitis. Int Wound J. 2015. doi: 10.1111/i wj.12433

10 SPECT in Children

Frederick D. Grant

10.1 Introduction

Soon after the availability of single-photon emission computed tomography (SPECT), it was used for imaging children.[1] As SPECT cameras became distributed more widely in the 1980s, pediatric applications became similar to those in the general population, although the clinical utility of SPECT in pediatrics has reflected the distribution of disease in children. Some SPECT studies are more likely to be performed in children: renal cortical imaging, splenic imaging, and tumor imaging with metaiodobenzylguanidine (MIBG); these will be the focus of this chapter.

SPECT is used for many other studies in pediatric nuclear medicine and may be performed for indications more common in children. For example, in children and young adults, skeletal scintigraphy may be performed for sports medicine indications (see Chapter 8). For other procedures such as brain SPECT or parathyroid SPECT, the indications and procedures in children are similar to those in adults (see Chapters 3 and 4). Other SPECT studies, such as myocardial perfusion imaging (see Chapter 5), are performed less frequently in children than in adults.

As in adults, the benefits of SPECT in children include improved lesion conspicuity due to greater image contrast[2] and the availability of cross-sectional images that can be coregistered with computed tomography (CT) and magnetic resonance imaging (MRI). However, in some pediatric situations, SPECT does not have a benefit over planar scintigraphy. In small children, the width of the camera bed may prevent rotating camera heads from being in close proximity to the organ(s) of interest. Thus, in children less than 1 year of age, planar images acquired with a pinhole collimator may provide more informative images than can be acquired with SPECT. The utility of hybrid SPECT/CT in pediatrics remains poorly defined, in part, due to concerns about radiation dose. On the other hand, newer techniques of SPECT image reconstruction[3] can be of particular interest in pediatrics. These methods of image processing can improve image quality while facilitating use of a smaller administered activity of radiopharmaceutical so that diagnostic accuracy can be improved while radiation dose is decreased.

10.2 Renal Cortical SPECT with ^{99m}Tc-DMSA

10.2.1 Indications

Renal cortical SPECT has a broad range of indications, mostly of particular interest in children and young adults.

- Cortical renal scintigraphy provides an accurate determination of differential renal function and can be an important part of the evaluation of patients with renal or urologic diseases.
- Renal SPECT can be used to identify functional cortical lesions, including scars, cysts, and dysplasia, and it has an important and evolving role in the evaluation of both acute pyelonephritis and the possible sequelae of inadequately treated kidney infections.
- Occasionally, cortical scintigraphy can be helpful in localizing a kidney in patients with a possible ectopic (e.g., pelvic) or congenitally absent kidney.

Correlation with renal ultrasound can be very helpful when interpreting renal SPECT, but coregistration of SPECT and CT images is rarely necessary.

10.2.2 Technique

Radiopharmaceutical

- Cortical renal scintigraphy is performed with technetium-99 m dimercaptosuccinic acid (^{99m}Tc-DMSA). After administration by intravenous injection, nearly all (90%) ^{99m}Tc-DMSA becomes protein bound[4] and clears from the blood pool with a half-life of slightly less than 1 hour.[5]
- Renal cortical uptake is approximately 40 to 50% by 1 hour and 70% by 24 hours,[4,5] with most ^{99m}Tc-DMSA accumulating in the epithelial cells of the proximal convoluted tubules.[6]
- The current harmonized guidelines recommend an administered activity of 1.85 MBq/kg (0.05 mCi/kg), with a minimum of 11.1 MBq (0.3 mCi) and a maximum of 111 MBq (3.0 mCi).[7]

Imaging

- Cortical scintigraphy is typically performed 2 to 4 hours after radiopharmaceutical administration. Uptake of ^{99m}Tc-DMSA is limited to the renal cortex, with no accumulation in the medulla; therefore, the pattern of ^{99m}Tc-DMSA uptake demonstrates the structure of the normal renal cortex.
- Although most ^{99m}Tc-DMSA is retained by the renal cortex, a small amount is excreted into the renal collecting system. In patients with substantial collecting system obstruction, tracer accumulation in the collecting system may interfere with imaging. In these patients, improved diagnostic accuracy and quantitation may be obtained by waiting even longer (up to 24 hours) before performing cortical scintigraphy.[8]
- Renal cortical scintigraphy can be acquired as static planar images or with SPECT. Planar renal scintigraphy is performed either with parallel-hole collimators or with pinhole collimators, which will provide a magnified and more detailed image of the kidney than available with planar parallel-hole collimators. However, pinhole images can be acquired in only limited projections (typically posterior and posterior oblique). Renal cortical SPECT using high-resolution or ultrahigh-resolution parallel-hole collimators provides higher quality images of the renal parenchyma than planar images acquired with either a parallel-hole or a pinhole collimator.[9] After reconstruction, SPECT can be displayed in three planes (transverse, coronal, and sagittal) or as rotating volume-rendered maximum intensity projection images (▶ Fig. 10.1). These two methods of image representation can be complementary when trying to identify and characterize lesions in the renal cortex.

Differential Renal Function

The relative distribution of tracer between the kidneys reflects differential renal blood flow and the mass of functional renal cortex.[10,11] Differential function is determined using regions of interest or volumes of interest to define renal cortex and background soft tissue. Separate regions can be applied to each moiety of a duplicated kidney. Accurate determination of renal size requires image-size calibration.

10.2.3 Pyelonephritis

Pyelonephritis is a urinary tract infection (UTI) involving the renal parenchyma. With appropriate therapy, pyelonephritis can resolve with no long-standing sequelae. However, delayed therapy can result in permanent renal cortical damage, which may increase the future risk of hypertension or chronic renal failure.[12] Renal scarring can be prevented by early antibiotic therapy.[13,14,15,16] Cortical renal SPECT can be used for both the initial evaluation of acute pyelonephritis and follow-up after resolution of the kidney infection (▶ Fig. 10.2).

- When used to evaluate patients with febrile UTI, ^{99m}Tc-DMSA scintigraphy has very high sensitivity and specificity for the early diagnosis and localization of cortical involvement,[17,18,19,20,21] particularly when imaged with SPECT.[9] Sites of infection will have decreased uptake of ^{99m}Tc-DMSA, and typically, during the acute infection, these cortical lesions will have poorly defined margins. Occasionally, focal sites of infection may appear to have increased volume compared to the normal renal cortex.
- If appropriate therapy is started (usually within approximately 48 hours) and there is successful treatment of the infection, the cortical abnormalities typically resolve with normalization of the scintigraphic abnormalities within 3 to 6 months, although long-term damage may be possible.[13] However, it is not clear that all renal cortical defects will persist and therefore have a clinical effect.[22] Rarely an infection may involve the entire renal parenchyma, which will appear as decreased ^{99m}Tc-DMSA uptake throughout the whole kidney.
- In the absence of prompt and appropriate therapy, a renal infection will produce permanent cortical damage or scarring.[13,14,15] On follow-up ^{99m}Tc-DMSA scintigraphy, regions of scar demonstrate clearly defined sharp margins with a corresponding loss of cortical volume. The typical cortical scar may appear wedge-shaped, although the appearance will depend on the location and age of the scar, as well as the degree of growth by the surrounding normal cortex.

10.2.4 Approaches to Imaging Recurrent Urinary Tract Infection

The role of renal cortical scintigraphy in the evaluation of recurrent UTI and suspected vesicoureteral reflux has evolved over the past decade.[23]

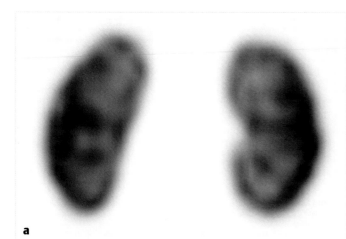

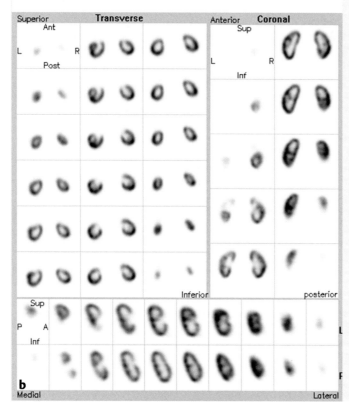

Fig. 10.1 Normal ^{99m}Tc-DMSA renal cortical SPECT. (a) A maximum intensity projection (MIP) image in the posterior projection demonstrates similar uptake, an indicator of similar differential function, in both kidneys. In each kidney, there is uniform tracer uptake throughout the cortex, with no focal cortical defects and no pelvicaliectasis. (b) Images acquired by SPECT and displayed in three planes, transverse (upper left), coronal (upper right), and sagittal (lower panels), confirm the absence of cortical lesions.

- Until recently, at most centers in North America, a child with a febrile UTI would be evaluated by the "bottom-up" approach.[14] The initial step has been an evaluation for possible vesicoureteral reflux. Detailed evaluation of the renal parenchyma was reserved for patients with repeated infections or breakthrough infections while on antibiotic prophylaxis.
- More recently, the "top-down" approach has gained favor among clinicians.[24] With this approach, the initial evaluation of a febrile UTI is focused on the kidney, and evaluation for reflux is performed only in patients with demonstrated renal involvement of the infection. There is variability in how the top-down approach has been implemented. Ideally, the top-down approach starts with renal cortical scintigraphy within 7 to 10 days of the febrile urinary infection. If evaluation is delayed, then signs of acute cortical infection may have resolved, and delayed

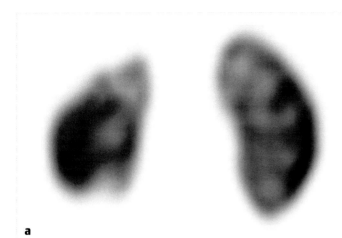

Fig. 10.2 99mTc-DMSA renal cortical SPECT in a 3-year-old girl with bilateral vesicoureteral reflux. (**a**) An MIP image (posterior projection) demonstrates an irregular cortical contour at both poles of the left kidney. (**b**) Images acquired by SPECT and displayed in three planes confirm moderate-sized cortical defects in both poles of the left kidney, which, in the absence of recent infection, likely represent scars due to prior UTIs.

imaging can give false reassurance that evaluation for vesicoureteral reflux is not needed.[24]

- Although renal cortical scintigraphy is more sensitive for identifying renal cortical injury,[19,25] some recent guidelines have allowed the use of renal ultrasound and have recommended that evaluation be performed only in patients with more than one febrile UTI.[15] However, these guidelines have been controversial because of concern that clinically important renal pathology or scarring will be missed.[26,27,28]

10.2.5 Morphological Renal Abnormalities

99mTc-DMSA cortical renal SPECT can have utility in the identification and characterization of morphological renal abnormalities.

- Renal SPECT can be complementary to renal ultrasound as each modality can identify findings not detected by the other. For example, cortical can be used to determine the relative renal function of each renal moiety and may demonstrate other findings, such as a duplicated renal collecting system or cortical thinning due to hydronephrosis (▶ Fig. 10.3).

- Occasionally, renal cortical SPECT will reveal a previously unappreciated renal anomaly, such as a horseshoe kidney or an ectopic kidney, and can be helpful for excluding an ectopic pelvic kidney in a patient with apparent renal agenesis (▶ Fig. 10.4).
- A renal cyst or neoplasm will appear as a region of nonfunctional cortex on cortical SPECT, and,

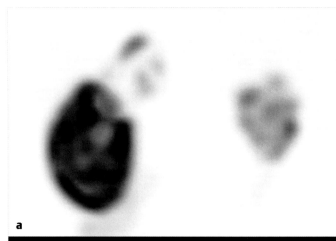

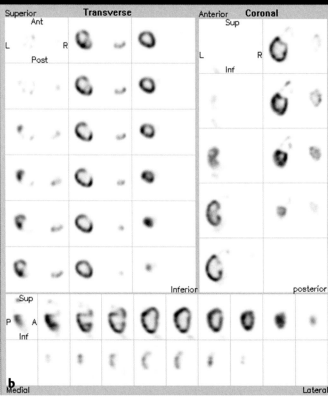

Fig. 10.3 ^{99m}Tc-DMSA renal cortical SPECT in a 1-year-old girl with bilateral duplex kidneys, with complete ureteral duplication, bilateral upper moiety ureteroceles, and right lower moiety megaureter. (a) An MIP image (posterior projection) demonstrates markedly decreased uptake in both upper moieties and heterogeneous uptake in the right lower moiety. (b) Images acquired by SPECT and displayed in three planes confirm uniform cortical uptake in the lower moiety of the left kidney. In the upper moiety of the left kidney and both moieties of the right kidney, marked cortical thinning with heterogeneous uptake likely reflects long-standing obstruction of urinary drainage.

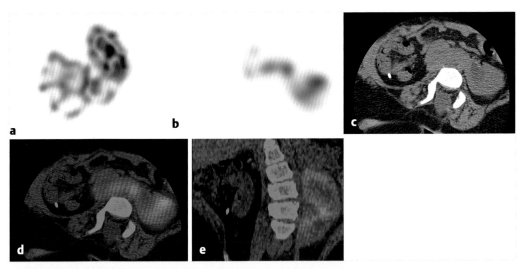

Fig. 10.4 ^{99m}Tc-DMSA renal cortical SPECT in a 12-year-old girl with myelodysplasia and a neurogenic bladder. (**a**) An MIP image (posterior projection) demonstrates cross-fused ectopia of two ptotic kidneys with heterogeneous cortical thinning. (**b**) SPECT image in the transverse plane shows heterogeneous renal cortical uptake. (**c**) A spine CT includes the renal moieties in the field of view. Coregistration of SPECT and CT in the (**d**) transverse and (**e**) coronal planes demonstrates multiple focal cortical defects consistent with widespread cortical scarring in both renal moieties.

conversely, cortical renal SPECT can be used to demonstrate normally functioning renal cortex and the absence of a tumor.[29,30]

- Renal SPECT is used for functional evaluation of multicystic dysplasia of the kidney (MCDK), one of the most common cystic renal disorders in infants and children. MCDK typically appears as a conglomerate of noncommunicating renal cysts, with no or little apparent renal parenchyma. However, there is wide variation in the extent of cortical involvement, and cortical SPECT can be used to assess the amount of functional renal cortex in a dysplastic kidney.
- Less commonly, cortical renal SPECT is used to assess residual and differential renal function in a patient with polycystic kidney disease.
- In teenagers and young adults being evaluated for hypertension, cortical renal SPECT is used to exclude postinfection or posttraumatic renal scarring as a secondary cause of hypertension.[31,32]

10.2.6 Correlative Studies

- Correlation with renal ultrasound is always important for accurate interpretation of renal cortical SPECT. Renal ultrasound has become the standard modality for anatomical imaging of the kidney due to its widespread availability and absence of ionizing radiation. For example, identification of a duplex renal collecting system or renal cyst can be performed easily with ultrasound. However, ultrasound does not have perfect sensitivity for these abnormalities, and renal SPECT is complementary with renal ultrasound.[19,25,33] For example, abnormalities of renal structure, such as a duplex collecting system or horseshoe kidney, may not always be perceived on a renal ultrasound, but may be clearly present on renal SPECT images. Renal ultrasound may detect only about half of significant renal scarring detected by cortical renal scintigraphy.[19,25,33] A normal renal ultrasound may not exclude significant genitourinary pathology,[34] and ultrasound rarely detects scarring that is not demonstrated by renal SPECT.
- In general, coregistration of renal SPECT with CT or MRI is not necessary, but correlation with available cross-sectional imaging, such as CT and MRI, can be helpful in complex cases.

10.3 Tumor Imaging with ^{123}I-MIBG

Neuroblastoma is the most common extracranial solid tumor in children.[35] Functional imaging with MIBG is an important part of tumor staging and patient management.[36,37,38] MIBG[39] is a catecholamine analogue that can be radiolabeled with either iodine-123 (^{123}I) or iodine-131 (^{131}I). It is a ligand of the norepinephrine transporter (NET), which facilitates reuptake of catecholamines, typically at autonomic nerve terminals. The NET is also expressed by nearly all neuroblastomas; therefore, radiolabeled MIBG can be used to localize and image these tumors.[40] In addition, ^{131}I-labeled MIBG is used as an investigational agent for tumor-specific radiotherapy of neuroblastoma and other neuroendocrine tumors expressing the NET.

10.3.1 Technique

Radiopharmaceutical

For ^{123}I-MIBG, the current harmonized guidelines[7] recommend an administered activity of 5.2 MBq/kg (0.14 mCi/kg) with a minimum of 37 MBq (1.0 mCi) and a maximum of 370 MBq (10.0 mCi).

Patient Preparation

Patent preparation is essential for MIBG scintigraphy to be technically adequate and clinically informative.[41,42] Patient preparation includes administering nonradioactive iodine to block uptake of unincorporated radioiodine by the thyroid gland and screening the patient's medication list for drugs that may interfere with the study. Although thyroid gland damage is not a concern with ^{123}I-MIBG, thyroid accumulation of ^{123}I could obscure sites of disease in the neck. Some guidelines suggest large doses of nonradioactive iodine, usually in the form of potassium iodide.[42] Many medications have the potential to interfere with MIBG scintigraphy, and lists of interfering drugs are available for reference.[41,43,44,45] For most of these compounds, specific interference with MIBG scintigraphy has not been demonstrated, but they are included as they are similar to drugs that have been reported to interfere with MIBG scans. Some medications need special mention. Labetalol has well-defined interference and must be stopped before performing MIBG scintigraphy.[43] Over-the-counter cough and cold remedies may contain interfering compounds, and patients and families should be advised to avoid these medications.[42] Most current clinical guidelines recommend that potentially interfering drugs be discontinued for 2 to 3 days before MIBG scintigraphy. However, neuroleptic drugs, such as phenothiazines, administered in depot form may interfere if administered up to 1 month before the imaging study. Ideally, all potentially interfering drugs are discontinued before MIBG imaging, but it may not be clinically appropriate to discontinue some medications, such as antihypertensive medications, necessary to control the symptoms of catecholamine excess or neuropsychiatric drugs. The decision to discontinue a prescription medication in preparation for an MIBG scan must be made after consultation with the referring or treating clinician.

Imaging

- ^{123}I-MIBG scintigraphy is performed 1 day after radiopharmaceutical administration and usually includes both whole-body planar imaging and SPECT or SPECT/CT (▶ Fig. 10.5). ^{123}I emits a substantial portion (~ 17%) of high-energy gamma emission that can penetrate a low-energy collimator, which will increase image noise and decrease the quality of the image. This effect is minimized by acquiring both planar and SPECT images with a medium-energy collimator.[46] Typically, diagnostic studies using ^{131}I-MIBG are also acquired 1 day after tracer administration. Although the longer half-life of ^{131}I makes later imaging possible, this is not usually done as improved image quality or diagnostic accuracy has not been demonstrated with delayed imaging. Imaging with ^{131}I-MIBG has other limitations that make it less desirable than ^{123}I-MIBG.[38,41] Due to higher energy gamma emission, a high-energy collimator is needed for ^{131}I-MIBG scintigraphy. However, many gamma cameras cannot perform SPECT with the heavier high-energy collimator. The radiation dose from ^{131}I-MIBG may be up to twenty times greater than with ^{123}I-MIBG. As a result, ^{131}I-MIBG is now used less frequently than ^{123}I-MIBG for diagnostic imaging.
- Correct interpretation of an MIBG scintigraphic study requires recognition of the normal patterns of physiological uptake of MIBG uptake.[37,38] Intense uptake in the liver and salivary glands is typical of MIBG. Variable levels of MIBG uptake are seen in the heart, lungs, and brown adipose tissue. MIBG typically includes a small amount of unincorporated radioiodine, which can be taken up by thyroid and gastric tissue. MIBG is excreted through both the bowel and the kidneys, and tracer accumulation in the bowel may obscure intra-abdominal pathology, especially on planar images.

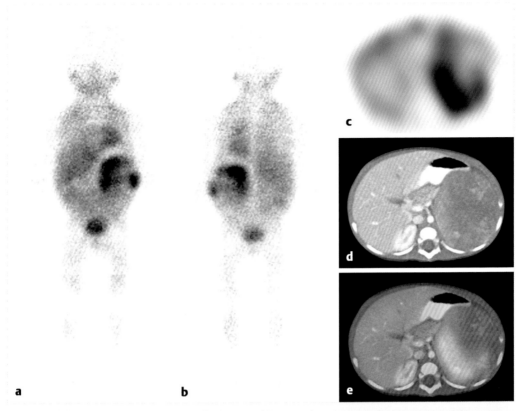

Fig. 10.5 ¹²³I-MIBG scan in an 18-month-old boy with neuroblastoma. Planar images in the (**a**) anterior and (**b**) posterior projections show heterogeneous intense uptake in the left upper quadrant. There is expected physiological uptake in salivary glands, supraclavicular brown adipose tissue, lungs, heart, and liver, with tracer excretion into the gastrointestinal and urinary tracts. (**c**) In the transaxial plane, SPECT shows a normal pattern of physiological uptake in the liver and a rim of intense uptake in the left upper quadrant. (**d**) A diagnostic CT shows a heterogeneous mass in the left upper quadrant. (**e**) Coregistration of SPECT and CT images confirms intense MIBG-avidity in the periphery of the mass. Absent uptake in lower-density regions in the center of the mass may reflect tumor necrosis.

- In addition to increasing sensitivity and contrast, SPECT can be essential for identifying and localizing sites of abnormal uptake. SPECT can detect sites of MIBG-avid disease that are not detected with planar images.[47] Hybrid imaging with SPECT/CT or software coregistration with CT or MR images can improve specificity by improving localization of abnormal tracer uptake or accumulation.[48] This can be helpful for localizing sites of disease as well as helping distinguish pathological from physiological tracer accumulation (▶ Fig. 10.5). For example, coregistered MIBG and CT/MR images can help discriminate pathological uptake in suprarenal soft tissue from excreted tracer accumulating in the renal collecting system (▶ Fig. 10.6).

10.3.2 Neuroblastoma

Neuroblastoma is the cause of approximately 15% of all pediatric cancer deaths.[35,38,49] Despite improved outcomes in patients with low-risk disease, patients with high-stage, high-risk disease continue to have a poor prognosis.[49,50] About half of patients will present with the finding of a primary tumor mass and half will present with metastatic disease. Most primary tumors occur in the abdomen, with half of all neuroblastomas arising from the adrenal medulla.[38,49] However, primary tumors can arise from neural crest tissue throughout the body.[50] A primary tumor is typically found upon physical examination or as an incidental imaging finding. Depending on the location, neuroblastoma occasionally presents with spinal cord compression or radiculopathy. With increased prenatal imaging, an increasing number of

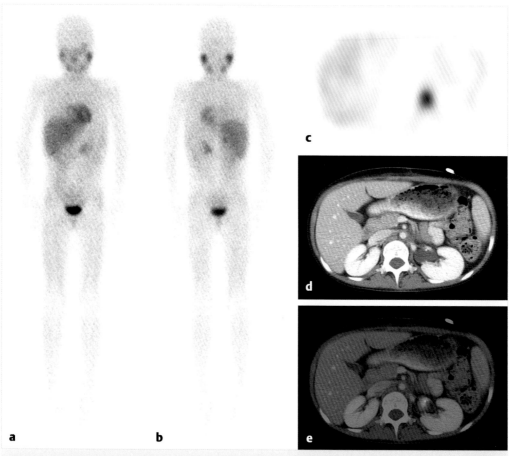

Fig. 10.6 A postoperative ^{123}I-MIBG whole-body scan in a 10-year-old girl with neuroblastoma demonstrates benign physiological tracer accumulation in the abdomen. After resection of a large abdominal neuroblastoma, a postoperative restaging whole-body scan in (**a**) anterior and (**b**) posterior projections shows tracer accumulation in the left face and left upper quadrant. There is expected physiological uptake in the salivary glands, heart, and liver, with tracer excretion into the gastrointestinal and urinary tracts. (**c**) In the transaxial plane, SPECT shows a small region of intense uptake in the left upper retroperitoneum. (**d**) A diagnostic CT of the abdomen shows no abnormal mass, but there is a dilated left renal pelvis. (**e**) Coregistration of SPECT and CT confirms tracer accumulation in urine in the dilated renal pelvis, with no findings to suggest MIBG-avid abdominal disease.

neuroblastomas are identified before birth. The other half of patients present with widespread hematogenous metastases to the skeleton, liver, or distant lymph nodes. Typically, these patients can present with systemic signs, such as fever, bone pain, or ecchymosis.[36,49] Rarely, patients with neuroblastoma will present with a paraneoplastic syndrome, such as the opsoclonus–myoclonus syndrome or severe diarrhea.[36,49]

Diagnostic Imaging

Initial evaluation of neuroblastoma is dependent on imaging. Although initial evaluation might be made with ultrasound, typically either CT or MRI is used to define the anatomical extent of the primary tumor mass.[36] In particular, MRI may be needed to define the extent of intraspinal spinal disease. However, due to the high sensitivity and specificity of ^{123}I-MIBG, it has become the primary imaging study for the staging of neuroblastoma.[38, 42] More than 95% of all primary tumors will demonstrate avidity for MIBG, which can be used to characterize the primary tumor and identify distant metastatic disease (▶ Fig. 10.6, ▶ Fig. 10.7).

^{123}I-MIBG SPECT will identify unsuspected skeletal or nodal metastatic disease not identified by other imaging studies.[42] Rarely, a known

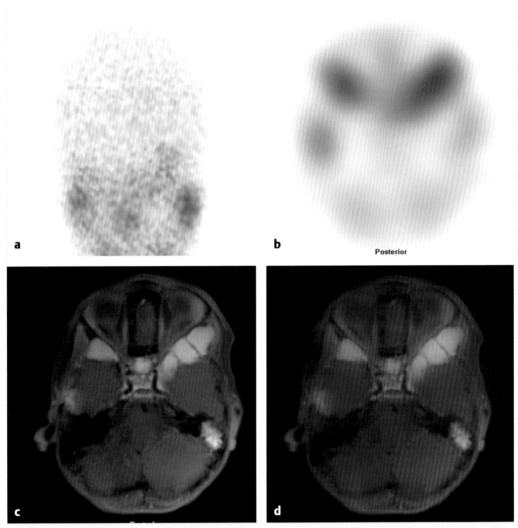

Fig. 10.7 ^{123}I-MIBG scan in a 10-year-old girl with neuroblastoma localizes disease in the skull base. (**a**) In the anterior projection of a whole-body sweep (see also ▶ Fig. 10.6a), there is an abnormal pattern of uptake, with increased uptake in the region of the orbits (left more prominent than right). (**b**) In the transaxial plane, SPECT shows abnormal uptake in the anterior skull base. (**c**) MRI of the skull base shows enhancing disease involving both wings of the sphenoid bone. (**d**) Coregistration of SPECT and contrast-enhanced MR images demonstrates the location and extension of MIBG-avid disease in the skull base.

neuroblastoma may not be MIBG-avid, and other methods, such as ^{111}In-pentetreotide SPECT[37] or fluorine-18 fluorodeoxyglucose (^{18}F-FDG) positron emission tomography/computed tomography (PET/CT), may be needed. Although some studies have suggested that ^{18}F-FDG PET/CT could be particularly useful for evaluating patients with low-stage neuroblastoma,[51] the role of ^{18}F-FDG in the routine imaging evaluation of neuroblastoma has not been determined. MIBG scintigraphy, particularly ^{123}I-MIBG, remains the standard imaging method for staging and assessing the response to therapy of neuroblastoma.[36,38,42]

Staging

The International Neuroblastoma Staging System became a standard for staging neuroblastoma in the 1990s.[52] However, this staging system was limited as it depended on surgical findings that precluded reliable preoperative staging. With further studies of neuroblastoma, a number of biological characteristics of the tumor that were associated with clinical prognosis were recognized. In addition to histological grade, these include MYCN oncogene status, chromosomal ploidy, and alterations in chromosome 1p and 11q.[50] A staging system developed by the International Neuroblastoma Risk Group[53] incorporates both imaging findings and biological characteristics of the tumor. This risk stratification approach for neuroblastoma has been adopted by the Children's Oncology Group.

Semiquantitative Scoring of MIBG-Avid Disease

In an effort to provide for consistent and reproducible interpretation of MIBG scans, a number of investigators have suggested semiquantitative scoring methods.[45,54,55,56] The Curie score[54] method of reporting MIBG scintigraphy correlates with clinical outcome[57] and has been used to assess response to therapy[58] by most multicenter trials of neuroblastoma therapy in North America.[45] The method developed by Lewington et al[56] was studied in a large SIOPEN study of neuroblastoma. All of these semiquantitative methods are limited somewhat as they use only planar images without incorporating diagnostic information provided by SPECT. Consequently, semiquantitative scoring of MIBG scintigraphy is usually performed only within clinical trials of neuroblastoma treatment.

10.3.3 Other Sympathochromaffin Tumors in Childhood

Children with sympathochromaffin tumors other than neuroblastoma can present with signs and symptoms of catecholamine excess, but less commonly may present with a tumor mass as an incidental finding on an unrelated radiological study or during screening of family members with a suspected hereditary syndrome.[59] By comparison, neuroblastoma rarely presents with symptoms of catecholamine excess, although blood catecholamine levels may be elevated mildly in some patients. ^{123}I-MIBG scintigraphy can be very helpful in the localization of paragangliomas and metastatic pheochromocytomas, but may have a sensitivity of less than 80%.[60,61] ^{111}In-pentetreotide scintigraphy with planar and SPECT imaging is less sensitive than ^{123}I-MIBG for the detection of sympathochromaffin tumors but may detect some MIBG-negative tumors.[62] ^{18}F-FDG PET is highly

sensitive, but not specific, for detecting sympathochromaffin tumors, but may be more sensitive than ^{123}I-MIBG for detecting sympathochromaffin tumors associated with mutations in the SDHB gene.[61]

10.4 Spleen Imaging with Damaged ^{99m}Tc-Labeled Red Blood Cells

Scintigraphic imaging of the spleen can be used to identify and localize splenic tissue and to evaluate the function of the spleen. Splenic uptake is seen with many radiopharmaceuticals, including ^{99m}Tc-labeled sulfur colloid. However, with ^{99m}Tc-labeled sulfur colloid, concurrent hepatic uptake of radiopharmaceutical can limit its utility for accurate imaging of the spleen. Heat-damaged ^{99m}Tc-labeled red blood cells demonstrate rapid and highly specific splenic sequestration that is not dependent solely on the phagocytic function of the reticuloendothelial system.[63,64] This pattern of uptake can be used to identify splenic tissue after trauma or surgery to localize splenic tissue in the setting of heterotaxy, to confirm functional asplenia in patients treated for immunological diseases (e.g., idiopathic thrombocytopenic purpura), and to assess splenic function in patients with suspected functional asplenia. Although these studies may be useful at any age, this broad range of indications makes SPECT of the spleen particularly useful in children and young adults.[65]

10.4.1 Technique

- *Preparation of heat-damaged, radiolabeled red cells* requires efficient radiolabeling of the cells and careful heat denaturing to produce cells that will be sequestrated rapidly and efficiently by the spleen. [99m]Tc labeling of the patients' red blood cells is accomplished most easily using a commercially available kit (e.g., Ultratag, Mallinckrodt) for in vitro ^{99m}Tc labeling of red blood cells that have been pretreated with stannous ions. In children, particularly, it is important to minimize the volume of blood used for the labeling procedure.[65] ^{99m}Tc-labeled red blood cells then are denatured by heating to 49.5°C for 20 minutes and then cooling in ice water for 1 minute.[66] After administration, up to 90% of the labeled red blood cells can undergo splenic sequestration.[63] Physically damaged or fragmented red blood cells will undergo phagocytosis in the reticuloendothelial system of both the liver and the spleen, and this increased hepatic uptake will decrease the specificity of the study. Therefore, to limit red blood cell damage by mechanical shearing, phlebotomy should be performed through the largest needle or indwelling catheter possible.

- *Scintigraphy* should be performed with a low-energy, high-resolution or ultrahigh-resolution collimator. SPECT can improve localization and increase diagnostic accuracy (▶ Fig. 10.8). In some cases, SPECT coregistration with CT or MRI or using SPECT/CT, if available, can be particularly useful (▶ Fig. 10.9).

10.4.2 Clinical Indications

Identifying/Localizing Splenic Tissue

Spleen scintigraphy can be used to locate an *accessory spleen* or identify *splenosis* due to regeneration of splenic tissue after surgery or trauma.[67,68] Prior studies[69,70] have demonstrated that the use of heat-damaged red blood cells is superior to ^{99m}Tc-labeled sulfur colloid for this indication. SPECT improves the diagnostic accuracy of these studies.[68,69] Identification of functioning splenic tissue may be sufficient, but, in some cases, hybrid SPECT/CT or software coregistration of SPECT and CT/MRI may be helpful. SPECT/CT or software fusion may be most helpful when assessing a mass lesion previously identified by CT or MRI. In these cases, demonstrating that the lesion of interest sequesters heat-damaged red blood cells is diagnostic of splenic tissue and can save the patient from additional imaging or an invasive diagnostic procedure. Although the most typical location of an accessory spleen is at the splenic hilum,[71] up to 17% of accessory spleens may be found within the pancreas.[71,72] An intrapancreatic accessory spleen is a particular diagnostic challenge, but sequestration of heat-damaged red blood cells within the mass can exclude neoplasm.[73,74]

In children and young adults, one common indication for spleen scintigraphy is the evaluation of patients with *heterotaxy*, who may present with either congenital *asplenia* or *polysplenia*.[64,75] Spleen scintigraphy can be sufficient to segregate patients with asplenia from polysplenia and to guide subsequent patient management. SPECT can be particularly useful for discriminating the multilobulated features of polysplenia from the configuration of a normal spleen (▶ Fig. 10.9). Spleen scintigraphy provides a lower radiation dose than a diagnostic CT,[64] and typically CT or SPECT/CT is not required for the evaluation of these patients.

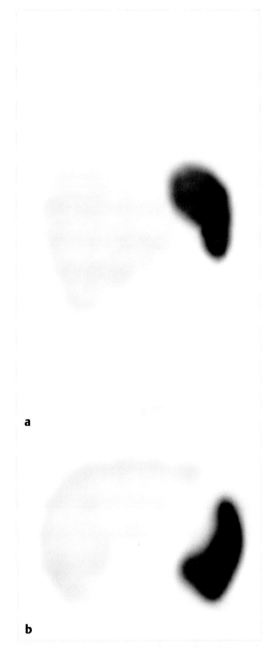

a

b

Fig. 10.8 ^{99m}Tc-labeled, heat-damaged red blood cell scan in a 3-year-old boy with a recent episode of sepsis. (a) An MIP image in the anterior projection demonstrates intense uptake in the expected location of the spleen in the left upper quadrant. There is mild uptake in the liver and excreted tracer in the bladder. (b) In the transaxial plane, SPECT demonstrates intense uptake in the spleen, which has the expected contour and is without focal defects. This confirms the location, size, and function of the spleen.

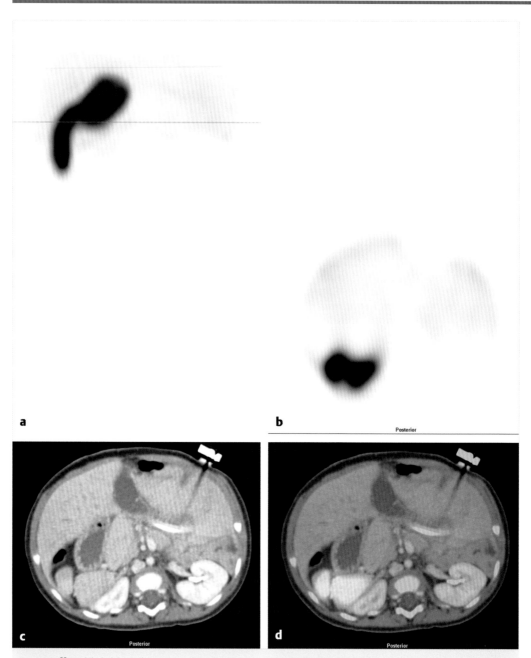

Fig. 10.9 ^{99m}Tc-labeled, heat-damaged red blood cell scan in a 1-year-old girl with heterotaxy syndrome. (**a**) An MIP image in the anterior projection demonstrates intense uptake in the right upper quadrant of the abdomen. There is mild uptake in the liver, which extends across the upper abdomen, and bone marrow. (**b**) In the transaxial plane, SPECT demonstrates an irregular pattern of intense uptake in the posterior right upper abdomen. (**c**) CT of the upper abdomen shows multiple soft tissue masses in the posterior right upper abdomen located posterior to the right-sided stomach and transverse liver. (**d**) Coregistration of SPECT and CT images confirms right-sided polysplenia with intact splenic function.

Evaluating Splenic Function

In recent years, spleen scintigraphy has found increased utility for the assessment of splenic immune function (▶ Fig. 10.8). Individuals with decreased or absent splenic function are at increased risk of overwhelming infection and sepsis, particularly with gram-positive bacteria.[76] Although overwhelming infection is rare, when it occurs, it is associated with a high mortality rate. Determining splenic function can help guide patient management, including immunization and prophylactic antibiotics.[76,77] SPECT or SPECT/CT with denatured [99mTc]-labeled red blood cells may provide the best current approach to assessing splenic function.[78] A wide range of diseases can be associated with decreased splenic function. The severity of splenic function varies among patients, and impairment of splenic function can change with disease activity.[78,79] Evaluation of splenic function with spleen scintigraphy can assist in assessing individual risk of hyposplenism-

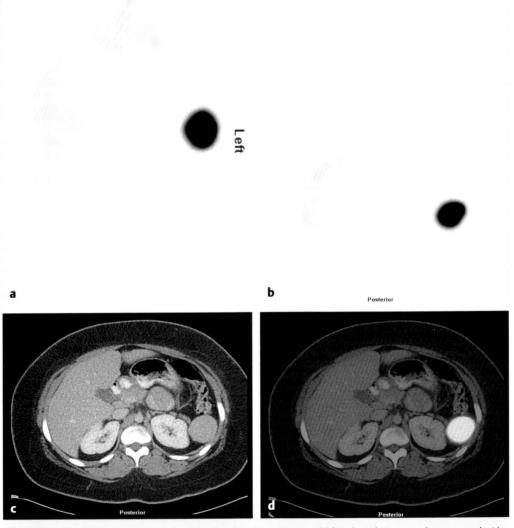

Fig. 10.10 [99mTc]-labeled, heat-damaged red blood cell scan in a 16-year-old female with Evans syndrome treated with splenectomy and recurrent thrombocytopenia. (**a**) An MIP image in the anterior projection demonstrates intense focal uptake in the left upper quadrant. (**b**) In the transaxial plane, SPECT demonstrates a circular region of intense uptake in the upper left abdomen. (**c**) CT of the upper abdomen shows a soft tissue mass in the left abdomen. (**d**) Coregistration of SPECT and CT images confirms a functioning splenule after splenectomy.

associated infections and help guide individual patient management.[78] Occasionally, spleen scintigraphy is used to evaluate splenic function in patients in whom hyposplenism is suspected due to recurrent sepsis with gram-positive organisms (▶ Fig. 10.8).[78]

In some immune-mediated diseases, such as immune thrombocytopenic purpura, splenectomy can be therapeutic. In a small number of patients, recurrent disease indicates the presence of a remnant accessory spleen or regeneration of splenic tissue (▶ Fig. 10.10). Spleen scintigraphy can be the imaging study of choice for confirming the presence of functional splenic tissue in these patients, and SPECT can be more sensitive than planar imaging.[68] SPECT and SPECT/CT are useful for localizing remnant or regenerated splenic tissue as its location within the abdomen can be uncertain.[68,69]

References

[1] Treves S, Hill TC, VanPraagh R, Holman BL. Computed tomography of the heart using thallium-201 in children. Radiology. 1979;132(3):707–710

[2] Jaszczak RJ, Coleman RE. Single photon emission computed tomography (SPECT). Principles and instrumentation. Invest Radiol. 1985;20(9):897–910

[3] Sheehy N, Tetrault TA, Zurakowski D, Vija AH, Fahey FH, Treves ST. Pediatric 99mTc-DMSA SPECT performed by using iterative reconstruction with isotropic resolution recovery: improved image quality and reduced radiopharmaceutical activity. Radiology. 2009;251(2):511–516

[4] Enlander D, Weber PM, dos Remedios LV. Renal cortical imaging in 35 patients: superior quality with 99mTc-DMSA. J Nucl Med. 1974;15(9):743–749

[5] Kawamura J, Hosokawa S, Yoshida O. Renal function studies using 99mTc-dimercaptosuccinic acid. Clin Nucl Med. 1979; 4(1):39–46

[6] Willis KW, Martinez DA, Hedley-Whyte ET, Davis MA, Judy PF, Treves S. Renal localization of 99mTc-stannous glucophetonate and 99mTc-stannous dimercaptosuccinate in the rat by frozen section autoradiography. The efficiency and resolution of technetium-99 m. Radiat Res. 1977;69(3):475–488

[7] Lassmann M, Treves ST, EANM/SNMMI Paediatric Dosage Harmonization Working Group. Paediatric radiopharmaceutical administration: harmonization of the 2007 EANM paediatric dosage card (version 1.5.2008) and the 2010 North American consensus guidelines. Eur J Nucl Med Mol Imaging. 2014;41(5):1036–1041

[8] Treves ST, Packard AB, Grant FD. Kidneys. In Treves ST, Fahey FH, Grant FD, eds. Pediatric Nuclear Medicine and Molecular Imaging. New York, NY: Springer;2014:283–334

[9] Applegate KE, Connolly LP, Davis RT, Zurakowski D, Treves ST. A prospective comparison of high-resolution planar, pinhole, and triple-detector SPECT for the detection of renal cortical defects. Clin Nucl Med. 1997;22(10):673–678

[10] Daly MJ, Jones W, Rudd TG, Tremann J. Differential renal function using technetium-99 m dimercaptosuccinic acid (DMSA): In vitro correlation. J Nucl Med. 1979;20(1):63–66

[11] Taylor A, Jr. Quantitation of renal function with static imaging agents. Semin Nucl Med. 1982;12(4):330–344

[12] Jacobson SH, Eklöf O, Eriksson CG, Lins LE, Tidgren B, Winberg J. Development of hypertension and uraemia after pyelonephritis in childhood: 27 year follow up. BMJ. 1989;299 (6701):703–706

[13] Miller T, Phillips S. Pyelonephritis: the relationship between infection, renal scarring, and antimicrobial therapy. Kidney Int. 1981;19(5):654–662

[14] Edefonti A, Tel F, Testa S, De Palma D. Febrile urinary tract infections: clinical and laboratory diagnosis, imaging, and prognosis. Semin Nucl Med. 2014;44(2):123–128

[15] American Academy of Pediatrics. Committee on Quality Improvement. Subcommittee on Urinary Tract Infection. Practice parameter: the diagnosis, treatment, and evaluation of the initial urinary tract infection in febrile infants and young children. Pediatrics. 1999;103(4, Pt 1):843–852

[16] Roberts KB, Subcommittee on Urinary Tract Infection, Steering Committee on Quality Improvement and Management. Urinary tract infection: clinical practice guideline for the diagnosis and management of the initial UTI in febrile infants and children 2 to 24 months. Pediatrics. 2011;128(3):595–610

[17] Handmaker H. Nuclear renal imaging in acute pyelonephritis. Semin Nucl Med. 1982;12(3):246–253

[18] Jakobsson B, Nolstedt L, Svensson L, Söderlundh S, Berg U. 99mTechnetium-dimercaptosuccinic acid scan in the diagnosis of acute pyelonephritis in children: relation to clinical and radiological findings. Pediatr Nephrol. 1992;6(4):328–334

[19] Tappin DM, Murphy AV, Mocan H, et al. A prospective study of children with first acute symptomatic E. coli urinary tract infection. Early 99mtechnetium dimercaptosuccinic acid scan appearances. Acta Paediatr Scand. 1989;78(6):923–929

[20] Yoo JM, Koh JS, Han CH, et al. Diagnosing acute pyelonephritis with CT, 99mTc-DMSA, and Doppler ultrasound: A comparative study. Korean J Urol. 2010;51(4):260–265

[21] Merrick MV, Uttley WS, Wild SR. The detection of pyelonephritic scarring in children by radioisotope imaging. Br J Radiol. 1980;53(630):544–556

[22] Moorthy I, Easty M, McHugh K, Ridout D, Biassoni L, Gordon I. The presence of vesicoureteric reflux does not identify a population at risk for renal scarring following a first urinary tract infection. Arch Dis Child. 2005;90(7):733–736

[23] Prasad MM, Cheng EY. Radiographic evaluation of children with febrile urinary tract infection: bottom-up, top-down, or none of the above? Adv Urol. 2012;2012:716739

[24] Herz DB. The top-down approach: an expanded methodology. J Urol. 2010;183(3):856–857

[25] Smellie JM, Rigden SPA, Prescod NP. Urinary tract infection: a comparison of four methods of investigation. Arch Dis Child. 1995;72(3):247–250

[26] Brandström P, Nevéus T, Sixt R, Stokland E, Jodal U, Hansson S. The Swedish reflux trial in children: IV. Renal damage. J Urol. 2010;184(1):292–297

[27] Juliano TM, Stephany HA, Clayton DB, et al. Incidence of abnormal imaging and recurrent pyelonephritis after first febrile urinary tract infection in children 2 to 24 months old. J Urol. 2013;190(4) Suppl:1505–1510

[28] Suson KD, Mathews R. Evaluation of children with urinary tract infection—impact of the 2011 AAP guidelines on the diagnosis of vesicoureteral reflux using a historical series. J Pediatr Urol. 2014;10(1):182–185

[29] Leonard JC, Allen EW, Goin J, Smith CW. Renal cortical imaging and the detection of renal mass lesions. J Nucl Med. 1979; 20(10):1018–1022

[30] Grüning T, Drake BE, Freeman SJ. Single-photon emission CT using (99m)Tc-dimercaptosuccinic acid (DMSA) for characterization of suspected renal masses. Br J Radiol. 2014;87(1039):20130547

[31] Rosen PR, Treves S. The efficacy of 99mTc screening of pediatric patients for renal etiologies in hypertension. J Nucl Med. 1983;24:22

[32] Fidan K, Kandur Y, Buyukkaragoz B, Akdemir UO, Soylemezoglu O. Hypertension in pediatric patients with renal scarring in association with vesicoureteral reflux. Urology. 2013;81(1):173–177

[33] Veenboer PW, Hobbelink MG, Ruud Bosch JL, et al. Diagnostic accuracy of Tc-99 m DMSA scintigraphy and renal ultrasonography for detecting renal scarring and relative function in patients with spinal dysraphism. Neurourol Urodyn. 2015;34(6):513–518

[34] Nelson CP, Johnson EK, Logvinenko T, Chow JS. Ultrasound as a screening test for genitourinary anomalies in children with UTI. Pediatrics. 2014;133(3):e394–e403

[35] Parodi S, Merlo DF, Ranucci A, et al. SETIL Working Group. Risk of neuroblastoma, maternal characteristics and perinatal exposures: the SETIL study. Cancer Epidemiol. 2014;38(6):686–694

[36] Kushner BH. Neuroblastoma: a disease requiring a multitude of imaging studies. J Nucl Med. 2004;45(7):1172–1188

[37] Pashankar FD, O'Dorisio MS, Menda Y. MIBG and somatostatin receptor analogs in children: current concepts on diagnostic and therapeutic use. J Nucl Med. 2005;46 Suppl 1:55S–61S

[38] Boubaker A, Bischof Delaloye A. MIBG scintigraphy for the diagnosis and follow-up of children with neuroblastoma. Q J Nucl Med Mol Imaging. 2008;52(4):388–402

[39] Vaidyanathan G. Meta-iodobenzylguanidine and analogues: chemistry and biology. Q J Nucl Med Mol Imaging. 2008;52(4):351–368

[40] Streby KA, Shah N, Ranalli MA, Kunkler A, Cripe TP. Nothing but NET: a review of norepinephrine transporter expression and efficacy of 131I-mIBG therapy. Pediatr Blood Cancer. 2015;62(1):5–11

[41] Bombardieri E, Giammarile F, Aktolun C, et al. European Association for Nuclear Medicine. 131I/123I-metaiodobenzylguanidine (mIBG) scintigraphy: procedure guidelines for tumour imaging. Eur J Nucl Med Mol Imaging. 2010;37(12):2436–2446

[42] Matthay KK, Shulkin B, Ladenstein R, et al. Criteria for evaluation of disease extent by (123)I-metaiodobenzylguanidine scans in neuroblastoma: a report for the International Neuroblastoma Risk Group (INRG) Task Force. Br J Cancer. 2010;102(9):1319–1326

[43] Khafagi FA, Shapiro B, Fig LM, Mallette S, Sisson JC. Labetalol reduces iodine-131 MIBG uptake by pheochromocytoma and normal tissues. J Nucl Med. 1989;30(4):481–489

[44] Solanki KK, Bomanji J, Moyes J, Mather SJ, Trainer PJ, Britton KE. A pharmacological guide to medicines which interfere with the biodistribution of radiolabelled meta-iodobenzylguanidine (MIBG). Nucl Med Commun. 1992;13(7):513–521

[45] Giammarile F, Chiti A, Lassmann M, Brans B, Flux G, EANM. EANM procedure guidelines for 131I-meta-iodobenzylguanidine (131I-mIBG) therapy. Eur J Nucl Med Mol Imaging. 2008;35(5):1039–1047

[46] Snay ER, Treves ST, Fahey FH. Improved quality of pediatric 123I-MIBG images with medium-energy collimators. J Nucl Med Technol. 2011;39(2):100–104

[47] Rufini V, Giordano A, Di Giuda D, et al. [123I]MIBG scintigraphy in neuroblastoma: a comparison between planar and SPECT imaging. Q J Nucl Med. 1995;39(4) Suppl 1:25–28

[48] Rozovsky K, Koplewitz BZ, Krausz Y, et al. Added value of SPECT/CT for correlation of MIBG scintigraphy and diagnostic CT in neuroblastoma and pheochromocytoma. AJR Am J Roentgenol. 2008;190(4):1085–1090

[49] Maris JM. Recent advances in neuroblastoma. N Engl J Med. 2010;362(23):2202–2211

[50] Brodeur GM. Neuroblastoma: biological insights into a clinical enigma. Nat Rev Cancer. 2003;3(3):203–216

[51] Sharp SE, Shulkin BL, Gelfand MJ, Salisbury S, Furman WL. 123I-MIBG scintigraphy and 18F-FDG PET in neuroblastoma. J Nucl Med. 2009;50(8):1237–1243

[52] Brodeur GM, Pritchard J, Berthold F, et al. Revisions of the international criteria for neuroblastoma diagnosis, staging, and response to treatment. J Clin Oncol. 1993;11(8):1466–1477

[53] Brisse HJ, McCarville MB, Granata C, et al. International Neuroblastoma Risk Group Project. Guidelines for imaging and staging of neuroblastic tumors: consensus report from the International Neuroblastoma Risk Group Project. Radiology. 2011;261(1):243–257

[54] Ady N, Zucker JM, Asselain B, et al. A new 123I-MIBG whole body scan scoring method—application to the prediction of the response of metastases to induction chemotherapy in stage IV neuroblastoma. Eur J Cancer. 1995;31A(2):256–261

[55] Suc A, Lumbroso J, Rubie H, et al. Metastatic neuroblastoma in children older than one year: prognostic significance of the initial metaiodobenzylguanidine scan and proposal for a scoring system. Cancer. 1996;77(4):805–811

[56] Lewington V, Bar-Sever Z, Lynch T, et al. Development of a new, semi-quantitative I-123 mIBG reporting method in high risk neuroblastoma. Eur J Nucl Med Mol Imaging. 2009;36:(S2):S375

[57] Yanik GA, Parisi MT, Shulkin BL, et al. Semiquantitative mIBG scoring as a prognostic indicator in patients with stage 4 neuroblastoma: a report from the children's oncology group. J Nucl Med. 2013;54(4):541–548

[58] Taggart DR, Han MM, Quach A, et al. Comparison of iodine-123 metaiodobenzylguanidine (MIBG) scan and [18F]fluorodeoxyglucose positron emission tomography to evaluate response after iodine-131 MIBG therapy for relapsed neuroblastoma. J Clin Oncol. 2009;27(32):5343–5349

[59] Waguespack SG, Rich T, Grubbs E, et al. A current review of the etiology, diagnosis, and treatment of pediatric pheochromocytoma and paraganglioma. J Clin Endocrinol Metab. 2010;95(5):2023–2037

[60] Wiseman GA, Pacak K, O'Dorisio MS, et al. Usefulness of 123I-MIBG scintigraphy in the evaluation of patients with known or suspected primary or metastatic pheochromocytoma or paraganglioma: results from a prospective multicenter trial. J Nucl Med. 2009;50(9):1448–1454

[61] Timmers HJ, Chen CC, Carrasquillo JA, et al. Comparison of 18F-fluoro-L-DOPA, 18F-fluoro-deoxyglucose, and 18F-fluorodopamine PET and 123I-MIBG scintigraphy in the localization of pheochromocytoma and paraganglioma. J Clin Endocrinol Metab. 2009;94(12):4757–4767

[62] Koopmans KP, Jager PL, Kema IP, Kerstens MN, Albers F, Dullaart RP. 111In-octreotide is superior to 123I-metaiodobenzylguanidine for scintigraphic detection of head and neck paragangliomas. J Nucl Med. 2008;49(8):1232–1237

[63] Groom AC, MacDonald IC, Schmidt EE. Splenic microcirculatory blood flow and function with respect to red blood cells. In: Bowdler AJ, ed. The Complete Spleen: Structure, Function, and Clinical Disorders. 2nd ed. Totowa, NJ: Humana Press; 2002:23–50

[64] Aburano T, Katada R, Shuke N, et al. Discordant splenic uptake of Tc-99 m colloid and Tc-99 m denatured RBC in candidiasis-endocrinopathy syndrome. Ann Nucl Med. 1997;11(4):335–338

[65] Ehrlich CP, Papanicolaou N, Treves S, Hurwitz RA, Richards P. Splenic scintigraphy using Tc-99m-labeled heat-denatured red blood cells in pediatric patients: concise communication. J Nucl Med. 1982;23(3):209–213

[66] Snowdon GM. A safe, simple method for preparing heat-damaged red cells for diagnosing splenic infarct or trauma. J Nucl Med Technol. 1998;26(3):204–205

[67] Hovius JWR, Verberne HJ, Bennink RJ, Blok WL. The (re)generation of splenic tissue. BMJ Case Rep. 2010;2010:56–78

[68] Ekmekçi Ş, Diz-Küçükkaya R, Türkmen C, Adalet I. Selective spleen scintigraphy in the evaluation of accessory spleen/splenosis in splenectomized/non-splenectomized patients and the contribution of SPECT imaging. Mol Imaging Radionucl Ther. 2015;24(1):1–7

[69] Gunes I, Yilmazlar T, Sarikaya I, Akbunar T, Irgil C. Scintigraphic detection of splenosis: superiority of tomographic selective spleen scintigraphy. Clin Radiol. 1994;49(2):115–117

[70] Williams G, Rosen MP, Parker JA, Kolodny GM. Splenic implants detected by SPECT images of Tc-99 m labeled damaged red blood cells. Clin Nucl Med. 2006;31(8):467–469

[71] Halpert B, Gyorkey F. Lesions observed in accessory spleens of 311 patients. Am J Clin Pathol. 1959;32(2):165–168

[72] Dodds WJ, Taylor AJ, Erickson SJ, Stewart ET, Lawson TL. Radiologic imaging of splenic anomalies. AJR Am J Roentgenol. 1990;155(4):805–810

[73] Ota T, Tei M, Yoshioka A, et al. Intrapancreatic accessory spleen diagnosed by technetium-99 m heat-damaged red blood cell SPECT. J Nucl Med. 1997;38(3):494–495

[74] Belkhir SM, Archambaud F, Prigent A, Chaumet-Riffaud P. Intrapancreatic accessory spleen diagnosed on radionuclide imaging. Clin Nucl Med. 2009;34(9):642–644

[75] Winer-Muram HT, Tonkin ILD. The spectrum of heterotaxic syndromes. Radiol Clin North Am. 1989;27(6):1147–1170

[76] Bisharat N, Omari H, Lavi I, Raz R. Risk of infection and death among post-splenectomy patients. J Infect. 2001;43(3):182–186

[77] Brigden ML, Pattullo A, Brown G. Pneumococcal vaccine administration associated with splenectomy: the need for improved education, documentation, and the use of a practical checklist. Am J Hematol. 2000;65(1):25–29

[78] de Porto AP, Lammers AJ, Bennink RJ, ten Berge IJ, Speelman P, Hoekstra JB. Assessment of splenic function. Eur J Clin Microbiol Infect Dis. 2010;29(12):1465–1473

[79] William BM, Corazza GR. Hyposplenism: a comprehensive review. Part I: basic concepts and causes. Hematology. 2007;12(1):1–13

11 Selected Interesting SPECT and SPECT/CT Cases

Samuel E. Almodóvar, Padma Manapragada, Katherine A. Zukotynski, and Chun K. Kim

11.1 Introduction

This chapter provides several illustrative cases in which single-photon emission computed tomography (SPECT) and/or SPECT/computed tomography (SPECT/CT) was helpful in achieving an accurate diagnosis. We have included two types of cases: (1) cases where SPECT and/or SPECT/CT is commonly performed in clinical practice but that illustrate points which have not been discussed elsewhere in this book and (2) cases for which the role of SPECT and/or SPECT/CT is not well established but rather is performed as needed. For example, SPECT and/or SPECT/CT is not commonly done for examinations requiring dynamic imaging (e.g., cholescintigraphy or gastrointestinal bleeding studies) but may be extremely valuable in certain cases.

11.2 Case 1: Incidental Retrosternal Goiter Found on Myocardial Perfusion SPECT

11.2.1 Clinical History and Imaging Findings

- An 80-year-old woman presented with shortness of breath.
- Technetium-99 m (^{99m}Tc)-sestamibi myocardial perfusion imaging (MPI) was performed

following pharmacological stress to evaluate for cardiac disease.
- SPECT images in short axis (SA), vertical long axis (VLA), and horizontal long axis (HLA) demonstrate normal myocardial perfusion (▶ Fig. 11.1 a).
- The raw data reveal a large area of increased radiotracer activity in the anterior mediastinum (*arrow*) that was confirmed to be a retrosternal goiter on surgery (▶ Fig. 11.1 b).

11.2.2 Teaching Points

- Careful attention should be paid to identify noncardiac as well as cardiac findings on MPI. In some cases, these findings may account for the patient's symptoms. Systematic review of the raw data is helpful not only to detect quality control issues but also to identify noncardiac incidental findings.
- Extracardiac thoracic uptake may be due to benign or malignant disease. For example, lung cancer, breast cancer, lymphoma, sarcoidosis, and vascular abnormalities may be identified, among other things. Thymic uptake, a retrosternal goiter, and skeletal uptake in multiple myeloma are some other conditions that can be seen by reviewing the raw data.[1,2]

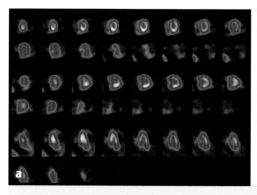
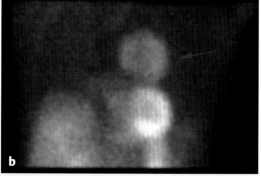

Fig. 11.1 (**a**) SPECT images in short axis, vertical long axis, and horizontal long axis demonstrate normal myocardial perfusion. (**b**) The raw data reveal a large area of increased radiotracer activity in the anterior mediastinum (*arrow*) that was confirmed to be a retrosternal goiter on surgery.

11.3 Case 2: Myocardial Viability Assessment with Thallium

11.3.1 Clinical History and Imaging Findings

- A 62-year-old woman presenting with ischemic cardiomyopathy and marked left ventricular contractile dysfunction underwent thallium-201 (^{201}Tl) SPECT for assessment of myocardial viability.
- Initial resting SPECT images (top row) on SA, VLA, and HLA demonstrate a large size, moderate to severe intensity perfusion defect in the anterior, apical, and inferolateral walls, corresponding to the vascular territory of the left anterior descending and left circumflex coronary arteries (▶ Fig. 11.2).
- Redistribution images at 4 hours (Fig. 11.2, bottom row) demonstrate significant redistribution of ^{201}Tl activity consistent with hibernating myocardium in both vascular territories. These findings suggest a high likelihood that this patient would benefit from a revascularization procedure.

11.3.2 Teaching Points

- "Hibernating" myocardium is viable tissue with contractile dysfunction due to hypoperfusion. Myocardial viability assessment is very important when planning a revascularization procedure in high-risk surgical patients. While fluorine-18 fluorodeoxyglucose (FDG) cardiac positron emission tomography (PET) is considered to be the gold standard test to identify hibernating myocardium, PET may not always be accessible, in which case ^{201}Tl SPECT may be an attractive alternative test.
- ^{201}Tl is a potassium analogue that is injected as thallous chloride and enters myocytes via active transport involving the Na + /K + adenosine triphosphate transport system. From the intracellular space, ^{201}Tl then washes back out into the systemic circulation. In general, ^{201}Tl clears more slowly from myocardium supplied by stenotic vessels than from myocardium that is normally perfused. Hypoperfused areas may continue to accumulate thallium intracellularly, with resultant redistribution.[3]

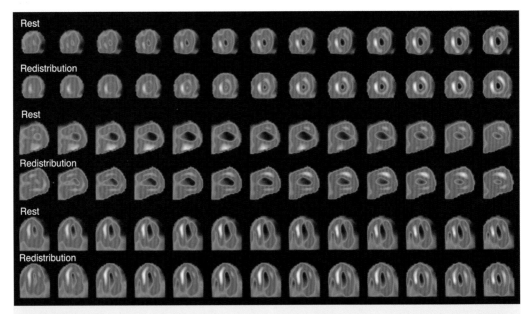

Fig. 11.2 Initial resting SPECT images (top row) on SA, VLA, and HLA demonstrate a large size, moderate to severe intensity perfusion defect in the anterior, apical, and inferolateral walls, corresponding to the vascular territory of the left anterior descending and left circumflex coronary arteries.

11.4 Case 3: Hepatic Hemangioma

11.4.1 Clinical History and Imaging Findings

- A 53-year-old man with left-sided abdominal pain had a diagnostic CT that showed a liver mass with features suggestive of but not definitive for a hepatic hemangioma.
- A ^{99m}Tc-labeled red blood cell (RBC) SPECT study was performed for further evaluation of the liver mass.
- SPECT images show a large area of abnormal radiotracer accumulation in the region of the left hepatic lobe corresponding to the mass on CT (▶ Fig. 11.3 a). The delayed radiotracer uptake is heterogeneous with relative photopenia centrally and intense radiotracer uptake peripherally.
- Fused diagnostic CT and SPECT images show radiotracer uptake predominantly along the periphery of the lesion (▶ Fig. 11.3 b). The scintigraphic appearance is consistent with a hepatic hemangioma.

11.4.2 Teaching Points

- Hemangiomas, focal nodular hyperplasia, and inflammatory pseudotumors of the liver are the common regenerative hepatic lesions. The most common benign hepatic tumor is the hemangioma, which is usually discovered incidentally and has an uncomplicated course. It is important to differentiate hemangiomas from other lesions, such as metastases, in order to avoid unnecessary investigations and/or treatment.
- Immediate ^{99m}Tc-RBC blood pool images often show decreased activity in a cavernous hemangioma. Heterogeneous activity is seen on imaging obtained 1 to 2 hours after radiotracer administration. Often there is increased activity peripherally and central photopenia related to thrombosis, fibrosis, and/ or necrosis.
- The specificity and positive predictive value of both planar and SPECT ^{99m}Tc-RBC blood pool imaging is virtually 100% in diagnosing hepatic hemangioma. Planar imaging alone can identify large lesions (e.g., > 3 cm) with a low overall sensitivity of 30 to 53%. The sensitivity of SPECT ^{99m}Tc-RBC blood pool imaging is higher but still heavily dependent on lesion

size and, to some degree, technique; overall sensitivity is 70 to 80% using single-head SPECT. Using multihead cameras, the sensitivity ranges from 17 to 20% for the detection of lesions < 1 cm, 65 to 80% for lesions 1 to 2 cm, and virtually 100% for lesions ≥ 1.4 cm.
- SPECT/CT improves the sensitivity further, especially when lesions are small or located adjacent to vascular structures.[4,5,6]

11.5 Case 4: Peritoneal Scintigraphy

11.5.1 Clinical History and Imaging Findings

- A 59-year-old man with end-stage renal disease on peritoneal dialysis presented with sudden onset of scrotal swelling and pain.
- Peritoneal scintigraphy was performed after injection of ^{99m}Tc-labeled sulfur colloid mixed with peritoneal dialysate into the peritoneal cavity.
- Initial planar images centered over the abdomen (left) and pelvis including the scrotum (right) show diffuse radiotracer activity in the peritoneal cavity and asymmetric radiotracer uptake extending inferiorly in the region of the scrotum (▶ Fig. 11.4 a).
- Coronal SPECT images show the radiotracer extending through the right inguinal canal into the scrotum (▶ Fig. 11.4 b). Focal photopenia surrounded by tracer within the right scrotum most likely represents the right testicle.
- Fused axial, sagittal, and coronal SPECT/CT images confirm radiotracer movement through the right inguinal canal into the scrotum consistent with an abnormal peritoneoscrotal communication and dialysate leak (▶ Fig. 11.4 c). Peritoneal dialysis was discontinued with initiation of hemodialysis, and the inguinoscrotal communication was surgically repaired.

11.5.2 Teaching Points

- A dialysate leak can occur as a result of a peritoneal membrane tear, where loss of peritoneal membrane integrity may be induced by increased intra-abdominal pressure when large volumes of dialysate are infused during peritoneal dialysis.

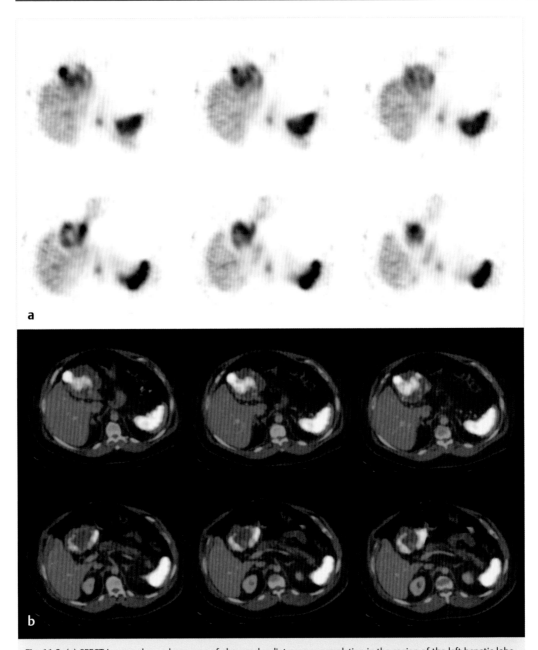

Fig. 11.3 (a) SPECT images show a large area of abnormal radiotracer accumulation in the region of the left hepatic lobe corresponding to the mass on CT. The delayed radiotracer uptake is heterogeneous with relative photopenia centrally and intense radiotracer uptake peripherally. (b) Fused diagnostic CT and SPECT images show radiotracer uptake predominantly along the periphery of the lesion. The scintigraphic appearance is consistent with a hepatic hemangioma.

- Dialysate leaks are classified as early and late based on the time of symptom onset following peritoneal catheter insertion.
- A dialysate may leak as follows:
  - Into the abdominal wall through a peritoneal defect, presenting as abdominal wall swelling.
  - Into the pleura via an abnormal peritoneal–pleural communication, causing a pleural effusion.

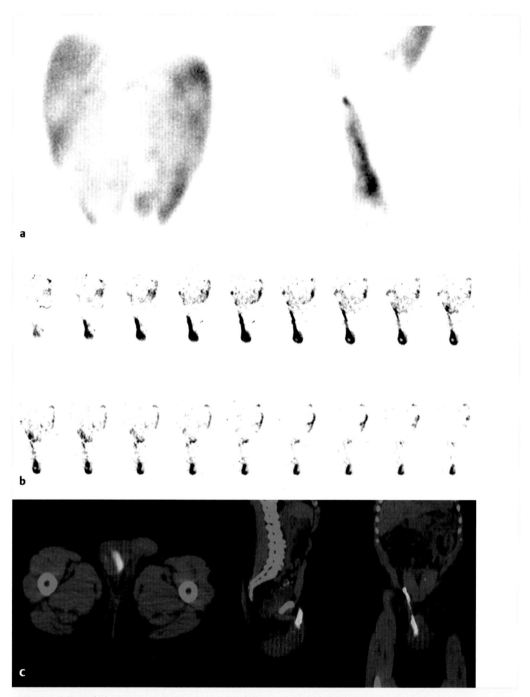

Fig. 11.4 (a) Initial planar images centered over the abdomen (left) and pelvis, including the scrotum (right), show diffuse radiotracer activity in the peritoneal cavity and asymmetric radiotracer uptake extending inferiorly in the region of the scrotum. (b) Coronal SPECT images show the radiotracer extending through the right inguinal canal into the scrotum. Focal photopenia surrounded by tracer within the right scrotum most likely represents the right testicle. (c) Fused axial, sagittal, and coronal SPECT/CT images confirm radiotracer movement through the right inguinal canal into the scrotum consistent with an abnormal peritoneoscrotal communication and dialysate leak. Peritoneal dialysis was discontinued with initiation of hemodialysis, and the inguinoscrotal communication was surgically repaired.

○ Into the scrotum through a patent processus vaginalis, presenting as inguinoscrotal swelling with pain.
○ At the catheter insertion or exit site, presenting as subfascial or subcutaneous swelling with or without pain.[7,8]
- An advantage of peritoneal scintigraphy is the ability to obtain delayed images, even up to 24 hours, allowing more time for the radiotracer to reach the leak or hernia. The addition of SPECT/CT can help pinpoint the exact location of the peritoneal leak. SPECT/CT can be useful in establishing an unequivocal diagnosis of peritoneal leak.[8]

11.6 Case 5: Pseudoaneurysm

11.6.1 Clinical History and Imaging Findings

- A 70-year-old man presented with coronary artery disease, peripheral vascular disease, and multiple prior vascular interventions.
- A ^{99m}Tc-HMPAO-labeled white blood cell (WBC) scan was performed for evaluation of unexplained fever.
- Whole-body planar images show mild asymmetric increased radiotracer activity in the region of the right femoral head and neck, which prompted further evaluation with SPECT/CT (▶ Fig. 11.5 a).
- Axial SPECT at the level of the hips shows focal activity in the right inguinal region (▶ Fig. 11.5 b).
- Fused SPECT/CT confirmed the increased radiotracer accumulation in the right inguinal region was in a pseudoaneurysm, consistent with an infected pseudoaneurysm (▶ Fig. 11.5 c).

11.6.2 Teaching Points

- Infected pseudoaneurysms can be challenging to diagnose and treat and can be associated with a risk of significant morbidity and mortality, including increased susceptibility to rupture. Noninfected pseudoaneurysms can be treated with minimally invasive procedures. Surgery has a major role in the treatment of infected pseudoaneurysms.
- Radiolabeled WBC studies are helpful for confirming the diagnosis of infection in these cases. Migration of the radiolabeled WBC to the

infected area is the basis for the diagnosis of infection on this examination.[9,10]

11.7 Case 6: Clinical Concern of Bile Leak

11.7.1 Clinical History and Imaging Findings

- A 66-year-old man presented with a history of cholecystectomy due to acute cholecystitis 13 years ago and chemotherapy for B-cell non-Hodgkin's lymphoma 12 years ago. One week before the hepatobiliary iminodiacetic acid (HIDA) scan shown in ▶ Fig. 11.6 was performed, the patient underwent laparoscopic lysis of extensive abdominopelvic adhesions and biopsy of a retropancreatic mass showing recurrent lymphoma. Following these procedures, the patient experienced persistent right upper quadrant (RUQ) pain and hyperbilirubinemia. An abdominal CT showed small-volume ascites, pneumobilia, a locule of gas, and a fluid collection in the RUQ.
- A ^{99m}Tc-mebrofenin HIDA scan was performed to evaluate for a biliary leak.
- Planar 60-minute dynamic anterior images show mildly decreased radiotracer and excretion into the biliary tract initially, with a gradual increase over approximately 30 minutes (▶ Fig. 11.6 a). The gallbladder is surgically absent. Vague, diffuse tracer activity that appeared below the right lobe of the liver (*arrows*) was felt to be atypical in appearance (somewhat wide and diffuse) for excreted radiotracer into the duodenum, and a bile leak could not be definitively excluded.
- SPECT/CT was performed for further evaluation (▶ Fig. 11.6 b). The vague diffuse activity below the right hepatic lobe seen on the planar images was found to be within the dilated duodenum. The mild and diffuse activity on planar images likely resulted from a combination of slow, decreased excretion of bile and dilatation of the duodenum. SPECT/CT showed no radioactivity outside the bowel (not all slices are shown here). No bile leak was identified.

11.7.2 Teaching Points

- Postoperative bile duct complications include bile leaks, common bile/hepatic duct injuries or

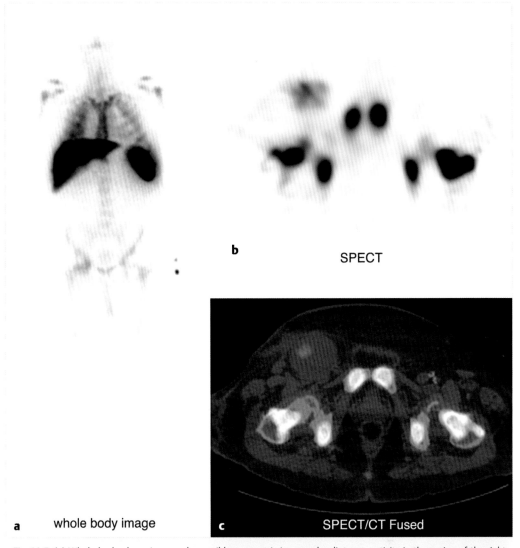

Fig. 11.5 (a) Whole-body planar images show mild asymmetric increased radiotracer activity in the region of the right femoral head and neck, which prompted further evaluation with SPECT/CT. (b) Axial SPECT at the level of the hips shows focal activity in the right inguinal region. (c) Fused SPECT/CT confirmed the increased radiotracer accumulation in the right inguinal region was in a pseudoaneurysm, consistent with an infected pseudoaneurysm.

strictures, retained biliary calculi, and obstruction.

- Bile leaks are best diagnosed by cholescintigraphy. When reviewing images, increasing image intensity often improves identification of a leak, if the amount of leak is small, and assessment of the extent of extravasation. Furthermore, the extent of the leak is often better identified on delayed images. However, planar images may be equivocal at times.

- SPECT/CT can be helpful to make the diagnosis of a suspected bile leak as well as to define the location and extent of a bile leak collection, which can guide therapy, such as drainage catheter placement. Although not routinely performed, in a small study including 32 patients who underwent both planar scintigraphy and SPECT/CT for a suspected bile leak, the sensitivity, specificity, and accuracy of SPECT/CT was 89, 100, and 97%, respectively, versus 78, 61, and

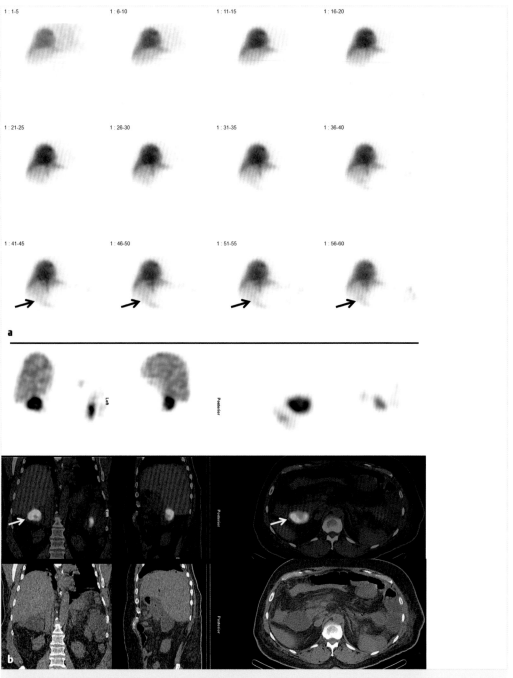

Fig. 11.6 (a) Planar 60-minute dynamic anterior images show mildly decreased radiotracer and excretion into the biliary tract initially, with a gradual increase over approximately 30 minutes. The gallbladder is surgically absent. Vague, diffuse tracer activity that appeared below the right lobe of the liver (*arrows*) was felt to be atypical in appearance (somewhat wide and diffuse) for excreted radiotracer into the duodenum, and a bile leak could not be definitively excluded. (b) SPECT/CT was performed for further evaluation. The vague diffuse activity below the right hepatic lobe seen on the planar images was found to be within the dilated duodenum (*arrow*). The mild and diffuse activity on planar images likely resulted from a combination of slow, decreased excretion of bile and dilatation of the duodenum. SPECT/CT showed no radioactivity outside the bowel (not all slices are shown here). No bile leak was identified.

66%, respectively, for planar imaging. In the preceding case, planar imaging was equivocal for a bile leak, which, in turn, could have led to more invasive procedures, such as exploratory laparotomy. SPECT/CT showed that there was no radiotracer outside the bowel; rather, the radiotracer was in the dilated duodenum, explaining the equivocal planar imaging findings.

- If a major leak is present, invasive procedures (e.g., reoperation, percutaneous transhepatic biliary drainage, or endoscopic sphincterotomy with placement of a stent or nasobiliary drainage catheter) may be required, whereas small, clinically insignificant leaks can heal spontaneously. Cholescintigraphy can be used to assess the effectiveness of such interventional procedures.[11,12,13]

11.8 Case 7: Bile Gastritis (Gastric Remnant)

11.8.1 Clinical History and Imaging Findings

- A 26-year-old woman presented with chronic abdominal pain and a history of multiple abdominal surgeries, including a laparoscopic Roux-en-Y gastric bypass for morbid obesity in 2009 and a laparoscopic cholecystectomy in 2011.
- ^{99m}Tc-Mebrofenin hepatobiliary scintigraphy was performed to rule out bile acid gastritis.
- Planar images show radiotracer excretion into the small intestine at 10 to 20 minutes (▶ Fig. 11.7 a). At 60 minutes, there is mild radiotracer activity within the epigastric region (*arrow*). The gallbladder is not seen, consistent with the history of prior cholecystectomy.
- SPECT/CT shows that the mild radiotracer activity seen on planar imaging at 60 minutes localizes to the lumen of the gastric remnant (▶ Fig. 11.7 b).

11.8.2 Teaching Points

- Bile reflux has been associated with chronic pain in patients post-Roux-en-Y gastric bypass for obesity.
- SPECT/CT provides both functional and anatomical evaluation and can be helpful in determining the precise anatomical location on CT of bile reflux seen on SPECT.

- We have found that SPECT/CT in addition to planar HIDA scans in patients with abdominal pain and a history of Roux-en-Y bypass surgery is helpful to identify bile reflux into the gastric remnant. Planar imaging may be sufficient in markedly abnormal cases. However, often it is difficult to ascertain on planar imaging alone if the activity seen in the epigastric region is in the gastric remnant (due to bile reflux from the afferent limb) or in the gastric pouch (due to reflux from the efferent limb, i.e., jejunum). SPECT/CT can provide definitive answers by localizing the functional abnormality seen on SPECT to the anatomical site involved on CT.[14,15]

11.9 Case 8: Intramuscular Bleeding in the Posterior Chest Wall

11.9.1 Clinical History and Imaging Findings

- A 52-year-old man presented with a history of mitral regurgitation, tricuspid regurgitation, atrial fibrillation, and chronic deep venous thrombosis post–mitral valve repair with an annuloplasty ring and a bovine pericardium patch, tricuspid valve repair with an annuloplasty ring, and a biatrial MAZE procedure. Postoperatively, therapeutic anticoagulation (heparin) was started, followed by a sudden precipitous drop in hematocrit. CT showed an asymmetric mass-like fluid collection in the left posterolateral chest wall, raising the question of a hematoma from active bleeding.
- ^{99m}Tc-RBC bleeding scan was performed to evaluate for active bleeding.
- Planar dynamic anterior and posterior images of the thorax as well as planar static anterior and posterior images 90 minutes following radiotracer administration were obtained (▶ Fig. 11.8 a). The static planar images show a large photopenic region in the left lateral hemithorax (*arrows*) corresponding to the fluid collection seen on CT. There was no significant radiotracer accumulation suggestive of active bleeding up to 90 minutes.
- Although the planar scintigraphy study was interpreted as negative for active bleeding, the hematocrit continued to drop after the study had been performed, and the patient returned for SPECT/CT the following day (▶ Fig. 11.8 b). The CT component of the SPECT/CT study

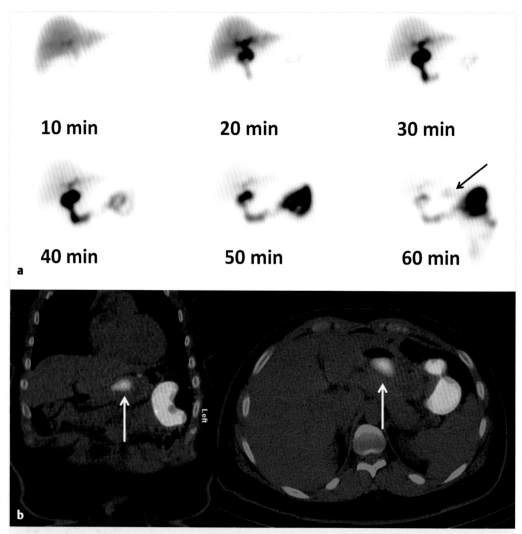

Fig. 11.7 (a) Planar images show radiotracer excretion into the small intestine at 10 to 20 minutes. At 60 minutes, there is mild radiotracer activity within the epigastric region (*arrow*). The gallbladder is not seen, consistent with the history of prior cholecystectomy. (b) SPECT/CT shows that the mild radiotracer activity seen on planar imaging at 60 minutes localizes to the lumen of the gastric remnant (*arrow*).

showed that the left lateral chest wall fluid collection was unchanged and had no radiotracer accumulation (*white arrows*). However, unexpected intense radiotracer accumulation was seen in the left posterior paraspinal muscles (*red arrow*), suggesting a site of active bleeding. Thus

SPECT/CT identified the site of active bleeding and explained the continued drop in hematocrit. This led to heparin being stopped.

- This bleeding site was likely missed on planar imaging because of superimposed blood pool activity in the chest.

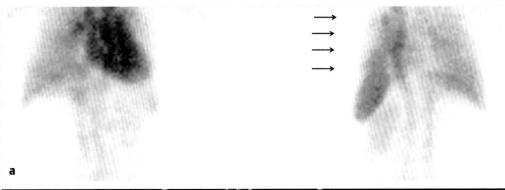

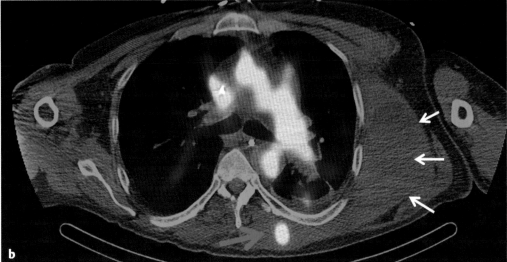

Fig. 11.8 (a) Planar dynamic anterior and posterior images of the thorax as well as planar static anterior and posterior images 90 minutes following radiotracer administration were obtained. The static planar images show a large photopenic region in the left lateral hemithorax (*arrows*) corresponding to the fluid collection seen on CT. There was no significant radiotracer accumulation suggestive of active bleeding up to 90 minutes. (b) Although the planar scintigraphy study was interpreted as negative for active bleeding, the hematocrit continued to drop after the study had been performed, and the patient returned for SPECT/CT the following day. The CT component of the SPECT/CT study showed that the left lateral chest wall fluid collection was unchanged and had no radiotracer accumulation (*white arrows*). However, unexpected intense radiotracer accumulation was seen in the left posterior paraspinal muscles (*red arrow*), suggesting a site of active bleeding. Thus SPECT/CT identified the site of active bleeding and explained the continued drop in hematocrit. This led to heparin being stopped.

11.9.2 Teaching Points

- An unexplained fall in hematocrit or blood pressure in a patient on heparin should prompt careful investigation for a site of active bleeding.
- In cases where active bleeding is suspected on clinical grounds and planar ^{99m}Tc-RBC scintigraphy does not show the site of active bleeding, SPECT/CT may be helpful to identify the site of active bleeding.[16]

11.10 Case 9: Large Bowel Bleeding versus Small Bowel Bleeding

11.10.1 Clinical History and Imaging Findings

- A 45-year-old man with a history of surgery for aortic dissection, placement of a mechanical aortic valve, multiple bowel resections for ischemic bowel, and chronic anticoagulation therapy presented with rectal bleeding and a drop in hematocrit 7 days following ileostomy reversal surgery.

- A ^{99m}Tc-RBC study was ordered to identify the site of active bleeding.
- Serial planar images from the ^{99m}Tc-RBC bleeding study demonstrate a curvilinear region of radiotracer in the right lower quadrant (▶ Fig. 11.9 a). Cine display of dynamic images (not shown) showed some to-and-fro movement of the radiotracer, but the origin of the active bleeding could not be definitively identified as being in the small bowel versus the large bowel.
- SPECT/CT showed radiotracer activity originating in the lumen of a dilated small bowel loop at the

site of the ileostomy reversal (▶ Fig. 11.9 b). The radiotracer activity was seen to extend to the left of midline in distal dilated small bowel loops, and this was subsequently confirmed on a diagnostic CT of the abdomen and pelvis.

11.10.2 Teaching Points

- When planar ^{99m}Tc-RBC scintigraphy suggests active bleeding but cannot conclusively identify the origin of the active bleeding, SPECT/CT may be very helpful to determine if the bleeding originates in the small versus the large bowel.[17,18]
- In the preceding case, we showed that SPECT/CT may be helpful in identifying active small bowel bleeding and may also improve the accuracy of

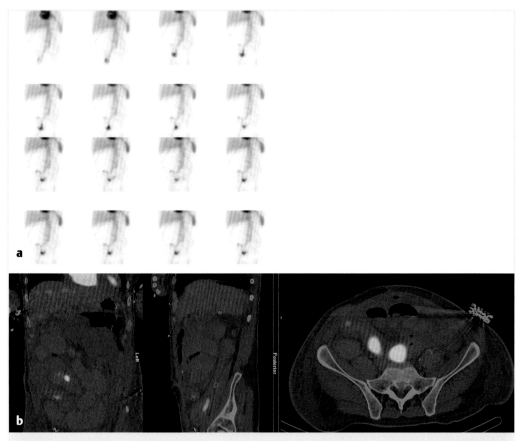

Fig. 11.9 (a) Serial planar images from the ^{99m}Tc-RBC bleeding study demonstrate a curvilinear region of radiotracer in the right lower quadrant. Cine display of dynamic images (not shown) showed some to-and-fro movement of the radiotracer, but the origin of the active bleeding could not be definitively identified as being in the small bowel versus the large bowel. (b) SPECT/CT showed radiotracer activity originating in the lumen of a dilated small bowel loop at the site of the ileostomy reversal. The radiotracer activity was seen to extend to the left of midline in distal dilated small bowel loops, and this was subsequently confirmed on a diagnostic CT of the abdomen and pelvis.

99mTc-RBC scintigraphy in active lower GI bleeding.

11.11 Case 10: Lymphocele

11.11.1 Clinical History and Imaging Findings

- A 74-year-old man presented with a right groin fluid collection following excision of a right inguinal mass.

- Filtered 99mTc sulfur colloid was divided into four injections: two intradermal injections into the dorsum of each foot.
- Sequential dynamic images (not shown) showed prompt drainage of radiotracer from the site of injection in both lower extremities, with localization of radiotracer in bilateral inguinal, external iliac, common iliac, and retroperitoneal lymph nodes.
- A selected static image shows prominent asymmetric radiotracer within the right inguinal region (▶ Fig. 11.10 a).

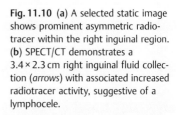

Fig. 11.10 (a) A selected static image shows prominent asymmetric radiotracer within the right inguinal region. (b) SPECT/CT demonstrates a 3.4 × 2.3 cm right inguinal fluid collection (*arrows*) with associated increased radiotracer activity, suggestive of a lymphocele.

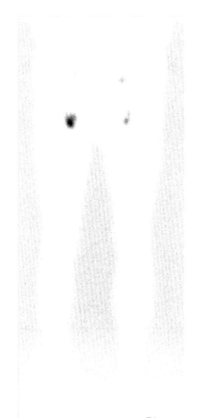

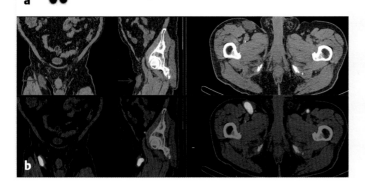

- SPECT/CT demonstrates a 3.4 × 2.3 cm right inguinal fluid collection with associated increased radiotracer activity, suggestive of a lymphocele (▶ Fig. 11.10 b).

11.11.2 Teaching Points

- Lymphoceles may be associated with surgical resection or sentinel lymph node biopsy.
- SPECT/CT may be helpful to identify postoperative lymphoceles and to clarify equivocal findings on planar scintigraphy.[19,20]

11.12 Case 11: Radioiodine Accumulation in a Renal Cyst

11.12.1 Clinical History and Imaging Findings

- A 42-year-old woman with well-differentiated papillary thyroid cancer, postthyroidectomy, received 154 mCi of ^{131}I for remnant ablation. The patient had very low thyroglobulin levels prior to radioiodine administration. A posttherapy scan was performed 7 days later.
- Whole-body planar images in anterior and posterior projections were obtained, demonstrating focal increased radiotracer uptake in the right neck, likely at a site of residual thyroid tissue (▶ Fig. 11.11 a). Additionally, there is focal radiotracer uptake projecting over the posteroinferior liver (*black arrow*). Elsewhere, there is normal biodistribution.
- Posterior planar spot view over the thorax and abdomen was obtained with markers placed over the suprasternal notch and the xiphoid process, as labeled (▶ Fig. 11.11 b). Focal radiotracer uptake persists, projecting over the posteroinferior liver (*white arrow*).
- SPECT images were fused to images from a previously acquired CT scan of the abdomen and pelvis (▶ Fig. 11.11 c). The focal radiotracer uptake seen on the planar images localizes to a cyst in the upper pole of the right kidney (*white arrow*).

11.12.2 Teaching Points

- Radioiodine uptake in renal cysts can be a pitfall of ^{131}I imaging. Different mechanisms have been proposed to explain radioiodine uptake in renal cysts, although a definitive mechanism has not

been established. These include (1) a process of active secretion and the presence of a communication between the cystic lesion and the main collecting system, as seen in a calyceal diverticulum, and (2) the presence of a human sodium-iodide symporter, although this has not been confirmed by histopathological finding or immunohistochemical analysis.[21]

11.13 Case 12: Focal Radioiodine Uptake at the Site of Dental Metal

11.13.1 Clinical History and Imaging Findings

- A 48-year-old man presented with differentiated thyroid cancer, status postthyroidectomy followed by radioiodine ablation treatment with 30 mCi of [131]I.
- Anterior planar images obtained 7 days after radioiodine ablation show focal increased activity in the thyroid bed (*solid arrow*), likely representing remnant thyroid tissue (▶ Fig. 11.12 a). In addition, there are two sites of focal increased activity in the region of the oral cavity/upper neck (*broken arrows*).
- SPECT, fused SPECT/CT, and CT images show these two sites of focal increased activity in the region of the oral cavity/upper neck localize to dental fillings within the mouth (▶ Fig. 11.12 b).

11.13.2 Teaching Points

- A whole-body radioiodine scan often shows increased uptake in the salivary glands as well as radioactivity in nasal secretion in the nasal region and salivary secretion in the oral cavity.
  - Radioactivity in salivary secretion in the oral cavity tends to be diffuse (rather than focal) and is generally seen within the first few days after administration of radioiodine. Therefore, the two sites indicated by broken arrows on the planar images would be atypical for physiological activity in salivary secretion, that is, too focal and intense, especially at 7 days.
  - Radioactivity in the salivary glands may persist for several days, but the intensity tends to diminish with time. For example, there is no radioactivity in the region of the parotid

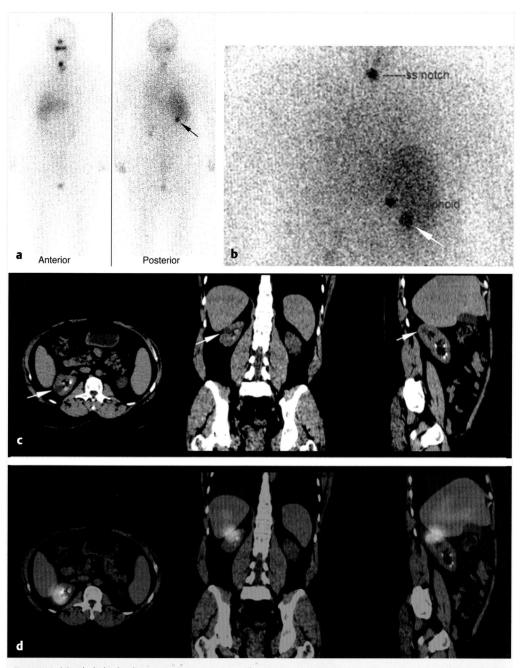

Fig. 11.11 (a) Whole-body planar images in anterior and posterior projections were obtained, demonstrating focal increased radiotracer uptake in the right neck, likely at a site of residual thyroid tissue. Additionally, there is focal radiotracer uptake projecting over the posteroinferior liver (*black arrow*). Elsewhere, there is normal biodistribution. (b) Posterior planar spot view over the thorax and abdomen was obtained with markers placed over the suprasternal notch and the xiphoid process, as labeled. Focal radiotracer uptake persists projecting over the posteroinferior liver (*white arrow*). (c,d) SPECT images were fused to images from a previously acquired CT scan of the abdomen and pelvis. The focal radiotracer uptake seen on the planar images localizes to a cyst in the upper pole of the right kidney (*white arrow*).

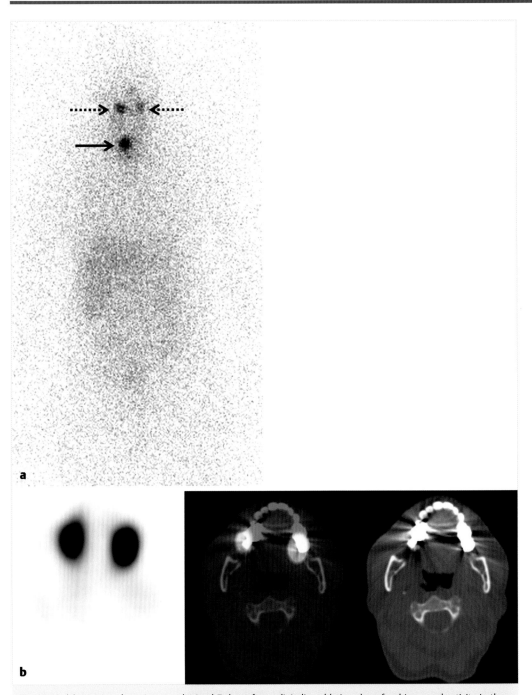

Fig. 11.12 (a) Anterior planar images obtained 7 days after radioiodine ablation show focal increased activity in the thyroid bed (*solid arrow*), likely representing remnant thyroid tissue. In addition, there are two sites of focal increased activity in the region of the oral cavity/upper neck (*broken arrows*). (b) SPECT, fused SPECT/CT, and CT images show these two sites of focal increased activity in the region of the oral cavity/upper neck localize to dental fillings within the mouth.

glands in the presented case, indicating complete washout by 7 days. Inflamed salivary glands may have persistent activity on delayed images due to prolonged salivary retention. While this possibility cannot be completely excluded on the planar images, it would be an unlikely explanation of the findings given the location (the two sites of focal activity on the planar images appear somewhat more medial than the typical location of the submandibular glands) and the intensity (very intense).

- Focal radioiodine activity in the region of the oral cavity is often due to partially reversible binding of radioiodine to dental metal.
- SPECT/CT increases the specificity of equivocal findings on planar scintigraphy.[22]

References

[1] Jones SE, Aziz K, Yasuda T, Gewirtz H, Scott JA. Importance of systematic review of rotating projection images from Tc99m-sestamibi cardiac perfusion imaging for noncardiac findings. Nucl Med Commun. 2008;29(7):607–613

[2] Gedik GK, Ergün EL, Aslan M, Caner B. Unusual extracardiac findings detected on myocardial perfusion single photon emission computed tomography studies with Tc-99 m sestamibi. Clin Nucl Med. 2007;32(12):920–926

[3] Dilsizian V, Bonow RO. Current diagnostic techniques of assessing myocardial viability in patients with hibernating and stunned myocardium. Circulation. 1993;87(1):1–20

[4] Krause T, Hauenstein K, Studier-Fischer B, Schuemichen C, Moser E. Improved evaluation of technetium-99m-red blood cell SPECT in hemangioma of the liver. J Nucl Med. 1993;34 (3):375–380

[5] Kim CK. Scintigraphic evaluation of the liver and biliary tract. In Gazelle SG, Saini S, Mueller PR, eds. Hepatobiliary and Pancreatic Radiology: Imaging and Interventions. New York, NY: Thieme; 1998:108–153

[6] Schillaci O, Danieli R, Manni C, Capoccetti F, Simonetti G. Technetium-99m-labelled red blood cell imaging in the diagnosis of hepatic haemangiomas: the role of SPECT/CT with a hybrid camera. Eur J Nucl Med Mol Imaging. 2004;31 (7):1011–1015

[7] Stuart S, Booth TC, Cash CJ, et al. Complications of continuous ambulatory peritoneal dialysis. Radiographics. 2009;29 (2):441–460

[8] Tun KN, Tulchinsky M. Pericatheter leak in a peritoneal dialysis patient: SPECT/CT diagnosis. Clin Nucl Med. 2012;37 (6):625–628

[9] Damodharan K, Beckett D. Endovascular management of an infected superficial femoral artery pseudoaneurysm. Cardiovasc Intervent Radiol. 2013;36(5):1411–1415

[10] Macedo TA, Stanson AW, Oderich GS, Johnson CM, Panneton JM, Tie ML. Infected aortic aneurysms: imaging findings. Radiology. 2004;231(1):250–257

[11] Sharma P, Kumar R, Das KJ, et al. Detection and localization of post-operative and post-traumatic bile leak: hybrid SPECT-CT with 99mTc-Mebrofenin. Abdom Imaging. 2012;37 (5):803–811

[12] Arun S, Santhosh S, Sood A, Bhattacharya A, Mittal BR. Added value of SPECT/CT over planar Tc-99 m mebrofenin hepatobiliary scintigraphy in the evaluation of bile leaks. Nucl Med Commun. 2013;34(5):459–466

[13] Kim CK, Joo JH, Lee SM. Liver and biliary tract. In Elgazzar AH, ed. The Pathophysiologic Basis of Nuclear Medicine. 3rd ed. Cham, Switzerland: Springer;2014:559–593

[14] Swartz DE, Mobley E, Felix EL. Bile reflux after Roux-en-Y gastric bypass: an unrecognized cause of postoperative pain. Surg Obes Relat Dis. 2009;5(1):27–30

[15] Schillaci O, Filippi L, Danieli R, Simonetti G. Single-photon emission computed tomography/computed tomography in abdominal diseases. Semin Nucl Med. 2007;37(1):48–61

[16] Antonelli D, Fares L, II, Anene C. Enoxaparin associated with hugh abdominal wall hematomas: a report of two cases. Am Surg. 2000;66(8):797–800

[17] Bentley BS, Tulchinsky M. SPECT/CT helps in localization and guiding management of small bowel gastrointestinal hemorrhage. Clin Nucl Med. 2014;39(1):94–96

[18] Schillaci O, Spanu A, Tagliabue L, et al. SPECT/CT with a hybrid imaging system in the study of lower gastrointestinal bleeding with technetium-99 m red blood cells. Q J Nucl Med Mol Imaging. 2009;53(3):281–289

[19] White I, Mills JK, Diggs B, Fortino Hima J, Ellis MC, Vetto JT. Sentinel lymph node biopsy for melanoma: comparison of lymphocele rates by surgical technique. Am Surg. 2013;79 (4):388–392

[20] Han DY, Cheng MF, Yen RF, Tzen KY, Wu YW. Postoperative lymphocele demonstrated by lymphoscintigraphy SPECT/CT. Clin Nucl Med. 2012;37(4):374–376

[21] Campennì A, Ruggeri RM, Giovinazzo S, Sindoni A, Santoro D, Baldari S. Radioiodine uptake in a renal cyst mimicking a metastasis in a patient affected by differentiated thyroid cancer: case report and review of the literature. Ann Nucl Med. 2014;28(5):472–476

[22] Burlison JS, Hartshorne MF, Voda AM, Cocks FH, Fair JR. SPECT/CT localization of oral radioiodine activity: a retrospective study and in-vitro assessment. Nucl Med Commun. 2013;34(12):1216–1222

Index

Note: Page numbers set **bold** or *italic* indicate headings or figures, respectively.